Social Determinants of Health, Diet, and Health Outcome

Social Determinants of Health, Diet, and Health Outcome

Guest Editor

Li Jiao

MDPI

Basel • Beijing • Wuhan • Barcelona • Belgrade • Novi Sad • Cluj • Manchester

Guest Editor
Li Jiao
Department of Medicine
Baylor College of Medicine
Houston, TX
USA

Editorial Office
MDPI AG
Grosspeteranlage 5
4052 Basel, Switzerland

This is a reprint of the Special Issue, published open access by the journal *Nutrients* (ISSN 2072-6643), freely accessible at: https://www.mdpi.com/journal/nutrients/special_issues/2352M68KR5.

For citation purposes, cite each article independently as indicated on the article page online and as indicated below:

Lastname, A.A.; Lastname, B.B. Article Title. *Journal Name* **Year**, *Volume Number*, Page Range.

ISBN 978-3-7258-5889-7 (Hbk)
ISBN 978-3-7258-5890-3 (PDF)
https://doi.org/10.3390/books978-3-7258-5890-3

Contents

About the Editor

Li Jiao

Li Jiao is a tenured Associate Professor of Medicine at the Baylor College of Medicine, Houston, TX. She has a long-standing interest in understanding how external environmental factors impact human health. Her research focuses on the molecular and nutritional epidemiologic of gastrointestinal cancers. She has explored how diet and lifestyle factors impact the body at the molecular and microenvironment level and has published a number of studies on the gut microbiota. Expanding her perspective, she has also explored how macroenvironmental factors, such as social and societal factors, shape dietary habits. Her unwavering goal is to promote healthy eating and lifestyle as strategies for disease prevention.

Preface

More than 20 years ago, my research centered on identifying genetic and modifiable risk factors for pancreatic and other gastrointestinal cancers. One of my findings indicated that a healthy lifestyle is associated with a lower risk of pancreatic cancer, with diet quality being an important component of one's lifestyle. This and other observations led me to further explore why and how diet impacts our health, which drew me towards the study of the gut microbiome.

As I delved deeper into how diet influences our health through modulating our internal microenvironment, I came across maps illustrating the striking geographic variation in disease burden. These images inspired me to guest edit this Special Issue, "Social Determinants of Health, Diet, and Health Outcome". In doing so, I aimed to bring together cutting-edge research on how the broad macroenvironment, where people live, work, and grow, interacts with diet choice to affect health.

This reprint includes research that examines the interrelationships among social determinants of health, diet, and health outcomes, contributed by researchers across the globe. These works underscore how multiple socioeconomic factors and social contexts profoundly shape what we eat, and in turn, our health. As shown in this reprint, SDOHs affect individuals across the life span. I therefore organized the articles to reflect this continuum, from research on pregnant women to research on the elderly.

I hope that future research can deepen our understanding of how both individual and societal factors shape diet and well-being. More public policies are needed to support those people who lack the privilege or resources to adopt healthy eating habits, who are often the same population who are more likely to bear a greater burden of chronic diseases.

I am sincerely grateful to all contributing authors for their important work. I also thank my husband for his support with coding-related tasks throughout the editing process.

Li Jiao
Guest Editor

nutrients

MDPI

Editorial

Social Determinants of Health, Diet, and Health Outcome

Li Jiao †

Baylor College of Medicine, Houston, TX 77030, USA; jiao@bcm.edu
† Current affiliation: Harris County Public Health, Houston, TX 77002, USA.

1. Introduction

This Special Issue delves into the intricate relationship between social determinants of health (SDOHs), diet, and health outcomes through 13 articles authored by scholars from 10 countries across five continents. The research examines how various socioeconomic factors, such as poverty, education level, occupation, geographic location, race/ethnicity, place of birth, immigration status, refugee status, and disability, affect food insecurity, diet quality, and food choices among different populations, including school-aged children, pregnant women, and the elderly. In low- and middle-income countries, food insecurity is associated with poverty, job instability, refugee status, and disability. In the U.S., geographic location and occupation influence food insecurity and dietary choices. Five articles in this Special Issue address health outcomes, linking food insecurity and poor diet to issues such as malnutrition, anemia in children, obesity, metabolic disorders, and cardiovascular diseases. Other factors like culture, climate, reginal conflict, dental hygiene, and social networks also impact food availability and diet quality. Stress and nutritional illiteracy might mediate the relationship between SDOHs and health outcomes. The authors advocate for interventions through policy, regulation, and health education, particularly for pregnant women, children, and the elderly, to mitigate the negative impacts of SDOHs on health. Future research could investigate the broader impacts of SDOHs and diet on preventable chronic diseases. Overall, this Special Issue highlights the critical connections between SDOHs, food insecurity, and diet qualities, emphasizing the need for comprehensive intervention to reduce health disparities and promote population health.

2. Social Determinants of Health, Food Insecurity, and Health Outcomes

Social determinants of health (SDOHs) are the non-medical conditions in which people are born, grow, work, live, worship, and age. Food insecurity occurs when households are, at times, unable to acquire adequate food for one or more members due to insufficient resources, such as finance [1]. Numerous studies have examined the relationship between food insecurity and socioeconomic status (SES), identifying contributing factors, including poverty [2], unemployment [3], immigration status [4], refugee status [5], disability [6], limited access to grocery stores, lack of transportation [7], and lower education levels [8,9]. This Special Issue highlights the association between these factors and food insecurity in Maputo City, southern Mozambique. In Peru, women's autonomy, immigration status, refugee status, and disability among Venezuelans were associated with unmet food needs. In the United States, children in urban areas were found to have a higher prevalence of food insecurity compared to their rural counterparts.

Malnutrition is a common consequence of food insecurity, particularly among the elderly, who may face challenges such as limited mobility and transportation. Malnutrition can lead to various health problems, including heart disease [10], type 2 diabetes, and certain cancers [11,12]. In Peru, low women autonomy was associated with a high prevalence of anemia in young children, highlighting this as an important social and public health issue in low- and middle-income countries (LMICs).

In summary, the findings from four studies in this Special Issue underscore the need for social inclusion, economic support, humanitarian aid, and improved access to safety nets for vulnerable populations in LMICs. Ensuring access to nutritious food is vital in reducing the burden of chronic diseases [13].

3. SDOHs, Dietary Quality, and Health Outcomes

Several studies have investigated the relationship between SDOHs and dietary quality, diversity, and food choices, focusing on factors such as race/ethnicity, place of birth, occupation, education, and geographic location. Below is a summary of key findings (Figure 1).

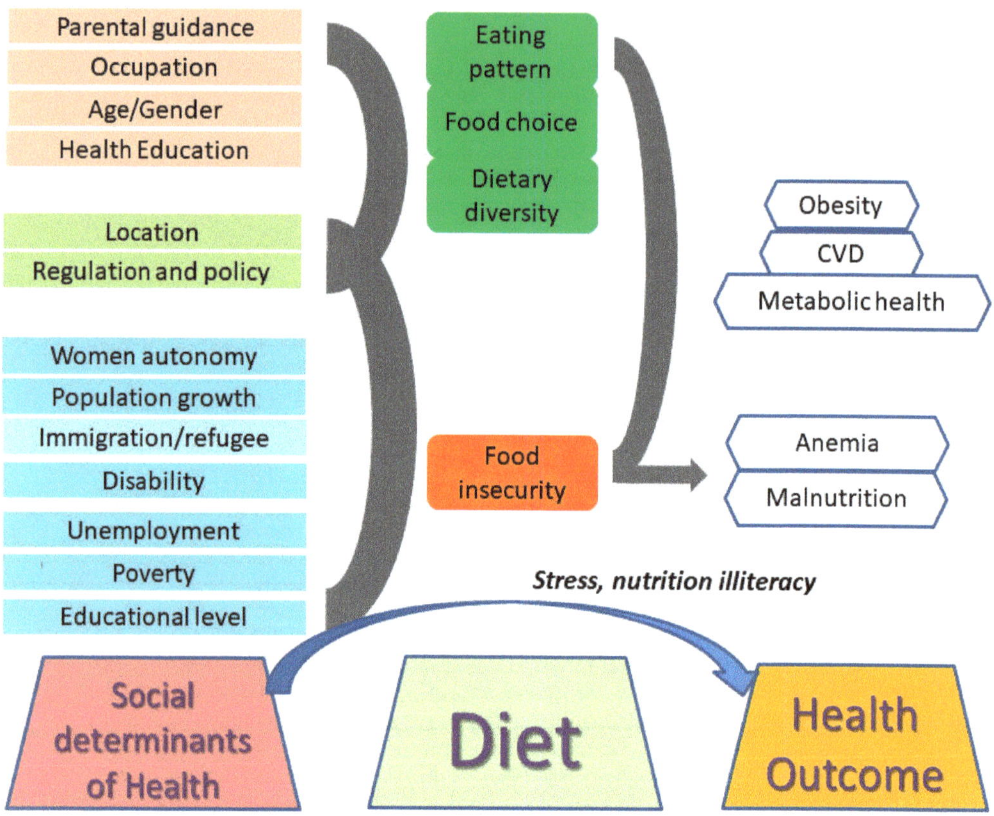

Figure 1. The SDOHs, diet, and health outcomes discussed in this special issue.

Race/Ethnicity and place of birth. One study found that U.S.-born non-Hispanic African American adults had lower diet quality than their foreign-born counterparts. Furthermore, foreign-born African American who had lived in the U.S. for less than 10 years had better diets than those who had been in the country for a longer period of time. This study highlighted the need for further research on dietary acculturation among immigrants and health in the U.S. [14].

Occupation. Mansouri et al. found that the unpredictable nature of emergency medical services (EMSs) poses barriers to maintaining a healthy diet. The barriers included fatigue, heavy workloads, lack of meal breaks, reliance on convenience food, and limited food options at work [15]. A previous study showed that hospital workers who skipped meals tended to make less healthy dietary choices, with those skipping breakfast having lower diet quality. Understanding how different occupations influence dietary habits could offer new opportunities for promoting healthy choices at work.

Geographic location and education levels. A study in Indonesia revealed that rural districts had a higher prevalence of inadequate fruit and vegetable consumption compared to urban areas, especially among females and older adults. Additionally, residents of districts with lower education levels consumed less fruits and vegetables. However, in the U.S., no significant differences in diet quality were observed between urban and rural areas.

Health outcome. Several studies have linked dietary habits to health outcomes. For example, obesity has been associated with unhealthy food choices related to occupation, nutrition illiteracy, and skipping breakfast in Greek children. Those who skipped breakfast also had poorer cardiorespiratory fitness, weaker handgrip strength, and worse metabolic health [16].

4. Other Factors and Diet Quality

Other factors, including climate change, political instability, regional conflicts, and the COVID-19 pandemic, have exacerbated food insecurity in Maputo City, southern Mozambique. Additionally, skipping breakfast, poor dental health in the elderly, cultural practices like eating together or alone in Japan, and peer influence among EMS providers in the U.S. have also been shown to affect food insecurity and diet quality. In a previous study in Spain, skipping breakfast has been associated with lower SES [17], highlighting its potential as an SDOH indicator.

5. SDOHs, Stress, and Health Outcomes

This Special Issue suggests that SDOHs influence health outcomes through stress and dietary choices. For instance, EMS is associated with stress, fatigue, and irregular eating patterns [15], which, when combined with reliance on snack-based foods, can further increase the risk of obesity, metabolic disturbance, diabetes, and cardiovascular disease (CVD). A review article discussed that pregnancy as a stress status [18] is often associated with increased consumption of high-fat and high-sugar foods and lower intake of healthy foods [19]. Moreover, "stress eating" can increase the risk of CVD in later life.

In summary, stress, whether directly or through its influence on dietary choice, can elevate the risk of chronic diseases. Additionally, other SDOHs, such as job instability, can also act as a chronic stressor that adversely impact health [20].

6. Policy and Regulation

Several studies in this Special Issue emphasize the role of policy and regulation in promoting healthy diets. For example, regulatory measures in Chile significantly reduced the purchase of sugar-sweetened beverages and unhealthy foods, shifting consumer behavior toward healthier products. One study underscores the need for further understanding how policies, such as taxes on unhealthy foods and beverages, could reduce the consumption of unhealthy products. In the U.S., adjusting shift schedules and revising organizational policies could support healthier eating habits among EMS providers and potentially reduce employee turnover costs for agencies. In Indonesia, policy recommendations include improving access to diverse and affordable fruit and vegetable options in rural and low-income areas and launching public health campaigns targeting females, older adults, and those with lower education levels. A Japanese study found that among older adults, personal dental health and cultural factors play a significant role in shaping dietary habits. This finding suggests that policymakers and regulators should consider cultural and health factors when developing nutritional guidelines for diverse elderly populations.

7. Potential Intervention: When and Where

Interventions targeting SDOHs aim to reduce the adverse effects of food and nutritional insecurity on health outcomes. Chronic non-communicable diseases (NCDs) often develop over time, making early education on nutrition literacy crucial. Several studies highlight the importance of influencing children through both parents and schools. For example, a Polish study found that childhood food restrictions were linked to lower levels of intuitive eating and higher levels of restrained eating in adulthood. Another study emphasized the critical role schools play in shaping children's health habits when healthy eating is not nurtured at home, as seen in obesity research in Saudi Arabia. This approach not only helps prevent childhood obesity but also has long-term benefits for the health of the population.

A review article in this Special Issue advocates for interventions during pregnancy to help women manage stress and adopt healthy dietary habit and lifestyles, which can prevent cardiovascular diseases later in life. Nutritional intervention during pregnancy supports fetal growth and contributes to epigenetic programming in the fetus [21], potentially influencing the risk of NCD in adults. Maternal nutrition's impact on offspring's risk of NCD in adulthood has been examined [22]. Furthermore, maternal diet can have a transgenerational effect and may profoundly impact the health of the population [23]. On the other hand, a mother's knowledge about nutrition can also be passed down to their children. Recently, in 2024, the U.S. Department of Agriculture made permanent increases to the cash value benefit for fruits and vegetables in the Special Supplemental Nutrition Program for Women, Infants, and Children (WIC) program. Such policies are crucial for improving health outcomes, closing nutrition gaps, and impacting health beyond the current generation.

In summary, promoting nutrition literacy and healthy eating habits should begin as early as possible as these interventions can significantly improve the health of the population.

8. Conclusions

SDOHs are recognized for having multiple factors related to health outcomes, such as the environment and access to health care. Diet is one pathway through which socioeconomic factors can impact health. Further research is needed to explore how social, political, and cultural factors relate to diet and health. Identifying effective intervention targets can help address health disparities due to SDOHs. Governmental and public agencies should promote collaboration across sectors—such as health, economic support, humanitarian aid, education, and municipalities—alongside families, schools, and communities to enhance healthy eating and reduce food insecurity. The collected studies have also shown gender differences in SDOHs and dietary habits and emphasize the need for a holistic and culture-sensitive approach to nutrition policy tailored to specific populations.

Conflicts of Interest: The author declares no conflict of interest.

References

1. U.S. Department of Agriculture. ERS Food Insequrity in the U.S. 2023. Available online: https://www.ers.usda.gov/topics/food-nutrition-assistance/food-security-in-the-u-s/ (accessed on 1 August 2024).
2. Vilar-Compte, M.; Burrola-Mendez, S.; Lozano-Marrufo, A.; Ferre-Eguiluz, I.; Flores, D.; Gaitan-Rossi, P.; Teruel, G.; Perez-Escamilla, R. Urban poverty and nutrition challenges associated with accessibility to a healthy diet: A global systematic literature review. *Int. J. Equity Health* **2021**, *20*, 40. [CrossRef]
3. Raifman, J.; Bor, J.; Venkataramani, A. Association Between Receipt of Unemployment Insurance and Food Insecurity Among People Who Lost Employment During the COVID-19 Pandemic in the United States. *JAMA Netw. Open* **2021**, *4*, e2035884. [CrossRef]
4. Choudhary, N.; Parthasarathy, D. Is migration status a determinant of urban nutrition insecurity? Empirical evidence from Mumbai city, India. *J. Biosoc. Sci.* **2009**, *41*, 583–605. [CrossRef] [PubMed]
5. Chevrier, J.; Lane, G.; Khakpour, M.; Vatanparast, H.; Batal, M. Food Security Among Syrian Refugee Families in Quebec, Canada. *Ecol. Food Nutr.* **2023**, *62*, 181–206. [CrossRef] [PubMed]
6. Coleman-Jensen, A.U. S food insecurity and population trends with a focus on adults with disabilities. *Physiol. Behav.* **2020**, *220*, 112865. [CrossRef] [PubMed]
7. Martinez, J.C.; Clark, J.M.; Gudzune, K.A. Association of personal vehicle access with lifestyle habits and food insecurity among public housing residents. *Prev. Med. Rep.* **2019**, *13*, 341–345. [CrossRef] [PubMed]

8. van der Velde, L.A.; Steyerberg, E.W.; Numans, M.E.; Kiefte-de Jong, J.C. Food insecurity status is of added value in explaining poor health: A cross-sectional study among parents living in disadvantaged neighbourhoods in the Netherlands. *BMJ Open* **2022**, *12*, e052827. [CrossRef] [PubMed]
9. Odoms-Young, A.; Brown, A.G.M.; Agurs-Collins, T.; Glanz, K. Food Insecurity, Neighborhood Food Environment, and Health Disparities: State of the Science, Research Gaps and Opportunities. *Am. J. Clin. Nutr.* **2024**, *119*, 850–861. [CrossRef]
10. Brandt, E.J.; Mozaffarian, D.; Leung, C.W.; Berkowitz, S.A.; Murthy, V.L. Diet and Food and Nutrition Insecurity and Cardiometabolic Disease. *Circ. Res.* **2023**, *132*, 1692–1706. [CrossRef]
11. Gundersen, C.; Ziliak, J.P. Food Insecurity And Health Outcomes. *Health Aff.* **2015**, *34*, 1830–1839. [CrossRef]
12. Thomas, M.K.; Lammert, L.J.; Beverly, E.A. Food Insecurity and its Impact on Body Weight, Type 2 Diabetes, Cardiovascular Disease, and Mental Health. *Curr. Cardiovasc. Risk Rep.* **2021**, *15*, 15. [CrossRef] [PubMed]
13. Campanera, M.; Gasull, M.; Gracia-Arnaiz, M. Food Security as a Social Determinant of Health: Tackling Inequalities in Primary Health Care in Spain. *Health Hum. Rights* **2023**, *25*, 9–21. [PubMed]
14. Adeyemi-Benson, O.S.; Roehll, A.M.; Flores, E.; Singleton, C.R. Differences in Nutrient Intake and Diet Quality among Non-Hispanic Black Adults by Place of Birth and Length of Time in the United States. *Nutrients* **2023**, *15*, 3644. [CrossRef]
15. Mansouri, T.; Ghanatios, G.; Hatzinger, L.; Barich, R.; Dampha, E.; Temple, J.L.; Clemency, B.M.; Hostler, D. Eating Patterns among Emergency Medical Service Providers in the United States: A Qualitative Interview Study. *Nutrients* **2022**, *14*, 4884. [CrossRef] [PubMed]
16. Gioxari, A.; Amerikanou, C.; Peraki, S.; Kaliora, A.C.; Skouroliakou, M. Eating Behavior and Factors of Metabolic Health in Primary Schoolchildren: A Cross-Sectional Study in Greek Children. *Nutrients* **2023**, *15*, 3592. [CrossRef] [PubMed]
17. Esquius, L.; Aguilar-Martinez, A.; Bosque-Prous, M.; Gonzalez-Casals, H.; Bach-Faig, A.; Colillas-Malet, E.; Salvador, G.; Espelt, A. Social Inequalities in Breakfast Consumption among Adolescents in Spain: The DESKcohort Project. *Nutrients* **2021**, *13*, 2500. [CrossRef] [PubMed]
18. Coppi, F.; Bucciarelli, V.; Solodka, K.; Selleri, V.; Zanini, G.; Pinti, M.; Nasi, M.; Salvioli, B.; Nodari, S.; Gallina, S.; et al. The Impact of Stress and Social Determinants on Diet in Cardiovascular Prevention in Young Women. *Nutrients* **2024**, *16*, 1044. [CrossRef] [PubMed]
19. Yau, Y.H.; Potenza, M.N. Stress and eating behaviors. *Minerva Endocrinol.* **2013**, *38*, 255–267.
20. Fricchione, G.L. The Challenge of Stress-Related Non-Communicable Diseases. *Med. Sci. Monit. Basic Res.* **2018**, *24*, 93–95. [CrossRef]
21. Fu, Q.; Cheung, W.A.; Majnik, A.V.; Ke, X.; Pastinen, T.; Lane, R.H. Adverse Maternal Environments Perturb Hepatic DNA Methylome and Transcriptome Prior to the Adult-Onset Non-Alcoholic Fatty Liver Disease in Mouse Offspring. *Nutrients* **2023**, *15*, 2167. [CrossRef]
22. Pullar, J.; Wickramasinghe, K.; Demaio, A.R.; Roberts, N.; Perez-Blanco, K.M.; Noonan, K.; Townsend, N. The impact of maternal nutrition on offspring's risk of non-communicable diseases in adulthood: A systematic review. *J. Glob. Health* **2019**, *9*, 020405. [CrossRef] [PubMed]
23. Jiang, W.; Han, T.; Duan, W.; Dong, Q.; Hou, W.; Wu, H.; Wang, Y.; Jiang, Z.; Pei, X.; Chen, Y.; et al. Prenatal famine exposure and estimated glomerular filtration rate across consecutive generations: Association and epigenetic mediation in a population-based cohort study in Suihua China. *Aging* **2020**, *12*, 12206–12221. [CrossRef] [PubMed]

nutrients

MDPI

Review

The Impact of Stress and Social Determinants on Diet in Cardiovascular Prevention in Young Women

Francesca Coppi [1], Valentina Bucciarelli [2], Kateryna Solodka [3], Valentina Selleri [4], Giada Zanini [4], Marcello Pinti [3,4], Milena Nasi [5], Beatrice Salvioli [6], Savina Nodari [7], Sabina Gallina [3,8] and Anna Vittoria Mattioli [3,6,*]

1 Department of Medical and Surgical Sciences for Children and Adults, University of Modena and Reggio Emilia, 41121 Modena, Italy; francesca.coppi@unimore.it
2 Cardiovascular Sciences Department, Azienda Ospedaliero-Universitaria delle Marche, 60166 Ancona, Italy; valentina.bucciarelli@ospedaliriuniti.marche.it
3 Istituto Nazionale per le Ricerche Cardiovascolari, 40126 Bologna, Italy; marcello.pinti@unimore.it (M.P.); sabina.gallina@unich.it (S.G.)
4 Department of Life Sciences, University of Modena and Reggio Emilia, 41121 Modena, Italy; valentina.selleri@unimore.it (V.S.); giada.zanini@unimore.it (G.Z.)
5 Department of Surgical, Medical and Dental Sciences, University of Modena and Reggio Emilia, 41121 Modena, Italy; milena.nasi@unimore.it
6 Department of Quality of Life Sciences, University of Bologna, 40126 Bologna, Italy; beatrice.salvioli@unibo.it
7 Department of Medical and Surgical Specialties, Radiological Sciences and Public Health, University of Brescia, 25123 Brescia, Italy; savina.nodari@unibs.it
8 Department of Neuroscience, Imaging and Clinical Sciences, "G. d'Annunzio" University of Chieti-Pescara, 66013 Chieti, Italy
* Correspondence: annavittoria.mattioli@unibo.it

Abstract: The prevention of cardiovascular diseases is a fundamental pillar for reducing morbidity and mortality caused by non-communicable diseases. Social determinants, such as socioeconomic status, education, neighborhood, physical environment, employment, social support networks, and access to health care, play a crucial role in influencing health outcomes and health inequities within populations. Social determinants and stress in women are interconnected factors that can significantly impact women's health and well-being. Pregnancy is a good time to engage young women and introduce them to beneficial behaviors, such as adopting essential life skills, especially diet, and learning stress management techniques. Stress influences diet, and women are more likely to engage in unhealthy eating behaviors such as emotional eating or coping with stress with food. Strong action is needed to improve women's lifestyle starting at a young age considering that this lays the foundation for a lower cardiovascular risk in adults and the elderly. The objective of this review is to examine cardiovascular primary prevention in young healthy women, focusing particularly on unresolved issues and the influence of social determinants, as well as the correlation with stressors and their influence on diet.

Keywords: women; cardiovascular risk; pregnancy; Life's Essential 8; monitoring; physical activity; diet

1. Introduction

Cardiovascular disease (CVD) in women presents with clinical pictures different from those in men; exposure to traditional risk factors is enriched with the action of risk factors specific to the female sex, and the response to drugs also seems to be influenced by the genetic differences. All this involves a different approach both in primary prevention and in the diagnosis and treatment of cardiovascular disease in women [1,2]. New evaluation algorithms have been introduced; however, since cardiovascular risk develops significantly after menopause, it is widely believed that women do not develop cardiovascular events before menopause [2]. This is not true because even women before menopause can develop cardiovascular (CV) events. This determines that prevention must start early as atherosclerosis is a slow and progressive phenomenon over time starting in the early stages of life [1–5].

Prevention of CVD presents both challenges and opportunities for disease prevention due to its multifaceted nature and significant impact on public health. The development of cardiovascular diseases is influenced by a multitude of risk factors and therefore requires global and multifaceted approaches. Subjects differ in their genetic predispositions, lifestyles, and environmental exposures, leading to variability in CVD risk profiles and responses to preventive interventions. Adapting prevention strategies to individual needs and characteristics can be difficult. The first obstacle is determined by the long period of development and latency of CVD, during which individuals can remain asymptomatic despite the progression of the underlying disease. This makes early diagnosis and intervention difficult [2,5].

Furthermore, socioeconomic factors such as income, education, access to healthcare, and living conditions significantly influence the risk and outcomes of cardiovascular disease. Addressing socioeconomic disparities in cardiovascular disease prevention requires addressing broader social determinants of health (SDOH) [1,2].

The objective of this review is to examine cardiovascular primary prevention in young healthy women, focusing particularly on unresolved issues and the influence of social determinants, as well as the correlation with stressors and their influence on diet. This review focuses on primary prevention in young women without any known heart disease and on the cardiovascular health of young, healthy women.

2. Gender Differences in CVD Prevention

2.1. The Long Journey of Atherosclerosis: Gender Differences

Although the clinical symptoms caused by atherosclerosis appear in middle and late adulthood, it is known that there is a long phase of development of the asymptomatic pathology, which begins in the first years of life, often during childhood. In most children, atherosclerotic vascular changes are mild and can be minimized or prevented with a healthy lifestyle [5–8].

Thus, events occurring in the early phases of life can profoundly impact future ASCVD (atherosclerotic cardiovascular disease) risk. For these reasons, ASCVD prevention should commence as early as possible to mitigate the onset of predisposing factors that could affect individual health later in life. Early detection and management of risk factors are essential in preventing or slowing the progression of atherosclerosis in young women and reducing the risk of cardiovascular events in adulthood and old age [4–8]. The initial stage of atherosclerosis is identified as a "fatty streak", commonly found in children and young individuals. These streaks comprise monocyte-derived macrophages and T lymphocytes, which are inflammatory cells that accumulate within arterial walls and serve as precursors to advanced atherosclerotic plaques [6]. The pathophysiological process involves multiple steps, starting with the inflammatory activation of endothelial cells [6–8]

Atherosclerosis and ischemic heart disease in women present unique challenges and considerations compared to men. While atherosclerosis, the buildup of plaque in the arteries, is a common underlying cause of ischemic heart disease in both genders, women often experience different manifestations, risk factors, and outcomes. Unlike men, women tend to develop a non-obstructive atherosclerotic disease in the phase of life preceding menopause due to the action of estrogen on the endothelial response [9].

Myocardial infarction with nonobstructive coronary arteries (MINOCA) is characterized by clinical evidence of acute myocardial infarction (AMI) with normal or near-normal coronary arteries on coronary angiography (stenosis < 50%) and without an alternative diagnosis for the acute presentation. Its prevalence ranges from 6% to 11% among all patients with AMI, with a predominance of young, nonwhite females with fewer traditional risks than those with obstructive coronary artery disease. MINOCA can be due to either epicardial causes such as rupture or fissuring of unstable nonobstructive atherosclerotic plaque, coronary artery spasm, spontaneous coronary dissection and cardioembolism, or other microvascular causes [10].

However, the perception of cardiovascular risk in young women is very poor leading to leading to poor effective prevention action [11,12].

2.2. Estrogens Prevent the CVD before Menopause

In the early stages, atherosclerosis may develop without causing significant narrowing or obstruction of the arteries. This stage may be asymptomatic and often goes undetected. However, even non-obstructive atherosclerosis can contribute to inflammation and plaque buildup in the arterial walls [5]. Estrogen, the primary female sex hormone, has both protective and potentially harmful effects on the cardiovascular system [11,12].

Before menopause, estrogen is believed to have a protective effect on the cardiovascular system, as it helps maintain healthy endothelium and vessels by promoting vasodilation, reducing endothelial dysfunction, and reducing vascular aging [9,13]. Estrogen also has antioxidant and anti-inflammatory properties that may reduce the risk of atherosclerosis [13,14]. However, after menopause, estrogen levels decline, leading to changes in lipid metabolism and increased inflammation, and promoting endothelial dysfunction and deposition of visceral fat in the abdomen [9,13,14].

This hormonal change contributes to the progression of atherosclerosis in post-menopausal women and the development of obstructive plaques, leading to a further increase in the risk of cardiovascular events [8,11–13].

2.3. Estrogen Is Not a Whole Story: The Impact of Lifestyle and (SDOH)

Overall, while estrogen plays a protective role in cardiovascular health before menopause, its decline after menopause may contribute to the progression of atherosclerosis and the development of obstructive ASCVD in women. Knowledge of these hormonal changes and their impact on the cardiovascular system is essential for developing effective prevention and treatment strategies for atherosclerosis in women [1,2]. The progression of atherosclerosis is influenced by both genetic predisposition and exposure to CV risk factors and environmental factors. Over time, atherosclerosis leads to plaque formation and to ASCVD such as ischemic heart disease, Ischemia with Non-Obstructed Coronary Arteries (INOCA), heart attack, stroke, or peripheral artery disease. Adopting a healthy lifestyle, including a balanced diet, regular physical activity, not smoking, and managing chronic conditions such as hypertension and diabetes, can help reduce the risk of developing atherosclerosis and its complications.

3. Strategies for CV Primary Prevention in Women

Effectively implementing primary prevention strategies in women poses significant challenges for various reasons. Firstly, there is a widespread belief that cardiovascular disease primarily affects women post-menopause, leading to a skewed perception of risk among young and adult women [11,15]. Secondly, women often face difficulties in adopting healthy lifestyles due to the multitude of social, familial, and occupational obligations they encounter in contrast to men [16,17]. Thirdly, the adoption of healthy habits, particularly physical activity, is heavily influenced by societal, environmental, and structural factors [1–3,18]. It is crucial to acknowledge that the development of atherosclerosis begins early in life, emphasizing the necessity for cardiovascular primary prevention to commence at a young age in women [4,5]. Pregnancy presents a unique opportunity to engage young women and guide them toward preventive behaviors [1,2,7,18–20].

Unsolved issues in cardiovascular prevention in young women encompass various challenges that persist despite advancements in healthcare. Some of these issues include awareness and perception of cardiovascular risk in young women, gender disparities, socioeconomic factors, lifestyle factors, and psychological and emotional health. Despite the increasing recognition of CVD as a significant health threat to women, there remains a lack of awareness among young women regarding their susceptibility to CVD and the importance of preventive measures [6,21]. Furthermore, women are often underrepresented in cardiovascular research, leading to a lack of understanding of how CVD manifests and progresses differently in women compared to men. This disparity may result in suboptimal prevention and treatment strategies tailored to women's unique risk factors and health needs [19,22]. Social determinants such as socioeconomic status, education, and access to healthcare significantly influence cardiovascular prevention efforts. Disparities in access to resources and healthcare services may exacerbate risk factors and hinder preventive measures for young women from disadvantaged backgrounds [1,17,19]. Providing access to quality healthcare, including preventive screenings and early intervention for risk factors such as high blood pressure and cholesterol, is crucial in safeguarding cardiovascular health in young women.

Mental health conditions such as stress, anxiety, and depression can impact cardiovascular health and exacerbate risk factors for CVD. Addressing the psychological well-being of young women and implementing effective stress management strategies are essential components of comprehensive cardiovascular prevention efforts [1,15–18].

Addressing these unsolved issues in cardiovascular prevention in young women requires a multifaceted approach that encompasses education, research, policy changes, and healthcare interventions tailored to the unique needs and challenges faced by this population. Encouraging healthy lifestyle habits such as regular physical activity, a balanced diet, stress management, and avoidance of tobacco and excessive alcohol use can significantly reduce the risk of developing CVD in young women. Additionally, addressing unique factors that affect women's cardiovascular health, such as pregnancy-related complications like gestational diabetes and pre-eclampsia, is essential.

3.1. *Pregnancy Stage Is a Good Time to Introduce Primary Prevention in Women*

Pregnancy is a challenging moment in the life of a young woman and is characterized by a series of both physical and psychological changes. While changes in physical conditions have been explored in several studies over time, attention to the psychological changes that can affect the body's responses has only recently increased [2–5].

The American Heart Association (AHA) proposed a consensus document regarding cardiovascular health in young women before pregnancy [19,20]. The pre-pregnancy period is indeed a critical time for interventions aimed at identifying and managing cardiovascular risk factors in individuals who are planning to conceive. This period of the woman's life offers an opportunity to address and modify risk factors that may contribute to adverse pregnancy outcomes and subsequent cardiovascular disease for both the mother and the offspring [20,21]. Pregnancy is a very critical moment in a woman's life and can be burdened by high levels of stress.

As suggested by the AHA consensus, one way to assess lifestyle factors and their impact on cardiovascular health is by evaluating Life's Simple 7 or Life's Essential 8 (LS8). Originally defined in 2010, the Life's Simple 7 framework includes seven key health factors: diet, physical activity, no smoking, body mass index, blood pressure, lipids, and blood sugar. This framework provides a comprehensive approach to assessing and promoting cardiovascular health. In a more recent update, sleep health was included as an eighth factor, resulting in the Life's Essential 8 framework [20–24].

Furthermore, the consensus document introduces and underlines the importance of the three pillars: stress/resilience, social determinants, and structural policies [20]. These determinants encompass aspects such as mental well-being, socio-economic factors, and access to healthcare and resources, which can influence an individual's overall health and well-being [20,23–26]. Stress, anxiety, and depression experienced by mothers during pregnancy harm the development of the fetus and increase the risk of cognitive, behavioral, and emotional difficulties in offspring [27]. At the same time, stress caused by external factors can influence the mother's lifestyle, especially aspects related to diet and physical activity. Stressful factors during pregnancy can be developing an unplanned or unwanted pregnancy, low economic level, poor support from family and friends, loneliness, and poor medical care support. These stressors can influence the mother's relationship with food with repercussions on the fetus. To this, we must add the risk of developing pregnancy-related pathologies.

3.2. Peripartum Cardiomyopathy

An example of a cardiovascular complication of pregnancy is peripartum cardiomyopathy (PPCM); it is a rare but serious condition characterized by the development of heart failure during the last month of pregnancy or within the first five months postpartum in women without pre-existing heart disease. The exact cause of PPCM is still not fully understood, but it is believed to involve a combination of genetic, hormonal, immunological, and environmental factors.

In the past, PPCM faced challenges in recognition and comprehension, resulting in a deficiency of standardized diagnostic criteria and treatment strategies. Frequently, PPCM was mistaken for other types of heart failure or disregarded due to its rarity and symptom overlap with typical pregnancy manifestations. This lack of awareness and comprehension notably hindered the timely detection and management of affected women, leading to increased rates of morbidity and mortality. The literature on PPCM, characterized by varied and occasionally contradictory discoveries, has posed difficulties for clinicians in providing confident guidance and treatment to patients [28].

The precise cause of PPCM remains elusive, yet it is considered to be multifaceted, involving genetic, environmental, and hormonal elements. This cardiomyopathy is defined by left ventricular systolic dysfunction and heart failure, manifesting in the absence of any other discernible cause. Theories surrounding its origin encompass myocardial inflammation, oxidative stress, and imbalances in angiogenesis. Additionally, PPCM is thought to be associated with the vascular and hormonal alterations inherent in pregnancy [28,29].

Prior research has indicated that many women diagnosed with PPCM experience partial or complete recovery of their left ventricular (LV) function. However, persistent LV systolic dysfunction can lead to adverse cardiac events such as life-threatening ventricular tachyarrhythmias, thromboembolic complications, and even mortality. The rate of recovery from PPCM appears to vary widely among individuals. Unfortunately, there are currently no specific and reliable predictors to determine whether myocardial recovery will occur. One of the factors contributing to the development of PPCM appears to be inflammation [30–33]. The link between inflammation and stress is very important and could be a good avenue to explore with future research.

4. SDOH and Stress in Women

SDOH are conditions in the environments where people are born, live, learn, work, play, worship, and age that affect a wide range of health, functioning, and quality-of-life outcomes and risks [34].

SDOH act by causing an increase in stress. Stress exerts a significant influence on women's behaviors across various life stages. Societal norms and gender expectations further compound this stress, creating substantial burdens related to caregiving responsibilities, professional duties, and conforming to societal standards of appearance and conduct. These stressors contribute to the risk of developing chronic non-communicable diseases in the future [1,2,21].

Stress can exert profound effects on the cardiovascular system through various physiological mechanisms, including the activation of the sympathetic nervous system, the hypothalamic–pituitary–adrenal (HPA) axis, and inflammatory pathways [25,35,36].

Chronic stress promotes the chronic inflammatory response in the body through the release of pro-inflammatory cytokines and activation of the immune cell system [29,31].

This chronic low-grade inflammation is associated with endothelial dysfunction, oxidative stress, and plaque formation in the arteries, contributing to the development and progression of atherosclerosis. Inflammatory processes in the cardiovascular system increase the risk of coronary and vascular artery disease [11,29,31,37,38].

Stress-induced activation of the sympathetic nervous system and HPA axis can induce endothelial dysfunction.

Endothelial dysfunction is characterized by reduced production of nitric oxide, a potent vasodilator. Impaired endothelial function contributes to vasoconstriction, inflammation, and thrombosis, further exacerbating cardiovascular risk [30–34].

4.1. *How Stress Influences Diet and Dietary Behavior in Women*

The impact of stress on cardiovascular health in women has been rediscovered in the COVID-19 pandemic and post-pandemic period [1,2,25]. Gender variations have been observed in brain activation, autonomic nervous system responses, cortisol secretion, endothelial dysfunction, inflammatory processes, and immune responses. Some studies suggest the amygdala's role in gender-specific cardiovascular events. Notably, a neuroimaging investigation revealed a correlation between preclinical carotid atherosclerosis and heightened amygdala reactivity [8,39,40].

Stress can have unique effects on women's health due to various physiological, hormonal, and social factors.

Women's hormonal fluctuations, particularly during menstruation, pregnancy, and menopause, can influence how they respond to stress. For example, fluctuations in estrogen and progesterone levels can affect mood and stress sensitivity.

Women are more prone to depression and anxiety, which can be exacerbated by stress. Hormonal changes, societal pressures, and caregiving responsibilities may contribute to this increased susceptibility [1]. Societal expectations and gender roles can influence how women experience and cope with stress. Balancing multiple roles such as caregiving, work, and household responsibilities can contribute to chronic stress in women.

Women may use different coping strategies to deal with stress compared to men. Seeking social support, talking about their feelings, and engaging in self-care activities such as exercise, mindfulness, and relaxation techniques are common coping mechanisms for women [1,8,25,41]. Women have a fragility largely determined by the poor socio-economic conditions that lead to incorrect lifestyles and a lack of prevention [1,8,20,25,41].

It is well known that stress can significantly influence dietary patterns and food choices, leading to both short-term and long-term effects on an individual's eating habits [41]. The impact of stress on diet is complex and can vary from person to person [42]. Many individuals under stress may turn to food for comfort, a phenomenon known as emotional eating. This often involves consuming high-calorie, sugary, or comfort foods as a way to cope with stress and negative emotions [42–46].

Furthermore, stress can induce food craving [47]. Food craving is characterized by a strong urge to consume a particular food. In Western cultures, these foods typically boast high palatability and are energy-dense, often containing high levels of sugar and/or fat. This craving experience encompasses various dimensions, including cognitive (such as thinking about food), emotional (like the desire to eat or mood changes), behavioral (such as seeking and consuming food), and physiological (including salivation) aspects [47].

These cravings may be linked to the brain's response to stress hormones [44,46–49]. Stress triggers the release of hormones, such as cortisol, which can impact metabolism and lead to weight gain, especially around the abdominal area. This hormonal response can influence the body's storage of fat [42,45].

Stress can lead to disruptions in normal eating patterns [41–46]. Some people may experience an increase in appetite and overeat, while others may lose their appetite and undereat. Both patterns can have consequences for overall health, especially during pregnancy.

4.2. Stress during Pregnancy and Its Relationship with Food

Several studies that have analyzed the impact of stress during pregnancy highlight the fundamental role of nurses who care for mothers in suggesting adequate nutrition and methods to reduce anxiety and stress [50,51].

Celik and coworkers investigated the stress, emotional eating, and weight bias levels in 210 Turkish pregnant women [50]. They found that pregnant women experience a moderate level of stress, emotional eating, and weight bias. There was a significant relationship between the weight bias score averages and the emotional eating and stress score averages of the pregnant women. The study underlines that nearly 1 in 2 pregnant women was overweight or obese, and when the body mass index level of the women increased, their weight stigma and emotional eating also increased. The authors underlined the importance of the nurse in providing training and counseling on how to deal with stress, stigma, and nutrition during pregnancy, in order to ensure the psychological adaptation of pregnant women to childbirth and the postpartum period, which they are at risk of in terms of stress and emotional problems. Bias factors are related to nutrition and weight [50].

Jackson H and coworkers evaluated pregnant women's recall of the nutritional advice provided by their healthcare during pregnancy [52]. They found that approximately half of the women enrolled in the survey recall receiving nutritional counseling during pregnancy and that 73% of women who were counseled on nutrition changed their behavior based on the recommendations received [52].

Pregnancy and nutrition are closely intertwined, as proper nutrition is essential for the health and well-being of both the mother and the developing baby. The first crucial point is a balanced and varied diet that includes a wide range of nutrients [45,53–56]. The diet should include fruits, vegetables, whole grains, lean proteins, dairy or plant-based alternatives, and healthy fats. It is important to avoid foods with empty calories and focus on nutrient-rich options [45,53–56]. Little information is available on the effect of stimulants such as coffee and caffeine during pregnancy. The guidelines indicate that a dosage of caffeine up to 200 mg per day is to be considered safe in women who are habitual consumers [57–60]. However, some studies link high caffeine intake with an increase in anxiety [61–64].

Many of the potential benefits attributed to coffee stem from the belief that it possesses antioxidant and anti-inflammatory properties [65]. The primary constituents of coffee believed to exert such effects include phenolic compounds, caffeine, diterpenes, trigonelline, and melanoidins [57,65]. Among these, the phenolic component is predominantly characterized by chlorogenic acids. Chlorogenic acids have been shown to elicit antioxidant effects by reducing the production of inflammatory mediators through various mechanisms [66]. The anti-inflammatory properties of coffee might also be influenced by its impact on the gut microbiota. Pre-clinical and human studies suggest that consuming coffee can lead to alterations in the composition and activity of the gut microbiota. This can result in changes to the balance among major microbial phyla favoring a profile associated with anti-obesity effects [67].

Social expectations require women to adopt a healthy lifestyle during pregnancy; however, no univocal behavior emerges in the various studies. The reduction in the consumption of coffee and tea appears frequent even if not supported by data highlighting side effects caused by moderate consumption of these drinks [68]. There are no studies that evaluate the consumption of energy drinks in young pregnant women; this is an interesting point to develop in the future considering the significant increase in the consumption of these caffeinated drinks [69,70].

A very controversial point is the impact of a vegan or vegetarian diet on cardiovascular health and prevention. These diets have been little studied compared to the Mediterranean diet [71]. The quality of the plant-based diet is an important feature. Individuals who follow a nutritious plant-based diet reportedly exhibit lower body mass index, reduced waist circumference, and decreased visceral fat compared to those adhering to less healthful plant-based diets [72]. Researchers have observed that the quality of the diet might hold greater significance than specific dietary patterns when comparing vegans, vegetarians, and omnivores, as there are no significant differences in adiposity values among these groups [73]. A recent meta-analysis on the vegetarian diet found that consuming a vegetarian diet was associated with significant improvements in low-density lipoprotein cholesterol (LDL-C), glycated hemoglobin (HbA1c), and body weight beyond the standard therapy in individuals at high risk of CVDs. However, the changes in LDL-C and HbA1c did not reach the clinical significance as per the cutoff target [74]. Few studies have been conducted on the effects of a vegetarian diet on cardiovascular risk in primary prevention. During pregnancy, blood docosahexaenoic acids (DHA) concentrations are often lower in vegetarians than in nonvegetarians; cord blood DHA is lower in infants of vegetarians [75]. When food access is satisfactory, infant birth weights and the duration of gestation are similar in vegetarian and nonvegetarian pregnancies [62], leading to the conclusion that with adequate nutrient intake, vegetarian and vegan diets are safe in pregnancy.

Stress can contribute to mindless or distracted eating, where individuals may eat without paying attention to hunger cues or the nutritional content of the food [75,76].

4.3. Perinatal Depression and Its Relationship with Food

Perinatal depression is defined as the onset of a major or minor depressive episode during pregnancy (antenatal depression), after childbirth (postpartum depression), or both [76].

Christian and coworkers explored the variations in eating disorders or depression symptoms among women at different stages of pregnancy and the impact of social determinants [77]. During pregnancy, eating disorder symptoms and various social and self-evaluative factors were uniquely linked to depression. Specifically, eating disorder symptoms, maladaptive perfectionism, social appearance anxiety, and self-compassion during pregnancy were significant predictors of postpartum depression, even after considering prenatal depression. Notably, during pregnancy, but not postpartum, a stronger association between eating disorders and depression symptoms was observed when social support and self-compassion were low and maladaptive perfectionism was high [77]. The authors suggest that targeting eating disorder symptoms and addressing social and self-evaluative factors in routine medical care and stepped-care interventions could enhance maternal mental healthcare and prevent postpartum depression [77]. The transition from pregnancy to postpartum represents a critical phase marked by numerous significant and abrupt changes. These include weight gain, alterations in appetite, fluctuations in hormones, and changes in social relationships. These biopsychosocial transformations, combined with increased social pressures and expectations surrounding pregnancy, such as the desire to appear "glowing" and the pressure to swiftly return to pre-pregnancy weight, contribute to the risk of experiencing alterations in eating behavior and depressive symptoms.

Support from healthcare professionals plays a fundamental role in helping women in the postpartum phase, reducing performance anxiety and expectations, and reducing the risk of developing depression. Moreover, a significant association between antenatal depression and the development of new CVD within 24 months postpartum exists [78–81].

Recent research has indeed highlighted the significant role of dietary and nutritional interventions in reducing depression, partly through their effects on the gut microbiota [82,83]. A diet rich in fruits, vegetables, whole grains, lean proteins, and healthy fats is associated with a lower risk of depression. These foods provide essential nutrients and antioxidants that support brain health and reduce inflammation, which is implicated in depression [41,84]. Conversely, diets high in processed foods, sugars, and unhealthy fats can contribute to inflammation and increase the risk of depression [41,84]. The gut microbiota, composed of trillions of microorganisms living in the digestive tract, plays a crucial role in brain health and mood regulation. Dietary patterns can influence the composition and diversity of the gut microbiota. A diet high in fiber and fermented foods, such as yogurt, kefir, sauerkraut, and kimchi, promotes the growth of beneficial gut bacteria, which can positively impact mood and reduce symptoms of depression [41,84]. Prebiotics are nondigestible fibers that serve as food for beneficial gut bacteria. Studies suggest that probiotic supplements and foods containing probiotics, such as yogurt and kefir, may have antidepressant effects by modulating the gut–brain axis and reducing inflammation [85]. Several studies have shown that omega-3 supplementation may reduce symptoms of depression and improve mood regulation. Omega-3 may also influence the gut microbiota composition, contributing to their antidepressant effects [86].

Some micronutrients, including vitamins B6, B12, folate, vitamin D, and magnesium, play key roles in neurotransmitter synthesis, mood regulation, and stress response. Deficiencies in these nutrients have been linked to an increased risk of depression.

The prevalence of vitamin D deficiency among pregnant women and newborns is a cause for serious concern as vitamin D plays a crucial role in hippocampal learning and memory for mothers and in neural cell growth for offspring as shown in preclinical studies [87,88]. Vitamin D acts as a neuroactive hormone, influencing the concentration of neuronal calcium ions, which are key to regulating neuroplasticity and mood [89,90].

A meta-analysis of nine longitudinal studies involving 8470 subjects revealed a noteworthy inverse association between serum 25(OH)D levels and the risk of postpartum depression, with a cutoff of 50 nmol/L [91]. However, a randomized controlled trial indicated that supplementation with 2000 IU vitamin D3 from 26 to 28 weeks of gestation up to childbirth significantly reduced depression scores [92]. These findings suggested that vitamin D supplementation during late pregnancy could be advantageous in mitigating perinatal depression [92,93].

Overall, dietary and nutritional interventions can have potent effects on reducing depression, partly through their interactions with the gut microbiota. Prolonged or chronic stress may affect the absorption of nutrients in the digestive system, potentially leading to nutrient deficiencies over time and inducing changes in the microbiota. The microbiota is a new cardiovascular risk factor that influences the absorption of fats and some drugs such as oral hypoglycemics and statins [94–96].

All this evidence supports the hypothesis that counseling in women plays an important role in maintaining and undertaking correct lifestyles [2,7,97]. The central component of the lifestyle is the diet, which is able to influence the other aspects of a healthy life such as obesity and sleep quality. The Academy of Nutrition and Dietetics identifies a balanced diet and adequate weight gain as two important components of a healthy pregnancy [98]. The amount of food a woman needs during pregnancy depends on a number of things including her body mass index, before pregnancy, the rate at which she gains weight, age, and appetite. All pregnant women should eat a variety of nutrient-rich foods each day [52–54,56,98].

These psychological conditions can have negative effects on the health of the mother during pregnancy and increase the risk of complications. Furthermore, they have a long-term effect that is reflected in the development of non-communicable diseases in adult women [24,99,100].

5. Proposed Intervention for Prevention in Young Women: The WEAR-Being Project

The WEAR-being project was designed to collect information on cardiovascular health in women in different age groups. For this end-point, young women and pre-menopausal women were selected. The goal is to gain information about cardiovascular health and how it is perceived in young women and women approaching menopause. The second objective of the study is to implement a lifestyle correction model that is personalized, responds to the needs of the individual woman, and is pursued through direct coaching carried out by expert and dedicated healthcare personnel. The third objective is to collect objective data through precise tools on the cardiovascular responses during the lifestyle modifications proposed by the trainers and verify whether this approach is effective.

The WEAR-being project addresses the global challenge of maintaining health in a rapidly changing society (HEALTH Cluster—Horizon Europe strategic plan) by providing lifestyle monitoring in a group of young women (30–40 years) compared with a control group of menopausal women (50–60 years). The devices will record data relating to daily physical activity, quality and duration of sleep, and vital signs. Information on calorie intake and diet quality will be entered manually by the subjects. The data collected will be managed through Big Data management techniques and will be analyzed using artificial intelligence and data mining techniques in order to establish personal trends and ranges of values in relation to the diet and activity carried out by the subject.

For this purpose, a 12-month monitoring study has been developed which will involve women. The women will be recruited through campaigns conducted on social media and through charity foundations that are very active in the area. The analysis will evaluate adherence to a correct lifestyle (diet, physical activity, and stress levels) and the control of bio-humoral parameters and vital parameters. For the objective assessment of lifestyle, the Life's Essential 8 evaluation score will be used. Women will be sent to dietary and lifestyle counseling sessions. The counseling sessions will be carried out in small groups and personalized and guided by specifically trained healthcare professionals. In young women, the need for good cardiovascular health will be highlighted in order to preserve the health of the fetus in the event of a pregnancy. Counseling dedicated to stress management will be introduced. The project is under evaluation by the local Ethics Committee. The study was developed in accordance with the Helsinki Declaration (www.wma.net (accessed on 1 December 2023)), and all patients will provide informed consent. The data will be processed in accordance with current privacy legislation. The goal is to promote awareness of good cardiovascular health even in young women. We have identified the Mediterranean Diet which is easily achievable in our country. The Mediterranean score and Life's Essential 8 score will also be calculated and compared in the same subject in order to verify an improvement in behavior and take personalized actions. To encourage subjects to increase physical activity, a wearable device monitoring activity (i.e., number of kilometers walking/day) will be used [101]. Over the past few years, wearable technologies have become increasingly common in everyday life. From an industry study conducted by Gartner, it has been found that the device market of wearables is continuously growing with an estimated spending of USD 81.5 billion in 2021 [102]. Wearable devices are a high-tech solution that can help us in the promotion of well-being, playing an important role in monitoring physical activity, diet and rhythms sleep, anxiety, and stress [103,104]. Furthermore, they allow the person wearing them to interact and monitor their body throughout the day, increasing awareness and active involvement in improving one's well-being. In a research study conducted by Business Insider, 75% of users agreed that wearable devices promote encouragement to take care of one's health, thereby promoting virtuous behavior [103,104]. Healthcare providers play a critical role in educating and supporting pregnant women in making healthy choices, monitoring weight gain during pregnancy, and managing any underlying health conditions. We aim to increase this attention towards young women. The WEAR-being project will contribute to stimulating awareness of the relevance of cardiovascular primary prevention in young women.

6. Conclusions

In conclusion, the social determinants of health have a strong impact on lifestyle, and women are more likely to adopt unhealthy behaviors in response to stress. Diet is an excellent tool to guide the trend toward healthy behaviors. To prevent chronic non-communicable disease, it is advisable to start primary prevention through correct lifestyles at a young age, and among women, a good time to intercept is pregnancy. Pregnancy can be a challenging factor in a woman's life because she is more exposed to stressful situations. Healthcare personnel, mainly nurses, play an important educational role in educating and supporting young women, especially from disadvantaged social backgrounds.

Author Contributions: Conceptualization, F.C., V.B., S.N., A.V.M. and S.G.; methodology, K.S., V.S., G.Z., M.P., M.N. and B.S.; software, V.S., G.Z. and V.B.; data curation, M.P. and M.N.; writing—original draft; preparation, all authors; supervision, S.N., A.V.M. and S.G.; funding acquisition, A.V.M. All authors have read and agreed to the published version of the manuscript.

Funding: This research was funded by Fondazione Carisbo, ref #20047 Grant Ricerca medica e alta tecnologia 2022—Progetto "WEARbeing—dispositivi medici e indossabili per la salute e il benessere" P-I-Anna Vittoria Mattioli.

Conflicts of Interest: The authors declare no conflicts of interest.

References

1. Vogel, B.; Acevedo, M.; Appelman, Y.; Bairey Merz, C.N.; Chieffo, A.; Figtree, G.A.; Guerrero, M.; Kunadian, V.; Lam, C.S.P.; Maas, A.H.E.M.; et al. The Lancet women and cardiovascular disease Commission: Reducing the global burden by 2030. *Lancet* **2021**, *397*, 2385–2438. [CrossRef] [PubMed]
2. Mattioli, A.V.; Moscucci, F.; Sciomer, S.; Maffei, S.; Nasi, M.; Pinti, M.; Bucciarelli, V.; Dei Cas, A.; Parati, G.; Ciccone, M.M.; et al. Cardiovascular prevention in women: Un update By the Italian Society of Cardiology Working Group On "Prevention, Hypertension and peripheral disease". *J. Cardiovasc. Med.* **2023**, *24* (Suppl. S2), e147–e155. [CrossRef] [PubMed]
3. Nathani, M.; Vogel, B.; Mehran, R. Closing the gap: Cardiovascular disease in women. *Climacteric J. Int. Menopause Soc.* **2024**, *27*, 16–21. [CrossRef] [PubMed]
4. Lloyd-Jones, D.M.; Hong, Y.; Labarthe, D.; Mozaffarian, D.; Appel, L.J.; Van Horn, L.; Greenlund, K.; Daniels, S.; Nichol, G.; Tomaselli, G.F.; et al. Defining and setting national goals for cardiovascular health promotion and disease reduction: The American Heart Association's Strategic Impact Goal through 2020 and beyond. *Circulation* **2010**, *121*, 586–613. [CrossRef] [PubMed]
5. D'Ascenzi, F.; Sciaccaluga, C.; Cameli, M.; Cecere, A.; Ciccone, M.M.; Di Francesco, S.; Ganau, A.; Imbalzano, E.; Liga, R.; Palermo, P.; et al. When should cardiovascular prevention begin? The importance of antenatal, perinatal and primordial prevention. *Eur. J. Prev. Cardiol.* **2021**, *28*, 361–369. [CrossRef] [PubMed]
6. Hong, Y.M. Atherosclerotic cardiovascular disease beginning in childhood. *Korean Circ. J.* **2010**, *40*, 1–9. [CrossRef] [PubMed]
7. Zanini, G.; Selleri, V.; Roncati, L.; Coppi, F.; Nasi, M.; Farinetti, A.; Manenti, A.; Pinti, M.; Mattioli, A.V. Vascular "Long COVID": A New Vessel Disease? *Angiology* **2024**, *75*, 8–14. [CrossRef] [PubMed]
8. Ross, R. Atherosclerosis—An inflammatory disease. *N. Engl. J. Med.* **1999**, *340*, 115–126. [CrossRef]
9. Nair, A.R.; Pillai, A.J.; Nair, N. Cardiovascular Changes in Menopause. *Curr. Cardiol. Rev.* **2021**, *17*, e230421187681. [CrossRef]
10. Foà, A.; Canton, L.; Bodega, F.; Bergamaschi, L.; Paolisso, P.; De Vita, A.; Villano, A.; Mattioli, A.V.; Tritto, I.; Morrone, D.; et al. Myocardial infarction with nonobstructive coronary arteries: From pathophysiology to therapeutic strategies. *J. Cardiovasc. Med.* **2023**, *24* (Suppl. S2), e134–e146. [CrossRef]
11. Mosca, L.; Hammond, G.; Mochari-Greenberger, H.; Towfighi, A.; Albert, M.A.; American Heart Association Cardiovascular Disease and Stroke in Women and Special Populations Committee of the Council on Clinical Cardiology; Council on Epidemiology and Prevention; Council on Cardiovascular Nursing; Council on High Bloo. Fifteen-year trends in awareness of heart disease in women: Results of a 2012 American Heart Association national survey. *Circulation* **2013**, *127*, 1254–1263. [CrossRef] [PubMed]
12. Lerner, D.J.; Kannel, W.B. Patterns of coronary heart disease morbidity and mortality in the sexes: A 26-year follow-up of the Framingham population. *Am. Heart J.* **1986**, *111*, 383–390. [CrossRef] [PubMed]
13. Taddei, S.; Virdis, A.; Ghiadoni, L.; Mattei, P.; Sudano, I.; Bernini, G.; Pinto, S.; Salvetti, A. Menopause is associated with endothelial dysfunction in women. *Hypertension* **1996**, *28*, 576–582. [CrossRef] [PubMed]
14. Signorelli, S.S.; Neri, S.; Sciacchitano, S.; Pino, L.D.; Costa, M.P.; Marchese, G.; Celotta, G.; Cassibba, N.; Pennisi, G.; Caschetto, S. Behaviour of some indicators of oxidative stress in postmenopausal and fertile women. *Maturitas* **2006**, *53*, 77–82. [CrossRef] [PubMed]
15. Maffei, S.; Meloni, A.; Deidda, M.; Sciomer, S.; Cugusi, L.; Cadeddu, C.; Gallina, S.; Franchini, M.; Scambia, G.; Surico, D.; et al. Cardiovascular Risk Perception and Knowledge among Italian Women: Lessons from IGENDA Protocol. *J. Clin. Med.* **2022**, *11*, 1695. [CrossRef] [PubMed]
16. Vlassoff, C. Gender differences in determinants and consequences of health and illness. *J. Health Popul. Nutr.* **2007**, *25*, 47–61. [PubMed]
17. Woodward, M. Cardiovascular disease and the female disadvantage. *Int. J. Environ. Res. Public Health* **2019**, *16*, 1165. [CrossRef] [PubMed]
18. Mattioli, A.V.; Coppi, F.; Bucciarelli, V.; Gallina, S. Cardiovascular risk stratification in young women: The pivotal role of pregnancy. *J. Cardiovasc. Med.* **2023**, *24*, 793–797. [CrossRef] [PubMed]
19. Humphries, K.H.; Izadnegahdar, M.; Sedlak, T.; Saw, J.; Johnston, N.; Schenck-Gustafsson, K.; Shah, R.U.; Regitz-Zagrosek, V.; Grewal, J.; Vaccarino, V.; et al. Sex differences in cardiovascular disease—Impact on care and outcomes. *Front. Neuroendocrinol.* **2017**, *46*, 46–70. [CrossRef]
20. Khan, S.S.; Brewer, L.C.; Canobbio, M.M.; Cipolla, M.J.; Grobman, W.A.; Lewey, J.; Michos, E.D.; Miller, E.C.; Perak, A.M.; Wei, G.; et al. Optimizing Prepregnancy Cardiovascular Health to Improve Outcomes in Pregnant and Postpartum Individuals and Offspring: A Scientific Statement from the American Heart Association. *Circulation* **2023**, *147*, e76–e91. [CrossRef]
21. Mehta, L.S.; Sharma, G.; Creanga, A.A.; Hameed, A.B.; Hollier, L.M.; Johnson, J.C.; Leffert, L.; McCullough, L.D.; Mujahid, M.S.; Watson, K.; et al. Call to action: Maternal health and saving mothers: A policy statement from the American Heart Association. *Circulation* **2021**, *144*, e251–e269. [CrossRef]

22. Lunova, T.; Komorovsky, R.; Klishch, I. Gender differences in treatment delays, management and mortality among patients with acute coronary syndrome: A systematic review and meta-analysis. *Curr. Cardiol. Rev.* **2023**, *19*, e300622206530. [CrossRef]
23. Agarwala, A.; Patel, J.; Stephens, J.; Roberson, S.; Scott, J.; Beckie, T.; Jackson, E.A.; American Heart Association Prevention Science Committee of the Council on Epidemiology and Prevention and Council on Cardiovascular and Stroke Nursing; Council on Clinical Cardiology; Council on Lifestyle and Cardiometabolic Health. Implementation of Prevention Science to Eliminate Health Care Inequities in Achieving Cardiovascular Health: A Scientific Statement from the American Heart Association. *Circulation* **2023**, *148*, 1183–1193. [CrossRef]
24. Wilkins, E.; Wickramasinghe, K.; Pullar, J.; Demaio, A.R.; Roberts, N.; Perez-Blanco, K.M.; Noonan, K.; Townsend, N. Maternal nutrition and its intergenerational links to non-communicable disease metabolic risk factors: A systematic review and narrative synthesis. *J. Health Popul. Nutr.* **2021**, *40*, 20. [CrossRef]
25. Mattioli, A.V.; Coppi, F.; Nasi, M.; Gallina, S. Stress and cardiovascular risk burden after the pandemic: Current status and future prospects. *Expert Rev. Cardiovasc. Ther.* **2022**, *20*, 507–513. [CrossRef]
26. Shibeshi, K.; Lemu, Y.; Gebretsadik, L.; Gebretsadik, A.; Morankar, S. Understanding Gender-Based Perception during Pregnancy: A Qualitative Study. *Int. J. Women's Health* **2023**, *15*, 1523–1535. [CrossRef] [PubMed]
27. Naaz, A.; Muneshwar, K.N. How Maternal Nutritional and Mental Health Affects Child Health During Pregnancy: A Narrative Review. *Cureus* **2023**, *15*, e48763. [CrossRef] [PubMed]
28. Safira, A.; Tjahjadi, A.K.; Adytia, G.J.; Waitupu, A.; Sutanto, H. Peripartum cardiomyopathy unveiled: Etiology, diagnosis, and therapeutic insights. *Curr. Probl. Cardiol.* **2024**, *49*, 102474. [CrossRef]
29. Arany, Z.; Elkayam, U. Peripartum cardiomyopathy. *Circulation* **2016**, *133*, 1397–1409. [CrossRef]
30. Tak, B.T.; Cay, S.; Pamukcu, H.E.; Ekizler, F.A.; Kafes, H.; Cetin, E.H.O.; Ulvan, N.; Ozeke, O.; Ozcan, F.; Topaloglu, S.; et al. Prognostic nutritional index as a novel marker for prediction of prognosis in patients with peripartum cardiomyopathy. *Medicine* **2020**, *99*, e19524. [CrossRef]
31. Sliwa, K.; Skudicky, D.; Bergemann, A.; Candy, G.; Puren, A.; Sareli, P. Peripartum cardiomyopathy: Analysis of clinical outcome, left ventricular function, plasma levels of cytokines and Fas/APO-1. *J. Am. Coll. Cardiol.* **2000**, *35*, 701–705. [CrossRef] [PubMed]
32. Mattioli, A.V.; Tarabini Castellani, E.; Vivoli, D.; Molinari, R.; Mattioli, G. Restoration of atrial function after atrial fibrillation of different etiological origins. *Cardiology* **1996**, *87*, 205–211. [CrossRef] [PubMed]
33. Adamson, D.L.; Nelson-Piercy, C. Managing palpitations and arrhythmias during pregnancy. *Heart* **2007**, *93*, 1630–1636. [CrossRef] [PubMed]
34. Available online: https://health.gov/healthypeople/priority-areas/social-determinants-health (accessed on 22 March 2024).
35. Koenig, H.G. Physical health consequences of psychological conditions. *Int. J. Psychiatry Med.* **2024**, *59*, 135–138. [CrossRef] [PubMed]
36. Lu, S.; Wei, F.; Li, G. The evolution of the concept of stress and the framework of the stress system. *Cell Stress* **2021**, *5*, 76–85. [CrossRef]
37. Cameli, M.; Lembo, M.; Sciaccaluga, C.; for the Working Groups of Echocardiography and Arterial Hypertension of Italian Society of Cardiology (SIC). Identification of cardiac organ damage in arterial hypertension: Insights by echocardiography for a comprehensive assessment. *J. Hypertens.* **2020**, *38*, 588–598. [CrossRef] [PubMed]
38. Kazemi, N.; Bordbar, A.; Bavarsad, S.S.; Ghasemi, P.; Bakhshi, M.; Rezaeeyan, H. Molecular Insights into the Relationship Between Platelet Activation and Endothelial Dysfunction: Molecular Approaches and Clinical Practice. *Mol. Biotechnol.* **2024**. [CrossRef] [PubMed]
39. Yang, H.J.; Koh, E.; Kang, Y. Susceptibility of Women to Cardiovascular Disease and the Prevention Potential of Mind-Body Intervention by Changes in Neural Circuits and Cardiovascular Physiology. *Biomolecules* **2021**, *11*, 708. [CrossRef]
40. Gianaros, P.J.; Hariri, A.R.; Sheu, L.K.; Muldoon, M.F.; Sutton-Tyrrell, K.; Manuck, S.B. Preclinical atherosclerosis covaries with individual differences in reactivity and functional connectivity of the amygdala. *Biol. Psychiatry* **2009**, *65*, 943–950. [CrossRef]
41. Coppi, F.; Farinetti, A.; Stefanelli, C.; Mattioli, A.V. Changes in food during the COVID-19 pandemic: The different roles of stress and depression in women and men. *Nutrition* **2023**, *108*, 111981. [CrossRef]
42. Ha, O.R.; Lim, S.L. The role of emotion in eating behavior and decisions. *Front. Psychol.* **2023**, *14*, 1265074. [CrossRef] [PubMed]
43. Legget, K.T.; Cornier, M.-A.; Sarabia, L.; Delao, E.M.; Mikulich-Gilbertson, S.K.; Natvig, C.; Erpelding, C.; Mitchell, T.; Hild, A.; Kronberg, E.; et al. Sex Differences in Effects of Mood, Eating-Related Behaviors, and BMI on Food Appeal and Desire to Eat: A Cross-Sectional Survey Study. *Nutrients* **2023**, *15*, 762. [CrossRef] [PubMed]
44. Borer, K.T. Why We Eat Too Much, Have an Easier Time Gaining Than Losing Weight, and Expend Too Little Energy: Suggestions for Counteracting or Mitigating These Problems. *Nutrients* **2021**, *13*, 3812. [CrossRef] [PubMed]
45. Li, D.L.; Hodge, A.M.; Cribb, L.; Southey, M.C.; Giles, G.G.; Milne, R.L.; Dugué, P.A. Body size, diet quality, and epigenetic ageing: Cross-sectional and longitudinal analyses. *J. Gerontol. Ser. A Biol. Sci. Med. Sci.* **2024**, *24*, glae026. [CrossRef]
46. Gilmartin, T.; Dipnall, J.F.; Gurvich, C.; Sharp, G. Identifying overcontrol and undercontrol personality types among young people using the five factor model, and the relationship with disordered eating behaviour, anxiety and depression. *J. Eat. Disord.* **2024**, *12*, 16. [CrossRef] [PubMed]
47. Rodríguez-Martín, B.C.; Meule, A. Food craving: New contributions on its assessment, moderators, and consequences. *Front. Psychol.* **2015**, *6*, 21. [CrossRef]

48. Langley, E.B.; O'Leary, D.J.; Gross, J.J.; Shiota, M.N. Breaking the Link between Negative Emotion and Unhealthy Eating: The Role of Emotion Regulation. *Affect. Sci.* **2023**, *4*, 702–710. [CrossRef]
49. You, Z.; Shan, L.; Cheng, S.; Xia, Y.; Zhao, Y.; Zhang, H.; Zhao, Z. Dietary intake patterns during pregnancy and excessive gestational weight gain: A systematic review and meta-analysis. *Food Funct.* **2023**, *14*, 5910–5920. [CrossRef] [PubMed]
50. Çelik, G.; Yılmaz, E.; Nazik, F.; Unver, H. Determination of distress, emotional eating and internalized weight bias levels of Turkish pregnant women. *J. Obstet. Gynaecol. J. Inst. Obstet. Gynaecol.* **2023**, *43*, 2153020. [CrossRef]
51. Mattioli, A.V.; Gallina, S. Early cardiovascular prevention: The crucial role of nurse-led intervention. *BMC Nurs.* **2023**, *22*, 347. [CrossRef]
52. Jackson, H.; Stickler, E.; Biddle, S.; Trilk, J.L. Do Pregnant Women Perceive Being Counseled about Nutrition by Healthcare Providers? A Cross-Sectional Study of the Recall and Satisfaction of Nutrition Counseling of Patients throughout the Course of Their Pregnancy. *Am. J. Lifestyle Med.* **2023**. [CrossRef]
53. World Health Organization. Sustainable Healthy Diets: Guiding Principles. 2019. Available online: https://www.who.int/publications/i/item/9789241516648 (accessed on 23 July 2022).
54. Truzzi, M.L.; Ballerini Puviani, M.; Tripodi, A.; Toni, S.; Farinetti, A.; Nasi, M.; Mattioli, A.V. Mediterranean Diet as a model of sustainable, resilient and healthy diet. *Prog. Nutr.* **2020**, *22*, 388–394.
55. Mattioli, A.V.; Coppi, F.; Migaldi, M.; Farinetti, A. Fruit and vegetables in hypertensive women with asymptomatic peripheral arterial disease. *Clin. Nutr. ESPEN* **2018**, *27*, 110–112. [CrossRef] [PubMed]
56. Singh, J.; Kaur, M.; Rasane, P.; Kaur, S.; Kaur, J.; Sharma, K.; Gulati, A. Nutritional management and interventions in complications of pregnancy: A systematic review. *Nutr. Health*, 2023; *published online ahead of print*. [CrossRef] [PubMed]
57. Mattioli, A.V.; Migaldi, M.; Farinetti, A. Coffee in hypertensive women with asymptomatic peripheral arterial disease: A potential nutraceutical effect. *J. Cardiovasc. Med.* **2018**, *19*, 183–185. [CrossRef] [PubMed]
58. Food Standards Australian and New Zealand. Available online: https://www.foodstandards.gov.au/consumer/generalissues/pages/caffeine.aspx#:~:text=It%20sets%20maximum%20permitted%20levels,is%20320%20mg%20per%20litre (accessed on 12 January 2024).
59. Coppi, F.; Bucciarelli, V.; Sinigaglia, G.; Zanini, G.; Selleri, V.; Nasi, M.; Pinti, M.; Gallina, S.; Mattioli, A.V. Sex Related Differences in the Complex Relationship between Coffee, Caffeine and Atrial Fibrillation. *Nutrients* **2023**, *15*, 3299. [CrossRef]
60. ESFA Journal "Scientific Opinion on the Safety of Caffeine". 2015. Available online: https://www.efsa.europa.eu/en/efsajournal/pub/4102 (accessed on 12 January 2024).
61. Klevebrant, L.; Frick, A. Effects of caffeine on anxiety and panic attacks in patients with panic disorder: A systematic review and meta-analysis. *Gen. Hosp. Psychiatry* **2022**, *74*, 22–31. [CrossRef]
62. Emokpae, M.A.; Brown, S.I. Effects of lifestyle factors on fertility: Practical recommendations for modification. *Reprod. Fertil.* **2021**, *2*, R13–R26. [CrossRef]
63. Caro, R.; Fast, J. Pregnancy Myths and Practical Tips. *Am. Fam. Physician* **2020**, *102*, 420–426.
64. Wikoff, D.; Welsh, B.T.; Henderson, R.; Brorby, G.P.; Britt, J.; Myers, E.; Goldberger, J.; Lieberman, H.R.; O'Brien, C.; Peck, J.; et al. Systematic review of the potential adverse effects of caffeine consumption in healthy adults, pregnant women, adolescents, and children. *Food Chem. Toxicol. Int. J. Publ. Br. Ind. Biol. Res. Assoc.* **2017**, *109 Pt 1*, 585–648. [CrossRef]
65. Grosso, G.; Godos, J.; Galvano, F.; Giovannucci, E.L. Coffee, Caffeine, and Health Outcomes: An Umbrella Review. *Annu. Rev. Nutr.* **2017**, *37*, 131–156. [CrossRef] [PubMed]
66. Godos, J.; Pluchinotta, F.R.; Marventano, S.; Buscemi, S.; Li Volti, G.; Galvano, F.; Grosso, G. Coffee components and cardiovascular risk: Beneficial and detrimental effects. *Int. J. Food Sci. Nutr.* **2014**, *65*, 925–936. [CrossRef] [PubMed]
67. Pan, M.H.; Tung, Y.C.; Yang, G.; Li, S.; Ho, C.T. Molecular mechanisms of the anti-obesity effect of bioactive compounds in tea and coffee. *Food Funct.* **2016**, *7*, 4481–4491. [CrossRef] [PubMed]
68. Hillier, S.E.; Olander, E.K. Women's dietary changes before and during pregnancy: A systematic review. *Midwifery* **2017**, *49*, 19–31. [CrossRef] [PubMed]
69. Temple, J.L.; Bernard, C.; Lipshultz, S.E.; Czachor, J.D.; Westphal, J.A.; Mestre, M.A. The Safety of Ingested Caffeine: A Comprehensive Review. *Front. Psychiatry* **2017**, *8*, 80. [CrossRef] [PubMed]
70. Mattioli, A.V.; Sabatini, S. Changes in energy drink consumption during the COVID-19 quarantine. *Clin. Nutr. ESPEN* **2021**, *45*, 516–517. [CrossRef] [PubMed]
71. Craig, W.J.; Mangels, A.R.; Fresán, U.; Marsh, K.; Miles, F.L.; Saunders, A.V.; Haddad, E.H.; Heskey, C.E.; Johnston, P.; Larson-Meyer, E.; et al. The Safe and Effective Use of Plant-Based Diets with Guidelines for Health Professionals. *Nutrients* **2021**, *13*, 4144. [CrossRef] [PubMed]
72. Ratjen, I.; Morze, J.; Enderle, J.; Both, M.; Borggrefe, J.; Muller, H.P.; Kassubek, J.; Koch, M.; Lieb, W. Adherence to a plant-based diet in relation to adipose tissue volumes and liver fat content. *Am. J. Clin. Nutr.* **2020**, *112*, 354–363. [CrossRef] [PubMed]
73. Mayra, S.; Ugarte, N.; Johnston, C.S. Health Biomarkers in Adults Are More Closely Linked to Diet Quality Attributes than to Plant-Based Diet Categorization. *Nutrients* **2019**, *11*, 1427. [CrossRef]
74. Wang, T.; Kroeger, C.M.; Cassidy, S.; Mitra, S.; Ribeiro, R.V.; Jose, S.; Masedunskas, A.; Senior, A.M.; Fontana, L. Vegetarian Dietary Patterns and Cardiometabolic Risk in People With or at High Risk of Cardiovascular Disease: A Systematic Review and Meta-analysis. *JAMA Netw. Open* **2023**, *6*, e2325658. [CrossRef]

75. Lakin, V.; Haggarty, P.; Abramovich, D.R.; Ashton, J.; Moffat, C.F.; McNeill, G.; Danielian, P.J.; Grubb, D. Dietary intake and tissue concentration of fatty acids in omnivore, vegetarian and diabetic pregnancy. *Prostaglandins Leukot. Essent. Fat. Acids* **1998**, *59*, 209–220. [CrossRef] [PubMed]
76. Leung, B.M.; Kaplan, B.J. Perinatal depression: Prevalence, risks, and the nutrition link–a review of the literature. *J. Am. Diet Assoc.* **2009**, *109*, 1566–1575. [CrossRef] [PubMed]
77. Christian, C.; Zerwas, S.C.; Levinson, C.A. The Unique and Moderating Role of Social and Self-Evaluative Factors on Perinatal Eating Disorder and Depression Symptoms. *Behav. Ther.* **2024**, *55*, 122–135. [CrossRef] [PubMed]
78. Albert, P.R. Why is depression more prevalent in women? *J. Psychiatry Neurosci.* **2015**, *40*, 219–221. [CrossRef] [PubMed]
79. Cattane, N.; Räikkönen, K.; Anniverno, R.; Mencacci, C.; Riva, M.A.; Pariante, C.M.; Cattaneo, A. Depression, obesity and their comorbidity during pregnancy: Effects on the offspring's mental and physical health. *Mol. Psychiatry* **2021**, *26*, 462–481. [CrossRef] [PubMed]
80. US Preventive Services Task Force; Curry, S.J.; Krist, A.H.; Owens, D.K.; Barry, M.J.; Caughey, A.B.; Davidson, K.W.; Doubeni, C.A.; Epling, J.W., Jr.; Grossman, D.C.; et al. Interventions to Prevent Perinatal Depression: US Preventive Services Task Force Recommendation Statement. *JAMA* **2019**, *321*, 580–587. [CrossRef] [PubMed]
81. Kuehner, C. Why is depression more common among women than among men? *Lancet Psychiatry* **2017**, *4*, 146–158. [CrossRef] [PubMed]
82. Bear, T.L.K.; Dalziel, J.E.; Coad, J.; Roy, N.C.; Butts, C.A.; Gopal, P.K. The role of the gut microbiota in dietary interventions for depression and anxiety. *Adv. Nutr.* **2020**, *11*, 890–907. [CrossRef]
83. Yang, Y.; Zhang, S.; Zhang, X.; Xu, Y.; Cheng, J.; Yang, X. The role of diet, eating behavior, and nutrition intervention in seasonal affective disorder: A systematic review. *Front. Psychol.* **2020**, *11*, 1451. [CrossRef]
84. Ross, F.C.; Mayer, D.E.; Gupta, A.; Gill, C.I.R.; Del Rio, D.; Cryan, J.F.; Lavelle, A.; Ross, R.P.; Stanton, C.; Mayer, E.A. Existing and Future Strategies to Manipulate the Gut Microbiota with Diet as a Potential Adjuvant Treatment for Psychiatric Disorders. *Biol. Psychiatry* **2024**, *95*, 348–360. [CrossRef]
85. Zidan, S.; Hilary, S.; Al Dhaheri, A.S.; Cheikh Ismail, L.; Ali, H.I.; Apostolopoulos, V.; Stojanovska, L. Could psychobiotics and fermented foods improve mood in middle-aged and older women? *Maturitas* **2024**, *181*, 107903. [CrossRef]
86. Dinu, M.; Lotti, S.; Mattioli, A.V.; Gensini, G.F.; Ambrosio, G.; Sofi, F. Effects of Omega-3 Fatty Acid Supplementation on Revascularization and Major Cardiovascular Events: A Systematic Review and Meta-Analysis. *Proceedings* **2023**, *91*, 199. [CrossRef]
87. Li, D.; Wang, K.; Yang, Z.; Li, H.; Wang, S. Vitamin d supplementation in mice with advanced maternal age and cognitive function of the offspring. *Am. J. Trans. Res.* **2021**, *13*, 7641–7653.
88. Liang, Q.; Cai, C.; Duan, D.; Hu, X.; Hua, W.; Jiang, P.; Zhang, L.; Xu, J.; Gao, Z. Postnatal vitamin d intake modulates hippocampal learning and memory in adult mice. *Front. Neurosci.* **2018**, *12*, 322097. [CrossRef]
89. de Abreu, D.F.; Eyles, D.; Feron, F. Vitamin D, a neuro-immunomodulator: Implications for neurodegenerative and autoimmune diseases. *Psychoneuroendocrinology* **2009**, *34*, S265–S277. [CrossRef] [PubMed]
90. Song, J.; Zhou, B.; Kan, J.; Liu, G.; Zhang, S.; Si, L.; Zhang, X.; Yang, X.; Ma, J.; Cheng, J.; et al. Gut microbiota: Linking nutrition and perinatal depression. *Front. Cell. Infect. Microbiol.* **2022**, *12*, 932309. [CrossRef]
91. Wang, J.; Liu, N.; Sun, W.; Chen, D.; Zhao, J.; Zhang, W. Association between vitamin d deficiency and antepartum and postpartum depression: A systematic review and meta-analysis of longitudinal studies. *Arch. Gynecol Obstet.* **2018**, *298*, 1045–1059. [CrossRef]
92. Vaziri, F.; Nasiri, S.; Tavana, Z.; Dabbaghmanesh, M.H.; Sharif, F.; Jafari, P. A randomized controlled trial of vitamin D supplementation on perinatal depression: In Iranian pregnant mothers. *BMC Pregnancy Childbirth* **2016**, *16*, 239. [CrossRef] [PubMed]
93. Kabuyanga, R.K.; Tugirimana, P.L.; Sifa, B.; Balezi, M.; Dikete, M.E.; Mitangala, P.N.; Elongi, J.P.M.; Kinenkinda, X.K.; Kakoma, J.S.Z. Effect of early vitamin D supplementation on the incidence of preeclampsia in primigravid women: A randomised clinical trial in Eastern Democratic Republic of the Congo. *BMC Pregnancy Childbirth* **2024**, *24*, 107. [CrossRef]
94. Ferenc, K.; Sokal-Dembowska, A.; Helma, K.; Motyka, E.; Jarmakiewicz-Czaja, S.; Filip, R. Modulation of the Gut Microbiota by Nutrition and Its Relationship to Epigenetics. *Int. J. Mol. Sci.* **2024**, *25*, 1228. [CrossRef]
95. Theofilis, P.; Vlachakis, P.K.; Oikonomou, E.; Tsioufis, K.; Tousoulis, D. Targeting the Gut Microbiome to Treat Cardiometabolic Disease. *Curr. Atheroscler. Rep.* **2024**. [CrossRef] [PubMed]
96. Aziz, T.; Hussain, N.; Hameed, Z.; Lin, L. Elucidating the role of diet in maintaining gut health to reduce the risk of obesity, cardiovascular and other age-related inflammatory diseases: Recent challenges and future recommendations. *Gut Microbes* **2024**, *16*, 2297864. [CrossRef] [PubMed]
97. Bucciarelli, V.; Mattioli, A.V.; Sciomer, S.; Moscucci, F.; Renda, G.; Gallina, S. The Impact of Physical Activity and Inactivity on Cardiovascular Risk across Women's Lifespan: An Updated Review. *J. Clin. Med.* **2023**, *12*, 4347. [CrossRef] [PubMed]
98. Academy of Nutrition and Dietetics. Available online: https://www.eatright.org/health/pregnancy/prenatal-nutrition/healthy-weight-during-pregnancy (accessed on 29 January 2024).
99. Mattioli, A.V.; Selleri, V.; Zanini, G.; Nasi, M.; Pinti, M.; Stefanelli, C.; Fedele, F.; Gallina, S. Physical Activity and Diet in Older Women: A Narrative Review. *J. Clin. Med.* **2022**, *12*, 81. [CrossRef] [PubMed]

100. Stephenson, J.; Heslehurst, N.; Hall, J.; Schoenaker, D.A.J.M.; Hutchinson, J.; Cade, J.E.; Poston, L.; Barrett, G.; Crozier, S.R.; Barker, M.; et al. Before the beginning: Nutrition and lifestyle in the preconception period and its importance for future health. *Lancet* **2018**, *391*, 1830–1841. [CrossRef] [PubMed]
101. Zhang, X.F.; Li, R.N.; Deng, J.L.; Chen, X.L.; Zhou, Q.L.; Qi, Y.; Zhang, Y.P.; Fan, J.M. Effects of mindfulness-based interventions on cardiovascular risk factors: An umbrella review of systematic reviews and meta-analyses. *J. Psychosom. Res.* **2024**, *177*, 111586. [CrossRef]
102. Tyler, J.; Won Choi, S.; Tewari, M. Real-time, personalized medicine through wearable sensors and dynamic predictive modeling: A new paradigm for clinical medicine. *Curr. Opin. Syst. Biol.* **2020**, *20*, 17–25. [CrossRef]
103. Meghan Rimol, Gartner Forecasts Global Spending on Wearable Devices to Total $81.5 Billion in 2021, STAMFORD, Conn. 12 January 2021. Available online: https://www.gartner.com/en/newsroom/press-releases/2021-01-11-gartner-forecasts-global-spending-on-wearable-devices-to-total-81-5-billion-in-2021 (accessed on 15 November 2023).
104. Latest Trends in Medical Monitoring Devices and Wearable Health Technology. Available online: https://www.businessinsider.in/latest-trends-in-medical-monitoring-devices-and-wearable-health-technology/articleshow/70907962.cms (accessed on 15 November 2023).

nutrients

MDPI

Article

Regional Variability in the Prevalence of Food Insecurity and Diet Quality among United States Children

Jayna M. Dave [1,*], Tzuan A. Chen [2,3], Alexandra N. Castro [1], Mamie White [1], Elizabeth A. Onugha [4,5], Sloane Zimmerman [6] and Debbe Thompson [1]

[1] USDA/ARS Children's Nutrition Research Center, Department of Pediatrics, Baylor College of Medicine, 1100 Bates Avenue, Houston, TX 77030, USA; alexandra.castro@bcm.edu (A.N.C.); mawhite@bcm.edu (M.W.); dit@bcm.edu (D.T.)

[2] Department of Psychological, Health, and Learning Sciences, University of Houston, 3657 Cullen Boulevard, Houston, TX 77204, USA; tchen3@central.uh.edu

[3] HEALTH Research Institute, University of Houston, 4349 Martin Luther King Boulevard, Houston, TX 77204, USA

[4] Renal Services, Texas Children's Hospital, 1102 Bates Avenue, Houston, TX 77030, USA; eaonugha@texaschildrens.org

[5] Department of Pediatrics—Nephrology, Baylor College of Medicine, 1102 Bates Avenue, Houston, TX 77030, USA

[6] Department of Pediatrics—Gastroenterology, Baylor College of Medicine, One Baylor Plaza, Houston, TX 77030, USA; sloane.zimmerman@bcm.edu

* Correspondence: jmdave@bcm.edu

Abstract: Understanding the association between food security status (FSS) and diet quality in children is crucial. This study investigated regional variability in FSS, participation in the federal nutrition assistance program (FNAP), and diet quality among US children. National Health and Nutrition Examination Survey (NHANES) data from 2013 to 2016 were analyzed. The association between FSS, FNAP participation, and diet quality (Healthy Eating Index—HEI-2015) was assessed using multiple linear/logistic regression models. The sample included 6403 children (mean age: 7.5 years; 51% male; 33% Hispanic). Within the sample, 13% reported child food insecurity, and 30% reported household food insecurity. Additionally, 90% participated in the FNAP, and 88% were enrolled in school lunch programs. Children in urban areas were significantly more likely to report household food insecurity than those in rural areas (29.15% vs. 19.10%). The overall HEI-2015 score was 48.2. The associations between child/household FSS and FNAP participation as well as between child/household FSS and diet quality did not differ by urban/rural residence status, irrespective of the children's age groups. There is a need for improvement in children's diet quality, regardless of age or urban/rural residence. The findings suggest that improving children's diets requires broader action as well as the prioritizing of children in urban areas experiencing food insecurity in future dietary interventions.

Keywords: food insecurity; diet quality; urban-rural differences; children; federal nutrition assistance program; NHANES

1. Introduction

Diet plays a vital role in children's overall health and well-being. A healthy diet provides children with the nutrients they need to grow and develop. Urban–rural differences in diet among US children have been well-documented, typically showing that rural children consume less nutritious diets than urban children [1–4].

Food security, the access by all people at all times to enough food for an active, healthy life, is one of the several conditions necessary for a population to be healthy and well-nourished [5]. Food insecurity, on the other hand, refers to the limited or uncertain availability of nutritionally adequate and safe foods and is strongly related to poverty [6].

As a result, food insecurity is associated with poor nutrient intake and increases the risk of obesity, diabetes, cardiovascular disease, anxiety, and depression [7–10]. In 2022, 12.8% of US households and 17.3% of households with children were food-insecure [6]. Households with incomes near or below the federal poverty line (i.e., below $24,600 annually for a household of four), single parents, individuals living alone, Black- and Hispanic-headed households, and households in suburban and rural areas experience higher rates of food insecurity than the national average [6]. Food insecurity also tends to be more prevalent in households with older children (5–17 years) than in households with younger children (0–4 years) [11].

Studies of children living in rural communities have shown a pattern of food consumption that is high in fat and sugar, and low in fruit and vegetables [12,13]. However, these studies lack a simultaneously obtained nationally representative sample of both urban and rural children. This limitation prevents an assessment of the relationship between urban/rural status and dietary behaviors. In addition, child poverty rates among children are higher in rural communities compared to their urban counterparts (~26% vs. 20%) [14]. Given the positive association between poverty and food insecurity, it is likely that food insecurity rates may be higher among rural children compared to urban children. However, no studies have specifically investigated the urban–rural differences in food security status among children.

The federal nutrition assistance programs (FNAPs) administered by the US Department of Agriculture aim to provide low-income households with access to food, promote a nutritious diet, offer nutrition education, and increase food security [5]. The five largest FNAPs intended to combat hunger and food insecurity are the Supplemental Nutrition Assistance Program (SNAP), the National School Lunch Program (NSLP), the Special Supplemental Nutrition Program for Women, Infants, and Children (WIC), the School Breakfast Program (SBP), and the Summer Food Service Program (SFSP). In 2022, approximately 46.7% of SNAP households, 41.9% of households receiving free or reduced-price school lunches, and 34.6% of WIC households experienced food insecurity [11]. Among households with children, food insecurity is most prevalent in low-income households that participate in SNAP and receive free or reduced-price lunches [11]. This suggests that those households with the greatest need for food assistance are more likely to participate in FNAP. Several studies have shown a significant association between participation in FNAP and lower rates of food insecurity in households with children, even after accounting for selection bias [15–19]. However, a USDA report showed a decrease in participation in all five major FNAPs between October 2016 and November 2017 [5], suggesting the need for the continued assessment of FNAP participation's impact on food insecurity. Federal data also revealed that rural SNAP participation rates are significantly greater than the urban participation rates [18,20].

Children from low-income, food-insecure households report poorer quality diets than those from households with higher-incomes. Food insecurity is linked to lower intakes of nutrient-dense foods such as fruits, vegetables, and whole grains and higher intakes of energy-dense foods [7,8,21]. These dietary patterns may lead to a net positive energy balance, increasing the risk of obesity and other diet-related chronic diseases. Moreover, households living in low-income neighborhoods, both urban and rural, may encounter difficulties in accessing affordable and nutritious foods [22,23]. Many low-income neighborhoods, particularly in rural areas, lack access to food retailers and are identified as food deserts, where fresh and affordable foods are in short supply [23]. This directly affects the dietary intake of children from low-income households who tend to purchase high-energy-dense and low-nutrient-dense foods [7,8,21]. Thus, it is imperative to continue to examine and understand how one's food security status relates to children's dietary intake, particularly in the context of a growing body of literature linking food insecurity to an increased risk of obesity.

Although the determinants of food insecurity in the US are well-researched, gaps in the literature exist, particularly concerning the urban–rural divide. Our research sought to fill this gap, examining the urban–rural differences in and associations between food security status, participation in FNAP, and dietary intake among children across different age groups, i.e., 2–5 years, 6–11 years, and 12–17 years of age.

2. Materials and Methods

2.1. Participants

This study employed data from the National Health and Nutrition Examination Survey (NHANES) from 2013 to 2016. A secondary analysis of the NHANES data was deemed exempt from review by the Baylor College of Medicine's Institutional Review Board. The NHANES, administered by the National Center for Health Statistics (NCHS) of the Centers for Disease Control and Prevention (CDC), is a cross-sectional, nationally representative survey of the non-institutionalized civilian population of the US. Details about each survey and their sampling designs can be found elsewhere [24]. Data from two survey cycles (2013–2014 and 2015–2016) containing information on food security status and dietary intake were employed to enhance the reliability and stability of estimates across subgroups [24]. The 2013–2016 NHANES included data on a total of 6685 children aged 2–17 years. Children between 2 and 17 years of age with reported food security status were included in the study. The participants with missing information on any of the independent or dependent variables were excluded from the analysis. The final sample included 6403 children, categorized into three age groups: 2–5 years old, 6–11 years old, and 12–17 years old. The NCHS Ethics Review Board of the CDC approved the NHANES protocols; all the participants provided informed consent prior to data collection.

2.2. Measures

2.2.1. Sociodemographic Variables

The sociodemographic variables in the NHANES were collected during the in-home interviews, using the computer-assisted personal interview system. Individuals who were at least 16 years old and emancipated minors were interviewed directly, while proxies provided information for survey participants under the age of 16. The demographic variables included age, gender, race/ethnicity, parent's marital and education status, and household income. The rural/urban status of the county of residence was determined based on its Urban Influence Code (UIC), as defined by the USDA's Economic Research Service. These codes were drawn from the 2013 Area Resource File, containing information about the characteristics of the 2142 counties in the US. Counties with UIC codes 1 or 2 were coded as urban, while those with other UIC codes (3–12, designated as nonmetropolitan codes by the USDA's ERS) were classified as rural [25,26]. The county of residence's urban–rural status is a restricted-use variable, and these data were accessed through the Research Data Center.

2.2.2. Food Security Status

The food security status was measured using the 18-item US Household Food Security Survey Module during the in-home interviews [27]. An adult provided responses to the 10 items pertaining to the entire household. An additional eight items were specific to households with children aged ≤17 years. Each question referenced the previous 12-month period. The data for food security status (household and child level) were coded using the USDA's coding guide. A score of 0–18 was created by summing the affirmative responses to the 18 questions, with higher scores indicating worse food insecurity. Consistent with the USDA's definitions and the existing literature, if the primary household respondent provided two or more affirmative responses to the child-specific questions, the children in the household were classified as food insecure [28]. The experiences of the entire household or children in the household were categorized into one of four food security categories (i.e., high, marginal, low, and very low) based on NHANES documentation [29]. High food security and marginal food security were merged as one category of food security; low and very low food security were merged to classify food insecurity.

2.2.3. Diet Quality—Healthy Eating Index-2015

A single 24 h dietary recall was collected for each participant using the USDA's automated multiple-pass method. For the participants aged <6 years old, a proxy answered the questions; for the children 6–8 years old, a proxy answered the questions with the child's assistance; the 9–11-year-old children answered the questions with the assistance of a proxy; and the participants aged 12 years or older answered the questions themselves. Diet quality was assessed using the Healthy Eating Index (HEI-2015) [30], which evaluates how closely an individual's dietary intake adheres to the Dietary Guidelines for Americans 2015–2020 [31,32]. The HEI-2015 was computed using the basic HEI scoring algorithm based on day 1 of the 24 h dietary recall data from the NHANES. The recall data were collected by trained interviewers. Only the weekday dietary data were employed to explore the association with HEI-2015. Furthermore, only the day 1 recall was utilized, due to a higher non-response rate and individuals tending to report a lower consumption on day 2 (possibly due to under-reporting or survey fatigue). This approach of utilizing only the day 1 recall has been used in previously published studies [33–35]. Additional information on the 24 h dietary recall procedure can be found elsewhere [36].

The HEI-2015 is a composite measure of thirteen dietary elements with nine adequacy components (i.e., total fruits, whole fruits, total vegetables, greens and beans, whole grains, dairy, total protein foods, seafood and plant proteins, and fatty acids) and four moderation components (i.e., refined grains, sodium, added sugars, and saturated fats). Detailed information about the HEI-2015 can be found elsewhere [30,37]. The scores on each component sum to a maximum score of 100. Higher scores for the adequacy components indicate greater intakes. For the moderation components, higher scores indicate lower intakes, as lower intakes are considered more desirable. For all the components, a higher score indicates a better-quality diet. A higher total score indicates a greater alignment of the diet with the Dietary Guidelines. HEI scores of <51, 51–80, and >80 indicate "poor diet", "needs improvement", and "good diet", respectively [37–39].

2.2.4. Federal Nutrition Assistance Program Participation

The FNAP includes SNAP, WIC, NSLP, SBP, SFSP, or any combination of these programs. SNAP, WIC, NSLP, SBP, SFSP participation was assessed with the following questions: "Do you/Does any member of your household currently receive SNAP or Food Stamp benefits?"; "Is (SP) now receiving benefits from the WIC program?"; "(Do you/Does SP) get these lunches free, at a reduced price, or (do you/does he/she) pay full price?"; "(Do you/Does SP) get these breakfasts free, at a reduced price, or (do you/does he/she) pay full price?"; and "(Do you/Does SP) get a free or reduced price meal at any summer program (he/she) attends?". The households with low socioeconomic statuses (SES) were eligible to participate in SNAP; if there were children attending school in these households, they were also eligible for free or reduced-price school meals. To address this, four FNAP participation categories were established. Participation in FNAP was then classified as either no participation or any participation.

2.2.5. Covariates

The covariates included age, sex, race/ethnicity, weight status, and family monthly poverty index. The primary respondent's age, sex, and race/ethnicity (Non-Hispanic White, Non-Hispanic Black, Hispanic, and Other Race) were reported in the NHANES Demographic Variables and Sample Weights Module, while their family's monthly poverty level index was included in the NHANES Income Questionnaire Module. The family monthly poverty level index, serving as an indicator for SES, represents a ratio of self-reported monthly income to poverty threshold. This index was chosen as it theoretically offers an equivalent SES measure that can be applied across different age groups. It serves as an economic measure to determine eligibility for certain federal benefits and programs (e.g., NSLP). Moreover, children from households with a family monthly poverty level index less than 1.85 are eligible for participation in some FNAP, including reduced-price lunches [40,41]. Body Mass Index (BMI), expressed as weight in kilograms divided by height in meters squared (kg/m^2), is a widely employed method for categorizing weight status. The cutoff criteria are based on the CDC's sex-specific 2000 BMI-for-age growth charts for the US [42]. One's weight status is categorized as underweight (BMI < 5th percentile), normal weight (BMI 5th to <85th percentile), overweight (BMI 85th to <95th percentile), and obese (BMI $\geq$ 95th percentile). The underweight children's data were combined with the normal weight group's data because of the small sample size for underweight children. All the covariates were self-reported and selected as potential confounding factors in the association between food insecurity and diet quality.

2.3. Data Analysis

The descriptive statistics of the participants' characteristics were computed for three age groups (i.e., 2–5, 6–11, and 12–17 years old). Rao-Scott Chi-square tests were conducted to examine the association of the participants' household/child food security status and urban/rural residence status for the overall sample and by the age groups. The analysis utilized sample-weighted data to accommodate the complex survey sampling methods (e.g., survey non-response, and post-stratification adjustment) used in the NHANES.

The final outcome models utilized the SAS SURVEYREG or SURVEYFREQ procedure to accommodate the complex, stratified, multistage probability cluster sampling design. In these final outcome models, the associations between participants' food security status and FNAP participation and the diet quality measures (including HEI-2015 and its 13 subcomponents) were assessed using multiple linear/logistic regression models. In addition, whether these associations were affected by the urban/rural residence status were examined by including the interaction term of the urban/rural residence and food security status. If significant interactions were detected, post hoc analyses were conducted. The covariates included in the final outcome model were age, sex, race/ethnicity, and family monthly poverty index. Those covariates and variables of interest were obtained directly or calculated from the NHANES datasets. For each outcome of interest (i.e., HEI-2015 and its 13 subcomponents), separate final outcome models were run, both for the entire sample and across the three age groups. All the analyses were performed using SAS 9.4. Statistical significance was designated at $p < 0.05$.

3. Results

Among the 6403 children included in the study, 27.33% were 2–5 years old, while 40.43% were 6–11 years old, and 32.23% were 12–17 years old (Table 1). The sex distribution was 51% males and 49% females, and most of the children were Hispanic (30.97–33.80%) and underweight or normal weight (59.03–71.95%) across each of the age groups. The reported child food insecurity ranged from 9.66% among the 2–5-year-old children to 14.77% in the 12–17-year-olds; the household food insecurity ranged from 26.19% among the 2–5-year-olds to 29.12% in the 12–17-year-olds. About 89% participated in SNAP, and about 90% participated in school meals programs.

Table 1. Descriptive statistics of participant characteristics by age group.

	All *n* = 6403	2–5 Years Old *n* = 1750	6–11 Years Old *n* = 2589	12–17 Years Old *n* = 2064
		Mean ± SD		
Age	7.51 ± 5.25	3.38 ± 1.14	8.44 ± 1.72	14.44 ± 1.68
BMI Percentile	19.81 ± 5.44	16.49 ± 1.85	18.79 ± 4.31	23.84 ± 6.19
Ratio of Family income to Poverty	1.88 ± 0.92	1.84 ± 0.91	1.87 ± 0.92	1.94 ± 0.92
		N (%)		
Gender				
Male	3266 (51.01)	903 (51.60)	1311 (50.64)	1052 (50.97)
Female	3137 (48.99)	847 (48.40)	1278 (49.36)	1012 (49.03)

Table 1. *Cont.*

	All n = 6403	2–5 Years Old n = 1750	6–11 Years Old n = 2589	12–17 Years Old n = 2064
Weight Status				
Underweight/Normal weight	3893 (63.70)	1172 (71.95)	1547 (62.05)	1174 (59.02)
Overweight	1048 (17.15)	250 (15.35)	431 (17.29)	367 (18.45)
Obese	1170 (19.15)	207 (12.71)	515 (20.66)	448 (22.52)
Ethnicity				
Non-Hispanic White	1730 (27.02)	486 (27.77)	698 (26.96)	546 (26.45)
Non-Hispanic Black	1556 (24.30)	432 (24.69)	632 (24.41)	492 (23.84)
Hispanic	2111 (32.97)	542 (30.97)	875 (33.80)	694 (33.62)
Others	1006 (15.71)	290 (16.57)	384 (14.83)	332 (16.08)
Child Food Security Status				
Child food security	5480 (87.08)	1552 (90.34)	2202 (86.35)	1726 (85.23)
Child food insecurity	813 (12.92)	166 (9.66)	348 (13.65)	299 (14.76)
Household Food Security Status				
Household food security	4535 (72.04)	1268 (73.81)	1837 (72.01)	1430 (70.58)
Household food insecurity	1760 (27.96)	450 (26.19)	714 (27.99)	596 (29.42)
Participation in Federal Nutrition Assistance Programs				
SNAP	2129 (89.68)	673 (90.21)	875 (89.74)	581 (88.97)
WIC	479 (49.33)	479 (49.33)	NA	NA
SBP	2143 (92.57)	187 (94.92)	1253 (92.95)	703 (91.30)
NSLP	2606 (87.66)	218 (92.77)	1407 (88.60)	981 (85.30)
SFSP	640 (34.32)	49 (35.51)	354 (34.40)	237 (33.95)
Any of the FNAP	3722 (72.60)	938 (77.78)	1619 (71.83)	1165 (69.89)

Notes. SNAP: Supplemental Nutrition Assistance Program; WIC: Women, Infants, and Children; SBP: School Breakfast Program; NSLP: National School Lunch Program; SFSP: Summer Food Service Program; BMI: Body Mass Index; SD: Standard deviation; NA: Not applicable.

A significant urban–rural difference was found in the household food security status among the children aged 6–11 years old (p = 0.003) (Table 2). The children living in urban areas were more likely to experience household food insecurity compared to the children living in rural areas (29.149% vs. 19.104%). However, there was no significant difference in child food security status by urban–rural residence.

Table 2. Urban–rural differences in food security status by different age groups.

	Urban			Rural			
Age Group	n	%	Weighted %	n	%	Weighted %	p-Value
Household Food Security status							
All							0.06
Household food security	3834	71.13	76.78	640	79.01	81.09	
Household food insecurity	1556	28.87	23.22	170	20.99	18.91	
2–5 years old							0.13
Household food security	1094	72.93	77.40	156	81.67	84.04	
Household food insecurity	406	27.07	22.60	35	18.33	15.96	
6–11 years old							<0.01
Household food security	1541	70.85	76.68	271	80.89	82.57	
Household food insecurity	634	29.15	23.32	64	19.11	17.43	
12–17 years old							0.54
Household food security	1199	69.91	76.47	213	75.00	78.54	
Household food insecurity	516	30.09	23.53	71	25.00	21.46	
Child Food Security Status							

Table 2. *Cont.*

	Urban			Rural			
Age Group	*n*	%	**Weighted %**	*n*	%	**Weighted %**	***p*-Value**
All							0.94
Child food security	4681	86.88	89.37	717	88.52	89.24	
Child food insecurity	707	13.12	10.63	93	11.48	10.76	
2–5 years old							0.44
Child food security	1350	90.00	91.60	176	92.15	93.53	
Child food insecurity	150	10.00	8.40	15	7.85	6.47	
6–11 years old							0.39
Child food security	1869	85.97	88.15	299	89.25	90.04	
Child food insecurity	305	14.03	11.85	36	10.75	9.96	
12–17 years old							0.33
Child food security	1462	85.30	89.12	242	85.21	86.63	
Child food insecurity	252	14.70	10.88	42	14.79	13.37	

The moderation effects of urban/rural residence status on the association between child/household food security status and the receipt of FNAP were not significant overall and across different children age groups.

Overall, the children had a poor diet quality (HEI-2015) of 48.17 ± 13.14 (Table 3). The children who were 2–5 years old had a slightly higher HEI-2015 score of 52.16 ± 12.97 compared to the children who were 6–11 years old (47.54 ± 12.90) and 12–17 years old (46.04 ± 12.92). However, this difference was not statistically significant. There were no significant differences in the HEI-2015 component scores by age groups. Additionally, the moderation effects of urban/rural residence status on the associations between child/household food security status and diet quality (i.e., HEI and 13 subcomponents) were not significant overall and across different children age groups. In other words, regardless of the children's age groups, the associations between child/family food security status and diet quality (i.e., HEI and 13 subcomponents) did not vary by urban–rural residency.

Table 3. Healthy Eating Index-2015 component and total scores by age group.

	Maximum Points	**All** *n* = 6403	**2–5 Years Old** *n* = 1750	**6–11 Years Old** *n* = 2589	**12–17 Years Old** *n* = 2064
		Mean ± SD			
Total HEI-2015 score	100	48.17 ± 13.14	52.16 ± 12.97	47.57 ± 12.90	46.04 ± 12.92
Total Vegetables	5	2.19 ± 1.60	2.07 ± 1.56	2.18 ± 1.57	2.28 ± 1.61
Greens and Beans	5	1.02 ± 1.87	1.03 ± 1.87	1.00 ± 1.85	1.03 ± 1.89
Total Fruits	5	2.54 ± 2.10	3.30 ± 1.98	2.48 ± 2.03	2.08 ± 2.11
Whole Fruits	5	2.30 ± 2.29	2.90 ± 2.28	2.28 ± 2.25	1.90 ± 2.25
Whole Grains	10	2.73 ± 3.29	3.02 ± 3.34	2.76 ± 3.23	2.51 ± 3.32
Dairy	10	6.66 ± 3.35	7.50 ± 3.16	6.68 ± 3.23	6.05 ± 3.49
Total Protein Foods	5	3.60 ± 1.57	3.42 ± 1.59	3.61 ± 1.53	3.71 ± 1.59
Seafood and Plant Proteins	5	1.62 ± 2.09	1.55 ± 2.06	1.66 ± 2.09	1.63 ± 2.12
Fatty Acids	10	3.99 ± 3.55	3.61 ± 3.49	3.91 ± 3.44	4.33 ± 3.67
Sodium	10	4.78 ± 3.37	5.53 ± 3.32	4.85 ± 3.29	4.19 ± 3.38
Refined Grains	10	4.97 ± 3.73	5.71 ± 3.67	4.69 ± 3.62	4.75 ± 3.81
Saturated Fats	10	5.41 ± 3.44	5.38 ± 3.40	5.31 ± 3.43	5.53 ± 3.49
Added Sugars	10	6.36 ± 3.27	7.14 ± 3.00	6.16 ± 3.24	6.05 ± 3.38
Energy kcal		1831.96 ± 821.58	1497.47 ± 585.40	1891.89 ± 740.56	1999.38 ± 966.03

Note: SD: Standard deviation.

4. Discussion

To our knowledge, this is one of the first studies to examine urban–rural differences in the association between food security status, participation in FNAP, and diet quality among children. An important finding of the study was the significant difference in household food security status among children aged 6–11 years, with urban-dwelling children displaying a higher prevalence of food insecurity compared to their rural counterparts. This divergence sheds light on the critical role of residence location in influencing household food security, particularly for this age group. However, no significant differences were observed in child food security status based on urban–rural residence, suggesting that the challenges of food insecurity may be more pronounced at the household level in urban areas for children in the 6–11 years age range. This aligns with a recent report highlighting that food insecurity was most prevalent in principal cities located within large urban areas compared to rural areas [43]. Nevertheless, this finding is contrary to some previous research findings [44–46], revealing that children living in rural areas have higher rates of food insecurity than children living in urban areas. However, it is also important to note that the difference in food insecurity status between urban and rural children was not statistically significant after controlling for other factors, such as household income and race/ethnicity. This suggests that the urban–rural difference in food insecurity may be due to other factors, such as access to healthy food and transportation. In fact, a recent study found that most families of teenagers drove a distance of 10 miles or less to grocery shop at least once a week [47]. Nonetheless, this disparity warrants the need for targeted interventions to address food security challenges, particularly in urban environments.

One key aspect of the study was to assess whether urban–rural residence status moderates the relationship between child/household food security status and participation in FNAP. However, no significant moderating effect was observed, both overall and when examined across different age groups of children. This suggests that the influence of food security on participation in these programs is consistent regardless of residence status. This study finding also indicates the importance of FNAP in addressing food security challenges and that FNAP may be effectively reaching children in need of food assistance across different geographic regions and age groups. In fact, federal data from 2017 indicate that, among those eligible for SNAP, participation rates are higher in rural areas (90%) relative to urban areas (82%), and this disparity in participation rates continues to widen [48].

One of the concerning findings of this study was the overall poor diet quality, as indicated by the HEI-2015 scores. While there were slight variations in the scores across different age groups, ranging from 46 to 52 out of 100, these differences were not statistically significant. Furthermore, this study found no significant disparities in the HEI-2015 component scores based on the different age groups, emphasizing the uniformity in diet quality challenges experienced by children across various age brackets, regardless of their urban or rural residence. Moreover, the scores tended to decrease with age, indicating poor adherence to the US Dietary Guidelines among children, regardless of age or geographic residence. In fact, the findings suggested that children showed the lowest adherence to recommendations for the consumption of greens and beans, while demonstrating the highest adherence to guidelines for total protein foods and dairy intake. Previous research using nationally representative samples has found similar results for children's diet quality in the US [49,50]. These study results underscore the significance of implementing strategies to enhance diet quality among US children, focusing on improving the access to and affordability of nutritious foods [51].

This study also explored whether urban–rural residence moderated the relationship between diet quality and food security status among children, a dimension not previously explored in depth. Interestingly, no significant moderation effects were detected, indicating that the impact of food security status on diet quality remains consistent regardless of residence. While previous research has primarily assessed the relationship between food security status on urban–rural residence and dietary intake, few studies have utilized a nationally representative sample to assess the relationship between urban–rural residency and dietary intake among children. These studies have yielded mixed results, with some reporting no significant differences in dietary intake [52] and others noting slight variations in fruit consumption between urban and rural adolescents [53]. Moreover, Euler et al. [2]

found that differences in reported dietary intake based on measures of rurality were minimal once SES and ethnicity were considered. This suggests that differences might be influenced by other community-level access factors or other social determinants of health. These findings suggest that strategies aimed at improving diet quality among children experiencing food insecurity should be implemented uniformly, irrespective of geographic location or age group.

This study's strengths lie in its utilization of a large nationally representative sample of the US population, which allows for robust conclusions regarding the associations being studied. The NHANES utilizes valid and reliable measures of diet, along with a standardized protocol for assessing weight and height. However, this study is constrained by its cross-sectional design, preventing causal inference. Another limitation is the lack of information regarding the timing of households' experiences of food insecurity relative to when they received food and nutrition assistance program(s) benefits. This limits the use of statistical analyses to tackle the issue of self-selection bias, a common problem in studies involving FNAP participation [54]. While our models accounted for potential confounding variables, there is a possibility that unmeasured or unobserved confounding factors could impact both FNAP and diet quality. This may partially explain the association between FNAP and diet quality. The assessment of dietary intake relied on a single 24 h dietary recall. This method is susceptible to bias and error due to day-to-day variation in eating habits and the tendency for people to underreport their food intake—a common issue in dietary intake data. Moreover, there is a potential for bias in diet assessment methods attributed to the utilization of a single dietary recall and the likelihood of measurement errors associated with self-reported dietary intake. Another limitation is the absence of an examination of differences in sex, race, or weight status in this study; however, they are important covariates and should be examined in future research. Despite the use of 2013–2016 data, diet quality was assessed using HEI-2015 instead of HEI-2010. Nonetheless, this is not a cause of concern, as multiple updates to school meal guidelines in 2012 align with HEI-2015 [55,56].

5. Conclusions

In conclusion, these findings underscore the complex interplay of factors affecting food security, diet quality, and the influence of geographic location. While differences were noted in household food security among children aged 6–11 years old, other aspects, including child food security, FNAP participation, and diet quality, exhibited uniform patterns across urban and rural settings and various age groups. These results emphasize the need for comprehensive, age-appropriate interventions to address food security and dietary challenges among children, with a focus on promoting healthier eating habits and reducing the risk of nutrition related health issues across diverse demographic and geographic contexts.

Author Contributions: Conceptualization, J.M.D.; methodology, J.M.D.; validation, J.M.D. and T.A.C.; formal analysis, T.A.C.; writing—original draft preparation, J.M.D.; writing—review and editing, J.M.D., T.A.C., A.N.C., M.W., E.A.O., S.Z. and D.T.; visualization, J.M.D.; supervision, J.M.D.; project administration, J.M.D. and T.A.C.; funding acquisition, J.M.D. All authors have read and agreed to the published version of the manuscript.

Funding: This work is a publication of the United States Department of Agriculture/Agricultural Research Service (USDA/ARS) Children's Nutrition Research Center, Department of Pediatrics, Baylor College of Medicine, Houston, Texas, and is funded, in part, with federal funds from the USDA/ARS under Cooperative Agreement no. 58-3092-0-001 (J.M.D.). The contents of this publication do not necessarily reflect the views or policies of the USDA nor does the mention of trade names, commercial products, or organizations imply endorsement from the U.S. government. This research was also supported by an internal grant funded by the Division of Research at the University of Houston awarded to T.A.C.

Institutional Review Board Statement: Data collection for the NHANES was approved by the NCHS Research Ethics Review Board (ERB). Analysis of de-identified data from the survey is exempt from the federal regulations for the protection of human research participants. Analysis of restricted data through the NCHS Research Data Center is also approved by the NCHS ERB.

Informed Consent Statement: Not applicable.

Data Availability Statement: The data analysis used publicly available data that can be accessed at https://wwwn.cdc.gov/nchs/nhanes/continuousnhanes/default.aspx?BeginYear=2013 (accessed on 31 January 2019).

Conflicts of Interest: The authors declare no conflicts of interest. The findings and conclusions in this paper are those of the author(s) and do not necessarily represent the views of the Research Data Center, the NCHS, or the CDC.

References

1. Crouch, E.; Abshire, D.A.; Wirth, M.D.; Hung, P.; Benavidez, G.A. Rural-urban differences in overweight and obesity, physical activity, and food security among children and adolescents. *Prev. Chronic. Dis.* **2023**, *20*, E92. [CrossRef]
2. Euler, R.; Jimenez, E.Y.; Sanders, S.; Kuhlemeier, A.; Van Horn, M.L.; Cohen, D.; Gonzales-Pacheco, D.; Kong, A.S. Rural-urban differences in baseline dietary intake and physical activity levels of adolescents. *Prev. Chronic. Dis.* **2019**, *16*, E01. [CrossRef] [PubMed]
3. Liu, J.; Bennett, K.J.; Harun, N.; Probst, J.C. Urban-rural differences in overweight status and physical inactivity among US children aged 10–17 years. *J. Rural Health* **2008**, *24*, 407–415. [CrossRef] [PubMed]
4. Neumark-Sztainer, D.; Wall, M.; Perry, C.; Story, M. Correlates of fruit and vegetable intake among adolescents. Findings from Project EAT. *Prev. Med.* **2003**, *37*, 198–208. [CrossRef] [PubMed]
5. Oliveira, V. The Food Assistance Landscape: FY 2017 Annual Report, EIB-190. Available online: https://www.ers.usda.gov/webdocs/publications/88074/eib-190.pdf?v=43174 (accessed on 2 November 2023).
6. Rabbitt, M.P.; Hales, L.J.; Burke, M.P.; Coleman-Jensen, A. Household Food Security in the United States in 2022, ERR-325. Available online: https://www.ers.usda.gov/webdocs/publications/107703/err-325.pdf?v=5285 (accessed on 3 November 2023).
7. Crawford, P.; Lamp, C.; Nicholson, Y.; Krathwohl, S.; Hudes, M.; Townsend, M. Food insecurity may be linked to childhood obesity in low-income Mexican-American families. *Calif. Agric.* **2007**, *61*, 106–111. [CrossRef]
8. Center on Hunger and Poverty and Food Research and Action Center. The Paradox of Hunger and Obesity in America. Available online: http://www.agnt.org/humane/hungerandobesity.pdf (accessed on 2 November 2023).
9. Gregory, C.A.; Coleman-Jensen, A. Food Insecurity, Chronic Disease, and Health Among Working-Age Adults, ERR-235. Available online: https://www.ers.usda.gov/webdocs/publications/84467/err-235.pdf?v=6980.4 (accessed on 6 November 2023).
10. Gunderson, C.; Ziliak, J.P. Food insecurity and health outcomes. *Health Aff.* **2015**, *34*, 1830–1839. [CrossRef] [PubMed]
11. Ralston, K.; Treen, K.; Coleman-Jensen, A.; Guthrie, J. Children's Food Security and USDA Child Nutrition Programs, EIB-174. Available online: https://www.ers.usda.gov/webdocs/publications/84003/eib-174.pdf?v=812 (accessed on 3 November 2023).
12. Davy, B.M.; Harrell, K.; Stewart, J.; King, D.S. Body weight status, dietary habits, and physical activity levels of middle school-aged children in rural Mississippi. *South Med. J.* **2004**, *97*, 571–577. [CrossRef]
13. Crooks, D.L. Food consumption, activity, and overweight among elementary school children in an Appalachian Kentucky community. *Am. J. Phys. Anthropol.* **2000**, *112*, 159–170. [CrossRef]
14. U.S. Department of Agriculture—Economic Research Service. Rural America at a Glance—2018 Edition, EIB-200. Available online: https://www.ers.usda.gov/webdocs/publications/90556/eib-200.pdf?v=8173.8 (accessed on 3 November 2023).
15. Arteaga, I.; Heflin, C. Participation in the National School Lunch Program and food security: An analysis of transitions into kindergarten. *Child. Youth Serv. Rev.* **2014**, *47*, 224–230. [CrossRef]
16. Huang, J.; Barnidge, E.; Kim, Y. Children receiving free or reduced-price school lunch have higher food insufficiency rates in summer. *J. Nutr.* **2015**, *145*, 2161–2168. [CrossRef]
17. Gundersen, C.; Kreider, B.; Pepper, J. The impact of the National School Lunch Program on child health: A nonparametric bounds analysis. *J. Econom.* **2012**, *166*, 79–91. [CrossRef]
18. Mabli, J. SNAP Participation and Urban and Rural Food Security. Prepared by Mathematica Policy Research for the U.S. Department of Agriculture, Food and Nutrition Service. Available online: https://www.mathematica.org/publications/snap-participation-and-urban-and-rural-food-security (accessed on 2 November 2023).
19. Ratcliffe, C.; McKernan, S.M.; Zhang, S. How much does the Supplemental Nutrition Assistance Program reduce food insecurity? *Am. J. Agric. Econ.* **2011**, *93*, 1082–1098. [CrossRef] [PubMed]
20. Bailey, J.M. Supplemental Nutrition Assistance Program and Rural Households. Available online: https://www.ruralhealth.us/NRHA/media/Emerge_NRHA/PDFs/snap-and-rural-households.pdf (accessed on 2 November 2023).
21. Kahn, R.; Sievenpiper, J.L. Dietary sugar and body weight: Have we reached a crisis in the epidemic of obesity and diabetes?: We have, but the pox on sugar is overwrought and overworked. *Diabetes Care* **2014**, *37*, 957–962. [CrossRef]

22. Bell, J.; Mora, G.; Hagan, E.; Rubin, V.; Karpyn, A. Access to Healthy Food and Why It Matters: A Review of the Research. Available online: https://www.policylink.org/resources-tools/access-to-healthy-food-and-why-it-matters (accessed on 2 November 2023).
23. Rural Health Information Hub. Rural Hunger and Access to Healthy Food: Why Do Food Deserts Exist in Rural Areas? Available online: https://www.ruralhealthinfo.org/topics/food-and-hunger#food-deserts (accessed on 2 November 2023).
24. Curtin, L.R.; Mohadjer, L.K.; Dohrmann, S.M.; Kruszon-Moran, D.; Mirel, L.B.; Carroll, M.D.; Hirsch, R.; Burt, V.L.; Johnson, C.L. National Health and Nutrition Examination Survey: Sample Design, 2007–2010. Vital and Health Statistics. Series 2, Number 160. Available online: http://www.cdc.gov/nchs/data/series/sr_02/sr02_160.pdf (accessed on 3 November 2023).
25. U.S. Department of Agriculture—Economic Research Service. Urban Influence Codes. Available online: https://www.ers.usda.gov/data-products/urban-influence-codes/ (accessed on 3 November 2023).
26. Centers for Disease Control and Prevention. National Health and Nutrition Examination Survey 1999–2018 Data Documentation, Codebook, and Frequencies: Appendix 1. 1999-2018 GCP Match Census 2010. Available online: https://wwwn.cdc.gov/Nchs/Nhanes/limited_access/GEO_2010.htm#Appendix_1._1999-2018_GCP_Match_Census_2010 (accessed on 7 November 2023).
27. Bickel, G.; Nord, M.; Price, C.; Hamilton, W.; Cook, J. Guide to Measuring Household Food Security, Revised 2000. Available online: https://fns-prod.azureedge.us/sites/default/files/FSGuide.pdf (accessed on 6 November 2023).
28. Gundersen, C.; Lohman, B.J.; Garasky, S.; Stewart, S.; Eisenmann, J. Food security, maternal stressors, and overweight among low-income US children: Results from the National Health and Nutrition Examination Survey (1999–2002). *Pediatrics* **2008**, *122*, e529–e540. [CrossRef] [PubMed]
29. National Center for Health Statistics. National Health and Nutrition Examination Survey 2015–2016 Data Documentation, Codebook, and Frequencies. Available online: https://wwwn.cdc.gov/Nchs/Nhanes/2015-2016/FSQ_I.htm (accessed on 6 November 2023).
30. National Cancer Institute—Division of Cancer Control and Population Sciences. Overview & Background of The Healthy Eating Index. Available online: https://epi.grants.cancer.gov/hei/ (accessed on 3 November 2023).
31. Kennedy, E.T.; Ohls, J.; Carlson, S.; Fleming, K. The Healthy Eating Index: Design and applications. *J. Am. Diet Assoc.* **1995**, *95*, 1103–1108. [CrossRef]
32. U.S. Department of Health and Human Services; U.S. Department of Agriculture. Dietary Guidelines for Americans 2015–2020. Available online: https://health.gov/sites/default/files/2019-09/2015-2020_Dietary_Guidelines.pdf (accessed on 6 November 2023).
33. Storey, M.L.; Anderson, P.A. Vegetable consumption and selected nutrient intakes of women of childbearing age. *J. Nutr. Educ. Behav.* **2016**, *48*, 691–696.e1. [CrossRef] [PubMed]
34. Powell, E.S.; Smith-Taillie, L.P.; Popkin, B.M. Added sugars intake across the distribution of US children and adult consumers: 1977–2012. *J. Acad. Nutr. Diet* **2016**, *116*, 1543–1550.e1. [CrossRef]
35. Mesirow, M.S.; Welsh, J.A. Changing beverage consumption patterns have resulted in fewer liquid calories in the diets of US children: National Health and Nutrition Examination Survey 2001–2010. *J. Acad. Nutr. Diet* **2015**, *115*, 559–566.e4. [CrossRef]
36. Centers for Disease Control and Prevention. National Health and Nutrition Examination Survey (NHANES): MEC In-Person Dietary Interviewers Procedures Manual. Available online: https://www.cdc.gov/nchs/data/nhanes/nhanes_05_06/dietary_mec.pdf (accessed on 3 November 2023).
37. Reedy, J.; Lerman, J.L.; Krebs-Smith, S.M.; Kirkpatrick, S.I.; Pannucci, T.E.; Wilson, M.M.; Subar, A.F.; Kahle, L.L.; Tooze, J.A. Evaluation of the Healthy Eating Index-2015. *J. Acad. Nutr. Diet* **2018**, *118*, 1622–1633. [CrossRef]
38. Krebs-Smith, S.M.; Pannucci, T.E.; Subar, A.F.; Kirkpatrick, S.I.; Lerman, J.L.; Tooze, J.A.; Wilson, M.M.; Reedy, J. Update of the Healthy Eating Index: HEI-2015. *J. Acad. Nutr. Diet* **2018**, *118*, 1591–1602. [CrossRef]
39. Acar Tek, N.; Yildiran, H.; Akbulut, G.; Bilici, S.; Koksal, E.; Gezmen Karadag, M.; Sanlier, N. Evaluation of dietary quality of adolescents using Healthy Eating Index. *Nutr. Res. Pract.* **2011**, *5*, 322–328. [CrossRef] [PubMed]
40. U.S. Department of Agriculture—Food and Nutrition Service. Child Nutrition Programs; Income Eligibility Guidelines. Available online: https://www.govinfo.gov/content/pkg/FR-2013-03-22/pdf/2013-06544.pdf (accessed on 3 November 2023).
41. U.S. Department of Agriculture—Food and Nutrition Service. Child Nutrition Programs; Income Eligibility Guidelines—Correction to Table. Available online: https://www.govinfo.gov/content/pkg/FR-2013-03-29/pdf/C1-2013-06544.pdf (accessed on 3 November 2023).
42. Centers for Disease Control and Prevention. NHANES National Youth Fitness Survey, NNYFS 2012 Data Documentation, Codebook, and Frequencies—Weight Status Classifications. Available online: https://wwwn.cdc.gov/Nchs/Nnyfs/Y_BMX.htm#:~:text=Weight%20status%20classification:%20BMI,%20expressed,criteria%20for%20children%20and%20adolescents (accessed on 18 December 2023).
43. Coleman-Jensen, A.; Rabbitt, M.P.; Gregory, C.A.; Singh, A. Household Food Security in the United States in 2021, ERR-309. Available online: https://www.ers.usda.gov/webdocs/publications/104656/err-309.pdf (accessed on 6 November 2023).
44. Hake, M.; Engelhard, E.; Dewey, A. Map the Meal Gap 2022: An Analysis of County and Congressional District Food Insecurity and County Food Cost in the United States in 2020. Available online: https://www.feedingamerica.org/sites/default/files/2022-07/Map%20the%20Meal%20Gap%202022%20Report.pdf (accessed on 3 November 2023).

45. Byker Shanks, C.; Andress, L.; Hardison-Moody, A.; Jilcott Pitts, S.; Patton-Lopez, M.; Prewitt, T.E.; Dupuis, V.; Wong, K.; Kirk-Epstein, M.; Engelhard, E.; et al. Food insecurity in the rural United States: An examination of struggles and coping mechanisms to feed a family among households with a low-income. *Nutrients* **2022**, *14*, 5250. [CrossRef]
46. Bowen, S.; Elliott, S.; Hardison-Moody, A. Rural Food Insecurity: A Longitudinal Analysis of Low-Income Rural Households with Children in the South. *Russell Sage Found. J. Soc. Sci.* **2022**, *8*, 50–77. [CrossRef]
47. Thompson, D.; Miranda, J.; Callender, C.; Dave, J.M.; Appiah, G.; Musaad, S.M.A. See me, hear me, know me: Perspectives on diet and physical activity influences among teens living in rural Texas communities. *Nutrients* **2023**, *15*, 4695. [CrossRef] [PubMed]
48. Vigil, A. Trends in Supplemental Nutrition Assistance Program Participation Rates: Fiscal Year 2010 to Fiscal Year 2017. Available online: https://fns-prod.azureedge.us/sites/default/files/resource-files/Trends2010-2017.pdf (accessed on 6 November 2023).
49. Thomson, J.L.; Tussing-Humphreys, L.M.; Goodman, M.H.; Landry, A.S. Diet quality in a nationally representative sample of American children by sociodemographic characteristics. *Am. J. Clin. Nutr.* **2019**, *109*, 127–138. [CrossRef] [PubMed]
50. Liu, J.; Rehm, C.D.; Onopa, J.; Mozaffarian, D. Trends in diet quality among youth in the United States, 1999–2016. *JAMA* **2020**, *323*, 1161–1174. [CrossRef]
51. U.S. Department of Agriculture; U.S. Department of Health and Human Services. Dietary Guidelines for Americans 2020–2025. Available online: https://www.dietaryguidelines.gov/sites/default/files/2020-12/Dietary_Guidelines_for_Americans_2020-2025.pdf (accessed on 3 November 2023).
52. Davis, A.M.; Bennett, K.J.; Befort, C.; Nollen, N. Obesity and related health behaviors among urban and rural children in the United States: Data from the National Health and Nutrition Examination Survey 2003–2004 and 2005–2006. *J. Pediatr. Psychol.* **2011**, *36*, 669–676. [CrossRef]
53. Liu, J.H.; Jones, S.J.; Sun, H.; Probst, J.C.; Merchant, A.T.; Cavicchia, P. Diet, physical activity, and sedentary behaviors as risk factors for childhood obesity: An urban and rural comparison. *Child. Obes.* **2012**, *8*, 440–448. [CrossRef]
54. Nord, M.; Golla, A.M. Does SNAP Decrease Food Insecurity? Untangling the Self-Selection Effect. Economic Research Report No. 85. Washington, DC: U.S. Department of Agriculture, Economic Research Service. 2009. Available online: https://www.ers.usda.gov/webdocs/publications/46295/10977_err85_1_.pdf?v=6686.2 (accessed on 20 November 2023).
55. Food and Nutrition Service—U.S. Department of Agriculture. Nutrition standards in the National School Lunch and School Breakfast Programs. Final Rule. *Fed. Regist.* **2012**, *77*, 4088–4167. Available online: http://www.gpo.gov/fdsys/pkg/FR-2012-01-26/pdf/2012-1010.pdf (accessed on 20 November 2023).
56. U.S. Department of Agriculture—Food and Nutrition Service. Nutrition Standards for School Meals. Available online: https://www.fns.usda.gov/cn/nutrition-standards-school-meals (accessed on 3 November 2023).

nutrients

MDPI

Article

Assessment of School Contributions to Healthy Eating, Physical Activity Education, and Support for Weight-Loss Attempts among Adolescents from Jazan, Saudi Arabia

Ibrahim M. Gosadi

Department of Family and Community Medicine, Faculty of Medicine, Jazan University, Jazan 82621, Saudi Arabia; gossady@hotmail.com

Abstract: This study evaluates the contribution of schools in Saudi Arabia towards the provision of education and support concerning weight management among adolescents. It also identifies adolescents who have attempted to lose weight and examines their preferred weight-loss methods and their sources of weight-loss support. This study is a cross-sectional investigation that targets adolescents in intermediate and secondary schools in Jazan, Saudi Arabia. Data was collected via a self-administered questionnaire that looked at the involvement of the school in the provision of education pertaining to weight control and the weight-loss experiences of students who had attempted to lose weight. The study involved 501 adolescents, 45% of whom had attempted to lose weight, where the most common methods for weight loss being reducing food consumption (77%), exercising (75%), and fasting (49%). The assessment of the schools' contributions indicated its suboptimal role in the provision of education concerning physical activity compared to education about eating habits. The most commonly reported sources of weight-loss support were the students' families (54%), followed by community facilities (44%). The least common sources were the students' schools (24%). These findings indicate that schools need to enhance their contribution to encouraging adolescents to adopt a healthy lifestyle, while also ensuring multi-sectorial collaboration with families and community members.

Keywords: adolescents; body weight; school; healthy eating; physical activity; weight loss; Jazan; Saudi Arabia

1. Introduction

Overweight and obesity is a public health concern in Saudi Arabia. According to the Saudi Ministry of Health, nearly 60% of Saudi adults are overweight or obese [1]. Changes in the dietary habits and physical activity levels of Saudis during the COVID-19 lockdown have also been found to be associated with weight gain [2]. Indeed, the impact of obesity in Saudi Arabia was reported as costing USD 3.8 billion during 2019, representing 4.3% of the total health expenditure in Saudi Arabia that year [3].

Overweight and obesity is a prevalent health issue among adolescents in the country. In a systematic review of studies published between 2002 and 2018, the assessed prevalence of overweight and obesity among adolescents in Saudi Arabia was between 22% and 48% and showed an upward trend over the last two decades [4]. In a more recent study, a sample of more than 351,000 children and adolescents aged between two and 19 years who had visited healthcare facilities in Saudi Arabia between 2016 and 2021 showed that 20.6% could be classified as overweight or obese, with obesity found to be higher among males [5]. This increased prevalence of overweight and obesity has been associated with the increased prevalence of chronic metabolic diseases in the country [6].

Several investigations have been conducted in Saudi Arabia to understand the determinants of overweight and obesity among Saudi adolescents and children. In a study that utilized a participatory approach to measure the perspectives of students, school staff,

Ministry of Education officials, and parents regarding school-related factors associated with obesity in girls aged between 13 and 15 years, it was concluded that offering affordable healthy food items (fruits and vegetables) and removing unhealthy food items (sweets and chocolate) from the school canteen, as well as more education about healthy foods, were important elements for school-based interventions aiming to reduce obesity [7].

In a study that involved a sample of 2696 students based in the south of Saudi Arabia and aged between 11 and 19 years, it was concluded that limited physical activity and exercise, either in general or during school activities, were associated with higher rates of obesity [8]. In a similar, more recent study that involved a sample of 471 male secondary school students aged between 14 and 18 years from Riyadh, Saudi Arabia, it was concluded that overweight and obese students' activity expenditure was nearly 500 min/week lower compared to students with normal body weight [9]. Furthermore, familial influence, such as having a parental history of obesity [10] or a reduced number of siblings [11], has been found to increase the risk of having a raised BMI among Saudi adolescents.

Early recognition and management of overweight and obesity among children and adolescents are important for reducing the negative health impacts and morbidities associated with these conditions [12]. Several national and international initiatives have been implemented to tackle childhood obesity. For example, the World Health Organization's Commission on Ending Childhood Obesity provided six main recommendations, including the promotion of healthy food intake, the promotion of physical activity, preconception and pregnancy care, early childhood diet and physical activity, and health for school-age children [13]. These efforts have been slow and inconsistent, however, as they have targeted the development of policies that require a multi-sectorial approach [14]. On a national level, the Saudi Guidelines for the Prevention and Management of Obesity were developed to provide evidence-based practices that target obesity in both adults and children [15].

The Saudi Guidelines for the Prevention and Management of Obesity provide recommendations for obesity prevention in children that include eating habit guidelines and the promotion of physical activity. The former involve specific dietary recommendations that encourage children to eat until they are full, consume regular meals including breakfast, and have a low consumption of salty and energy-dense foods. They also recommend that children consume five portions of fruits and vegetables a day, eat in sociable settings, and do not have easy access to food that is not suitable for children.

To promote physical activity in children and adolescents, the guidelines recommend reducing screentime to less than two hours a day and ensuring a minimum of one hour of active play. It is also suggested that the whole family should be involved in increasing the physical activity levels of children. If a child or adolescent is not able to maintain their body weight or prevent weight gain, referral to a specialist is advised, especially if there may be an eating disorder, poor body image, depression or anxiety, the presence of a comorbidity or underlying medical issue, or if there is a need for pharmacological or surgical intervention for weight management [15].

The Saudi Guidelines for the Prevention and Management of Obesity also recommend developing sustainable school-based interventions for proper prevention of overweight and obesity among children and adolescents. These interventions should consider an intersectorial approach that includes their families. Unfortunately, there is limited information regarding the involvement of schools in Saudi Arabia in the provision of school-based interventions aimed at weight management in children and adolescents. In a recent study by Al-Daghri et al. [16], which was conducted in Riyadh, Saudi Arabia, and involved a sample of 363 adolescents aged between 12 and 18 years, an intervention was developed that aimed to reduce the body weight of the adolescents by 5% or more. The intervention involved the provision of educational materials about healthy eating and the promotion of physical activity via educational sessions provided in the classroom. After 12 months, a significant reduction in BMI was found in the adherent groups compared to the non-adherent groups [16].

Although the current weight-management guidelines in Saudi Arabia recommend school-based interventions for tackling childhood obesity, the provision of such interventions is extremely limited. Furthermore, studies that assess the involvement of schools in Saudi Arabia in the promotion of healthy eating and physical activity are also limited. The contribution of schools in Saudi Arabia, via the established official educational program, towards the prevention of overweight and obesity among adolescents is currently unknown. Therefore, the current study measures the contribution of schools in the Jazan region, in the southwest of Saudi Arabia, towards the provision of education concerning the prevention of overweight and obesity among adolescents. It also identifies adolescents who have attempted to lose weight and examines their preferred weight-loss methods and their sources of weight-loss support.

2. Materials and Methods

2.1. Study Design and Settings

This investigation used a cross-sectional design to sample adolescents studying in intermediate and secondary schools in Jazan, Saudi Arabia. Data collection was initiated after securing ethical approval from the Standing Committee for Scientific Research of Jazan University (approval number REC-44/06/446, dated December 2022). Data were collected via an online platform, and an online information sheet explaining the study was shared with parents. The parents who agreed that their children could take part in the study allowed their children to complete the online questionnaire.

2.2. Data Collection Tool

A self-administered questionnaire collected information about the participants' demographics, their reported body weight and height, the involvement of their schools in the provision of educational materials related to weight control, their body weight satisfaction, and the experiences of participants who had tried to lose weight. The sections of the questionnaire that measured the participants' perceptions of their weight, their methods of weight loss, and the involvement of their schools in providing education related to weight control, were adopted from the Global School-based Student Health Survey.

The participants were asked about any education they had received concerning healthy eating, the benefits of consuming fruits and vegetables, methods for maintaining a healthy body weight, the risks of eating salty and energy-dense foods, sport in school, the benefits of physical activity, or the prevention of injury when taking part in sporting activities [17]. The participants were also asked if they were satisfied with their weight and about their intentions concerning their weight. A filtering question was used to identify participants who had tried to lose weight during the last three years, with those answering positively directed to another section of the questionnaire that examined their methods for weight loss

2.3. Data Collection Process

The questionnaire was converted to an online format using Google Forms and a weblink was generated to distribute the data information sheet and the questionnaire to the parents of the participants. The parents were recruited by advertising the study in WhatsApp groups, which are a popular method of communication in school and work settings in Saudi Arabia [18].

The consenting parents were asked to give the questionnaire to their children to complete. They were also asked to share the weblink with their relatives and friends to help achieve the target sample size. Sample size estimation was conducted via the StatCal function of Epi Info. As no previous studies have used the Global School-based Student Health Survey to measure the contribution of schools towards weight management education among adolescents, it was estimated that 50% of the sample would have received relevant education. The target sample size was 480 participants, assuming a prevalence of 50% with a 5% margin of error, 95% confidence interval, and 25% refusal to participate.

The expected frequency of 50% was selected for sample size estimation as it produced the maximum sample size according to the selected sample size parameters.

2.4. Data Analysis

Data analysis was performed using the IBM Statistical Package for the Social Sciences, version 24.0. Frequencies and proportions were used to summarize the binary and categorical data, while means, medians, standard deviations, and interquartile ranges were used to describe continuous data depending on their distribution. A standard Chi-square test investigated the relationship between BMI levels and the intention to lose weight across the sample.

BMI levels were calculated by entering the participants' reported weight and height into the BMI Percentile Calculator for Child and Teen from the Centers for Disease Control and Prevention. The participants were then classified as underweight, normal-weight, or overweight/obese. The chi-square test looked at the relationship between the participants who had tried to lose weight in the previous three years and their BMI, body weight satisfaction, and education level. A p-value of <0.05 was used to indicate statistical significance.

3. Results

The total number of participants who completed the questionnaire was 501. The majority of the sample were female (61%) with a mean age of 16 years (SD = 1.9). More than half of the participants lived in urban areas (54%), and the majority were secondary school students (67%). When asked about their family, 86.5% of participants indicated that they were living with both of their parents, and more than half (57%) indicated that they had up to four siblings. Over half (60%) of the sample had a normal body weight, while nearly one quarter (24%) were overweight or obese. The most frequently reported medical condition was asthma (6.2%), followed by dental illnesses (5.4%). Finally, half of the sample (51%) reported that one or both of their parents had a chronic disease. See Table 1 for complete demographic information.

Table 2 shows the participants' responses regarding the provision of education related to healthy eating and physical activity in their schools. Overall, the majority of participants (76%) reported receiving education about healthy eating. However, only 63% reported receiving education during the school year regarding how to maintain a healthy weight. Furthermore, fewer participants reported receiving education about the benefits of physical activity compared to education about healthy eating. This suggests schools in the Jazan region have low engagement in education related to the benefits of physical activity.

Table 3 displays the satisfaction of the students concerning their body weight, perception of their body weight, and their intentions concerning modifications to their body weight. More than half of the sample were satisfied with their body weight (58%), while 211 adolescents indicated that they were not satisfied (42%). When the students were asked how they would describe their body weight, the majority believed that their body weight was normal (51%). When the students were asked about their intentions concerning their body weight, nearly half of the sample indicated that they intend to modify their body weight, 22% reported that they need to make an effort to maintain their body weight, while 29% reported that they intend to do nothing about their body weight. Finally, when the adolescents were asked about their attitude about body weight, the majority indicated that body weight is important, and is important for disease prevention. However, fewer adolescents indicated that having a normal body weight would make them proud or increase their confidence.

Table 1. Demographic characteristics, BMI categories, and family history of chronic diseases for 501 intermediate and secondary school students from Jazan, Saudi Arabia.

Variables	Frequency [Proportion]
Gender	
Male	197 [39.3%]
Female	304 [60.7%]
Residence area	
Rural	230 [45.9%]
Urban	271 [54.1%]
Education level	
Intermediate	166 [33.1%]
Secondary	335 [66.9]
Living with the parents *	
With both parents	428 [86.5%]
With the father only	10 [2%]
With the mother only	57 [11.4%]
Number of siblings in the family	
4 or less	287 [57.3%]
More than 4	214 [42.7%]
BMI category *	
Underweight	75 [15.6%]
Normal	291 [60.4%]
Overweight or obese	116 [24%]
Diagnosis with a chronic disease	
Frequent dental illness	27 [5.4%]
Mental illness	9 [1.8%]
Obesity	21 [4.2%]
Asthma	31 [6.2%]
Sickle cell disease	13 [2.6%]
Diabetes	5 [1%]
Parental history of chronic disease	259 [51.7%]

* 19 missing cases for BMI, 6 missing cases for living with the parents' status.

Table 2. Responses of 501 intermediate and secondary school students from Jazan, Saudi Arabia, regarding education in school related to healthy eating and physical activity.

Statement	Percentage Who Responded with "Yes"
During this school year, were you taught in any of your classes that healthy eating can help you be healthy and strong?	383 [76.4%]
During this school year, were you taught in any of your classes about the benefits of eating more fruits and vegetables?	350 [69.9%]
During this school year, were you taught in any of your classes how to maintain a healthy weight?	315 [62.9%]
During this school year, were you taught in any of your classes about the risks related to eating too many foods that are high in fat, sugar, or salt?	333 [66.5%]
During this school year, were you keen to take part in the sports classes provided by the school?	288 [57.5%]
During this school year, were you taught in any of your classes how to develop a physical fitness plan for yourself?	257 [51.3%]
During this school year, were you taught in any of your classes about preventing injury during physical activity?	273 [54.5%]
During this school year, were you taught in any of your classes about the benefits of physical activity?	340 [67.9%]
During this school year, were you taught in any of your classes about the opportunities for physical activities in your community?	273 [54.5%]

Table 3. Satisfaction with and perceptions of body weight among 501 intermediate and secondary school students from Jazan, Saudi Arabia.

Statement	Frequency [Proportion]
Are you satisfied with your body weight?	
Yes.	290 [57.9%]
No.	211 [42.1%]
How would you describe your body weight?	
My body weight is low.	72 [14.4%]
My body weight is normal.	258 [51.5%]
My body weight is high.	171 [34.1%]
Attitudes toward body weight:	
Having a normal body weight is important.	436 [87%]
Having a normal body weight is beneficial for disease prevention.	371 [74.1%]
Body weight is important for body image improvement.	373 [74.5%]
I feel proud when I have a normal body weight.	230 [45.9%]
Having a normal body weight increases confidence.	319 [63.7%]
Intentions towards their body weight:	
To do nothing.	144 [28.7%]
To increase their body weight.	60 [12%]
To reduce their body weight.	188 [37.5%]
To maintain their body weight.	109 [21.8%]

Slightly fewer than half of the participants (45%) reported attempting to lose weight. Figure 1 shows the frequencies of the selected methods for weight loss. The majority (77%) tried to lose weight by reducing their food consumption, exercising, or fasting. A small number of participants (9%) reported consulting a physician about losing weight, while under 10% reported using medication, artificial sweeteners, herbal medication, induced vomiting, or surgery for weight loss. Table 4 displays perceptions of weight-loss support among the participants who attempted to lose weight. The most common source of support when trying to lose weight was the participants' families (54%), followed by community facilities (44%). The least common source of support was the participants' schools (24%).

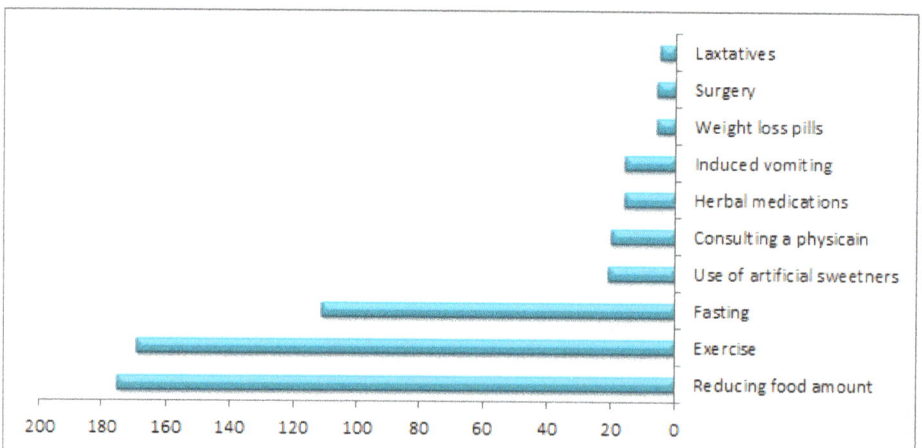

Figure 1. Preferences of 226 adolescents from Jazan, Saudi Arabia, regarding their weight-loss choices during the previous three years.

Table 4. Perceptions of weight-loss support among 226 intermediate and secondary school students from Jazan, Saudi Arabia.

Statement	Frequency of Agreement [Proportion]		
	Agree	Neutral	Do Not Agree
Receipt of family support.	121 [53.5]	66 [28%]	40 [17%]
Receipt of friend support.	93 [41.2%]	75 [33.2%]	58 [25.7%]
Receipt of school support.	54 [23.9%]	78 [34.5%]	94 [41.6%]
Receipt of relative and community support.	74 [32.7%]	72 [31.9%]	80 [35.4%]
Availability of community facilities supporting weight loss.	99 [43.8%]	59 [26.1%]	68 [30.1%]

Table 5 shows the distribution of the participants according to their attempt to lose weight, their gender, education level, BMI category, and satisfaction with their weight. It was found that participants at secondary school, participants classified as overweight or obese, and participants who were not satisfied with their weight were more likely to have attempted to lose weight in the last three years ($p < 0.05$). Interestingly, six participants (8%) classified as underweight and 121 (41.6%) classified as normal-weight had also tried to lose weight in the last three years. This suggests low body weight satisfaction among underweight and normal-weight participants. Finally, there was no significant difference between genders in relation to weight-loss attempts.

Table 5. Associations between weight-loss attempts, gender, education level, BMI category, and weight satisfaction in 501 adolescents from Jazan, Saudi Arabia.

Variables	Attempt to Lose Weight Frequency [Proportion]		
	No	Yes	*p* Value
Gender			0.46
Male	104 [52.8%]	93 [47.2%]	
Female	171 [56.3%]	133 [43.8%]	
Education level			0.01
Intermediate	105 [63.3%]	61 [36.7%]	
Secondary	170 [50.7%]	165 [49.3%]	
BMI category *			<0.001
Underweight	69 [92%]	6 [8%]	
Normal	170 [58.4%]	121 [41.6%]	
Overweight or obese	24 [20.7%]	92 [79.3%]	
Body weight satisfaction			<0.001
Yes	215 [74.1%]	75 [25.9%]	
No	60 [28.4%]	151 [71.6%]	

* 19 missing cases for BMI.

4. Discussion

This study investigated the provision of education related to the prevention of overweight and obesity in adolescents and the methods used by adolescents who had attempted to lose weight. The assessment of the schools' contributions to educating their students about weight management indicated that they were less likely to provide education about the benefits of physical activity compared to education about healthy eating habits.

Just under half of the participants reported being unsatisfied with their body weight, with a similar amount reporting that they believed they had a normal body weight. About 45% had attempted to lose weight during the previous three years, with the most common methods being reducing food consumption, fasting, and exercising. When asked about their sources of support when trying to lose weight, the most frequently reported source was their family, while the least reported source was their school. Interestingly, a number of students who were classified as underweight or normal-weight adolescents had tried to lose weight in the past three years, which suggests they had low body weight satisfaction.

There is a limited number of studies looking at the influence of schools on the eating behaviors and physical activity levels in Saudi adolescents. In a study that assessed the eating habits of 1149 elementary school students from Jeddah, Saudi Arabia, it was found that 56% consumed food and beverages from the school canteen. However, no information regarding their choice of food and beverages or their body weight was provided [19]. A similar study looked at the breakfast intake of elementary school students in Jeddah and found that 80% of the students skipped breakfast for reasons such "as not feeling hungry" and "waking up late" [20].

The current study showed that some adolescents had attempted to lose weight despite having a normal body weight or even being underweight, suggesting that they had misperceptions about their body weight. This is similar to the findings of a study by AsSaigal et al. that measured the body weight perceptions of 270 male secondary school students in the Qassim region of Saudi Arabia. They found that 35% perceived their weight incorrectly, with 18.4% of overweight and obese students perceiving their weight as normal, 53% of the underweight students also perceiving their weight as normal, and 20% of the normal-weight students perceiving themselves as overweight [21].

The attempts of adolescents who are normal-weight or underweight to lose weight can be explained by several notions related to human behavior. Adolescents, during school year and during their development, can be subjected to peer pressure and the associated body-weight shaming and stigmatization, making them more inclined to adopt harmful weight loss measures. Additionally, body weight misperception among adolescents can be influenced by the body weight norm in communities which favor individuals who are thin. Though not measured in the current study, recent evidence indicates that body image among adolescents is further affected by the impact of social media, motivating adolescents, especially girls, to weigh less and may eventually lead to the development of unhealthy eating behaviors and eating disorders [22]. This idea is supported by the findings of the current study, in which some adolescents who attempted to lose weight reported the use of induced vomiting, weight loss pills, herbal medications, and a minority of the adolescents reported consulting a physician for weight loss attempt.

Attempts to lose weight among adolescents, as well as unhealthy dieting, has been explained by several different types of factors, such as body image dissatisfaction (individual), the absence of positive adult role models (familial), and a poor school involvement (environmental) [23]. Interestingly, the adolescents in the current study showed positive attitudes toward weight loss, with the main reasons for having a normal body weight being related to health and the prevention of disease. These results are similar to the findings of a systematic review of the motivators for weight loss among adolescents, where the most common motivators were related to the desire to improve health and self-esteem [24]. Although overweight and obesity among adolescents can be managed in a clinical setting by health professionals [25], it should be noted that only a small number of the adolescents in the current study who had attempted to lose weight reported consulting a physician.

This study found that families are a more common source of support for weight loss compared to other institutions such as schools. This is similar to the results of other studies, which have shown that parental involvement can be a motivating factor for adolescents. In a study looking at 49 American adolescents who had attempted to lose weight, it was concluded that younger adolescents were more likely to be motivated to lose weight if their parents were involved compared to older adolescents [26]. The current study indicates that friends, schools, and communities are less likely to provide weight-loss support, indicating the presence of barriers to weight loss. In a review that examined weight victimization among adolescents, it was reported that this acted as a barrier to physical activity due to humiliation by others and the resulting insecurity [27].

The current study identified several different methods used by adolescents when trying to lose weight, with the most common being reducing food intake and exercising.

This is similar to the findings of the American National Health and Nutrition Examination Survey, which indicated that exercising was the most frequently used method of weight loss among adolescents aged between 16 and 19 years [28]. Similarly, adolescents from Mauritius aged between 13 and 18 years were most likely to try reducing their consumption of energy-dense foods, increasing their consumption of fruits and vegetables, and exercising to lose weight [29].

The current study found that weight-loss attempts were more likely in secondary school adolescents compared to the younger, intermediary school adolescents, suggesting that age influences the likelihood of a student attempting to lose weight. Nonetheless, the study by Rancourt et al., which assessed success of weight loss initiation and maintenance among adolescents with overweight and obesity, indicated that adolescents at a younger age were more likely to initiate weight loss attempt when their parents were involved. Nonetheless, Rancourt et al. also reported that older adolescents were more likely to initiate weight loss on their own, even with less parental involvement [25]. Although there is some variability in the association between age and weight loss attempts identified in our study and the findings of the Rancourt et al. study, it must be noted that the study by Rancourt et al. was restricted to a small sample of adolescents who were overweight or obese while our study recruited a lager sample with variable levels of BMIs, including some adolescents classified as normal-weight or underweight who attempted to lose weight.

Interestingly, gender was not found to influence whether or not a student attempted to lose weight. These findings are similar to those of a large-scale European study by Dzielsa et al., which involved a sample of more than 600,000 adolescents from 26 European countries and compared weight-loss behavior in 2001/2002 to that in 2017/2018. They found that girls were more likely to engage in weight-loss behavior in 2001/2002, but that this gender difference reduced over time, with more boys attempting to lose weight during 2017/2018 [30]. In contrast, a UK-based study that compared weight-loss attempts between two periods (1997/1998 and 2015/2016) indicated that the number of these attempts increased over time and were more common among girls [31].

The current findings indicate that nearly 58% of the recruited adolescents were satisfied with their body weight. Nonetheless, among those who reported being satisfied with their body weight, 63 adolescent students (22% of the those who are satisfied) declared their wish to alter their body weight. It is possible to argue that the identified 63 adolescents may exhibit lower satisfaction levels in comparison to the majority of the satisfied adolescents who did not wish to alter their body weight. However, this was not measured in the current study since satisfaction was assessed via binary answering options (yes, no). Furthermore, satisfaction levels can be associated with different factors such as age, gender, BMI level, body composition, and appearance. This suggests the need for further research to assess satisfaction levels (such as utilizing five-point Likert scales, and to identify the factors associated with the satisfaction level and the intention to alter body weight among the adolescents).

Adolescents in Saudi Arabia spend a very significant part of their lives in schools. The education system and school environment are directly involved with the mental, emotional, and physical well-being of adolescents. It is possible to argue that any public health intervention targeting adolescents would not succeed without the optimal involvement of schools. Overweight and obesity during adolescence is rather critical due to its long-term impact and the raised risk of developing chronic non-communicable diseases during a later phase of life. Therefore, schools should invest in enhancing their communication with young people, especially during the developmental changes the adolescents are experiencing.

Enhancement of the communication of schools with young people can be implemented on several levels. Firstly, in a country that is witnessing a rise in the incidence of lifestyle-influenced chronic diseases such as obesity, diabetes, and hypertension, education about healthy eating and physical activity should be a core part of the curricular activities delivered to the students. Secondly, schools should provide tailored extracurricular activities for adolescents who are suffering from raised BMIs or are at risk of developing obesity. These curricular and extracurricular activities should be provided by teachers who themselves are adherent to a healthy lifestyle to act as role models to the adolescents, and they should be well-trained communicators with young people in a manner that addresses the emotional and psychological considerations associated with the development of adolescents. Success of the school's communication with its adolescents via curricular and extracurricular activities should create a culture in schools that reduces stigma associated with body weight and body image and motivate the adolescents to engage in a healthy lifestyle.

The current study has several strengths and weaknesses. The main strengths are associated with the utilization of an online platform to enhance the ability to reach adolescents in different weight categories. Additionally, this study was able to identify adolescents who had attempted to lose weight without seeking help from a healthcare professional. The study's main weaknesses are associated with the likelihood of selection bias due to its online approach and possible measurement bias in relation to the self-reported heights and weights of the participants. Nonetheless, the findings regarding the prevalence of abnormal BMIs and the presence of misperceptions about body weight among adolescents are similar to those reported in the literature locally and internationally.

Additionally, this study assessed schools' contribution to the education of adolescents about healthy eating, physical activity, and their support of weight-loss without involving their teachers or the relevant stakeholders in the education system. Targeting the teachers and the relevant stakeholders is important to ensure objective assessment of school's contribution to adolescents' health. This indicates an area for further research to perform an objective assessment of the school's contribution to a healthy lifestyle in adolescents, via assessing the opinions of the teachers and education system stakeholders concerning healthy lifestyle education among the students. Finally, this study targeted adolescents in one region in Saudi Arabia. Although the education system is unified in the country under the umbrella of the Saudi Ministry of Education, and the teaching system is similar in all regions of the country, it must be noted that the findings of the current study have limited generalizability and further research is required in other regions to assess schools' contributions towards the education of adolescents about healthy lifestyles.

5. Conclusions

The findings of the current study suggest a suboptimal involvement of schools in the south of Saudi Arabia when promoting healthy eating behaviors and physical activity among students. Furthermore, some adolescents reported not being satisfied with their body weight, which partially explains why some of those classified as underweight or normal-weight had attempted to lose weight in the past three years. Among the adolescents who attempted to lose weight, the most frequently reported source of support was their family. This indicates the need to enhance schools' contributions to supporting the adoption of healthy lifestyles. Furthermore, governmental and public agencies should establish collaboration between different sectors, such as the health, education, and municipality sectors, as well as families and communities, to tackle body weight abnormality among adolescents and enhance the adolescents' knowledge about healthy eating, physical activity, and weight loss.

Funding: This research did not receive any specific grant from any funding agency.

Institutional Review Board Statement: The study was approved by the Research Ethics Committee of Jazan University, Saudi Arabia (IRB Approval number REC-44/06/446, dated December 2022).

Informed Consent Statement: Informed consent was obtained from all subjects' parents involved in the study.

Data Availability Statement: The data presented in this study are available on request from the corresponding author.

Conflicts of Interest: The author declares no conflict of interest.

References

1. Saudi Ministry of Health. World Health Survey. 2019. Available online: https://www.moh.gov.sa/en/Ministry/Statistics/Population-Health-Indicators/Documents/World-Health-Survey-Saudi-Arabia.pdf (accessed on 7 October 2023).
2. Abdulsalam, N.M.; Khateeb, N.A.; Aljerbi, S.S.; Alqumayzi, W.M.; Balubaid, S.S.; Almarghlani, A.A.; Ayad, A.A.; Williams, L.L. Assessment of Dietary Habits and Physical Activity Changes during the Full COVID-19 Curfew Period and Its Effect on Weight among Adults in Jeddah, Saudi Arabia. *Int. J. Environ. Res. Public Health* **2021**, *18*, 8580. [CrossRef] [PubMed]
3. Malkin, J.D.; Baid, D.; Alsukait, R.F.; Alghaith, T.; Alluhidan, M.; Alabdulkarim, H.; Altowaijri, A.; Almalki, Z.S.; Herbst, C.H.; Finkelstein, E.A.; et al. The economic burden of overweight and obesity in Saudi Arabia. *PLoS ONE* **2022**, *17*, e0264993. [CrossRef] [PubMed]
4. Habbab, R.M.; Bhutta, Z.A. Prevalence and social determinants of overweight and obesity in adolescents in Saudi Arabia: A systematic review. *Clin. Obes.* **2020**, *10*, e12400. [CrossRef]
5. AlEnazi, S.; AlAjlan, R.; AlKhalaf, H.; Abolfotouh, M.; Alharbi, O.; Alfawaz, R.; Aldebasi, B.; Alghnam, S. Prevalence of Obesity among Children and Adolescents in Saudi Arabia: A Multicenter Population-Based Study. *Saudi J. Med. Med. Sci.* **2023**, *11*, 19–25. [CrossRef]
6. Gosadi, I.M. Assessment of the environmental and genetic factors influencing prevalence of metabolic syndrome in Saudi Arabia. *Saudi Med. J.* **2016**, *37*, 12–20. [CrossRef] [PubMed]
7. Almughamisi, M.; O'Keeffe, M.; Harding, S. Adolescent Obesity Prevention in Saudi Arabia: Co-identifying Actionable Priorities for Interventions. *Front. Public Health* **2022**, *10*, 863765. [CrossRef]
8. Mahfouz, A.A.; Abdelmoneim, I.; Khan, M.Y.; Daffalla, A.A.; Diab, M.M.; Al-Gelban, K.S.; Moussa, H. Obesity and related behaviors among adolescent school boys in Abha City, Southwestern Saudi Arabia. *J. Trop. Pediatr.* **2008**, *54*, 120–124. [CrossRef]
9. Alhowikan, A.M.; Alsharqawy, N.E.; Alazmaa, N.N.; Saeed, A.I.; Alhazzani, Y.A.; Alhowaish, N.Y.; Yahya, A.F.B.; Alhozaimi, Z.A.; Aleid, N.E.; Alhussain, M.H. Lifestyle habits and obesity indices among male adolescents in Riyadh, Saudi Arabia. *Sci. Rep.* **2023**, *13*, 12099. [CrossRef]
10. Aljassim, H.; Jradi, H. Childhood overweight and obesity among the Saudi population: A case-control study among school children. *J. Health Popul. Nutr.* **2021**, *40*, 15. [CrossRef]
11. Alshaikh, A.A.; Alqahtani, A.S.; FA, A.A.; Al Hadi, A.M.; Alqahtani, M.M.M.; Alshahrani, O.M.; Albraik, M.A.; Alamri, S.A.; Ghazy, R.M. Examining the Impact of Socioeconomic Factors and Lifestyle Habits on Obesity Prevalence among Male and Female Adolescent Students in Asser, Saudi Arabia. *Cureus* **2023**, *15*, e43918. [CrossRef]
12. Hampl, S.E.; Hassink, S.G.; Skinner, A.C.; Armstrong, S.C.; Barlow, S.E.; Bolling, C.F.; Avila Edwards, K.C.; Eneli, I.; Hamre, R.; Joseph, M.M.; et al. Clinical Practice Guideline for the Evaluation and Treatment of Children and Adolescents with Obesity. *Pediatrics* **2023**, *151*, e2022060640. [CrossRef]
13. Wold Health Organization. Report of the Commission on Ending Childhood Obesity: Implementation Plan: Executive Summary. 2017. Available online: https://iris.who.int/handle/10665/259349?locale-attribute=ar&show=full (accessed on 7 October 2023).
14. Lister, N.B.; Baur, L.A.; Felix, J.F.; Hill, A.J.; Marcus, C.; Reinehr, T.; Summerbell, C.; Wabitsch, M. Child and adolescent obesity. *Nat. Rev. Dis. Primers* **2023**, *9*, 24. [CrossRef] [PubMed]
15. Saudi ministry of Health. Saudi Guidelines on the Prevention and Management of Obesity. 2016. Available online: https://www.moh.gov.sa/Ministry/About/Health%20Policies/008.pdf (accessed on 7 October 2023).
16. Al-Daghri, N.M.; Amer, O.E.; Khattak, M.N.K.; Hussain, S.D.; Alkhaldi, G.; Alfawaz, H.A.; Elsaid, M.A.; Sabico, S. Attendance-Based Adherence and Outcomes of Obesity Management Program in Arab Adolescents. *Children* **2023**, *10*, 1449. [CrossRef]
17. World Health Organization. Global School-Based Student Health Survey. 2021. Available online: https://www.who.int/teams/noncommunicable-diseases/surveillance/systems-tools/global-school-based-student-health-survey (accessed on 7 October 2023).
18. Ryani, M.A.; Alshahrani, A.; Khmees, R.A.; Gosadi, I.M. Assessment of the Association Between Use of WhatsApp for Work-Related Purposes and Levels of Depression, Anxiety, and Stress Among Healthcare Workers from Jazan, Saudi Arabia. *Psychol. Res. Behav. Manag.* **2023**, *16*, 713–725. [CrossRef] [PubMed]
19. Jabri, L.; Al-Rasheedi, A.A.; Alsulaimani, R.A.; Al-Hazzaa, H.M. Breakfast Eating Habits and Lifestyle Behaviors among Saudi Primary School Children Attending Public Versus Private Schools. *Children* **2021**, *8*, 134. [CrossRef] [PubMed]
20. Al-Hazzaa, H.M.; Al-Rasheedi, A.A.; Alsulaimani, R.A.; Jabri, L. Anthropometric, Familial- and Lifestyle-Related Characteristics of School Children Skipping Breakfast in Jeddah, Saudi Arabia. *Nutrients* **2020**, *12*, 3668. [CrossRef] [PubMed]
21. AsSaigal, O.A.; Alguefly, S.; El-Mosaad, Y.M.; Al Saigul, A.M. Secondary School Male Students Perception Towards Their Weight, Almethnab Town, Qassim, Saudi Arabia. *Cureus* **2021**, *13*, e20370. [CrossRef]
22. Morris, A.M.; Katzman, D.K. The impact of the media on eating disorders in children and adolescents. *Paediatr. Child. Health* **2003**, *8*, 287–289. [CrossRef]
23. Paediatric Child Health. Dieting in adolescence. *Paediatr. Child. Health* **2004**, *9*, 487–503. [CrossRef]
24. Silva, D.F.O.; Sena-Evangelista, K.C.M.; Lyra, C.O.; Pedrosa, L.F.C.; Arrais, R.F.; Lima, S. Motivations for weight loss in adolescents with overweight and obesity: A systematic review. *BMC Pediatr.* **2018**, *18*, 364. [CrossRef] [PubMed]
25. Steinbeck, K. Adolescent overweight and obesity—How best to manage in the general practice setting. *Aust. Fam. Physician* **2007**, *36*, 606–612.

26. Rancourt, D.; Jensen, C.D.; Duraccio, K.M.; Evans, E.W.; Wing, R.R.; Jelalian, E. Successful weight loss initiation and maintenance among adolescents with overweight and obesity: Does age matter? *Clin. Obes.* **2018**, *8*, 176–183. [CrossRef]
27. Skogen, I.B.; Båtevik, F.O.; Krumsvik, R.J.; Høydal, K.L. Weight-Based Victimization and Physical Activity Among Adolescents with Overweight or Obesity: A Scoping Review of Quantitative and Qualitative Evidence. *Front. Sports Act. Living* **2022**, *4*, 732737. [CrossRef]
28. McDow, K.B.; Nguyen, D.T.; Herrick, K.A.; Akinbami, L.J. Attempts to Lose Weight among Adolescents Aged 16-19 in the United States, 2013–2016. *NCHS Data Brief* **2019**, *340*, 1–8.
29. Bhurtun, D.D.; Jeewon, R. Body Weight Perception and Weight Control Practices among Teenagers. *ISRN Nutr.* **2013**, *2013*, 395125. [CrossRef]
30. Dzielska, A.; Kelly, C.; Ojala, K.; Finne, E.; Spinelli, A.; Furstova, J.; Fismen, A.S.; Ercan, O.; Tesler, R.; Melkumova, M.; et al. Weight Reduction Behaviors among European Adolescents-Changes from 2001/2002 to 2017/2018. *J. Adolesc. Health* **2020**, *66*, S70–S80. [CrossRef] [PubMed]
31. Ahmad, A.; Little, M.; Piernas, C.; Jebb, S. Trends in weight loss attempts among children in England. *Arch. Dis. Child.* **2022**, *107*, 896–901. [CrossRef] [PubMed]

nutrients

MDPI

Article

Retrospective Reports of Parental Feeding Practices and Current Eating Styles in Polish Adults

Aleksandra Małachowska * and Marzena Jeżewska-Zychowicz

Department of Food Market and Consumer Research, Institute of Human Nutrition Sciences, Warsaw University of Life Sciences (SGGW-WULS), Nowoursynowska 159C, 02-776 Warsaw, Poland; marzena_jezewska_zychowicz@sggw.edu.pl

* Correspondence: aleksandra_malachowska@sggw.edu.pl; Tel.: +48-608-448-606

Abstract: The role of childhood food experiences (CFEs) in determining future eating behaviors remains unclear. The aim of the study was to examine the link between CFEs and selected eating styles (ESs), i.e., intuitive (IE), restrained (ResEat) and external (ExtEat) eating, among 708 Polish adults aged 18–65 (477 women and 231 men). CFEs were measured with the Adults' Memories of Feeding in Childhood questionnaire. Polish versions of the Intuitive Eating Scale-2 and Dutch Eating Behavior Questionnaire were used to assess ESs. Mann-Whitney U test was used to compare ESs scores between those with lower and higher CFEs. In the total sample, "Restrictions" and "Pressure and Food Reward" parental feeding practices favored lower IE, while "Healthy Eating Guidance" and "Monitoring" practices predisposed higher levels of IE in adulthood. "Restrictions" were found to correlate with greater chances of ResEat, whereas "Healthy Eating Guidance" was linked with lower probability of ResEat. "Pressure and Food Reward" and "Monitoring" were associated with higher score for ExtEat. "Restrictions", "Child Control", "Monitoring" and "Healthy Eating Guidance" practices were differently linked to ESs in women and men. The findings suggest that education programs for parents should focus on the long-term consequences of feeding practices.

Keywords: parental feeding practices; childhood food experiences; eating style; intuitive eating; external eating; restrained eating

1. Introduction

Childhood food experiences (CFEs) stem from diverse parental feeding practices (PFPs), such as pressuring to eat, teaching about nutrition, applying restrictions, monitoring a child's food intake or using food as a reward [1,2]. PFPs can greatly influence a child's eating, predisposing to favorable or unfavorable behaviors [3]. There is an ongoing debate on whether dietary behaviors established during early childhood (birth to 6 years) and middle childhood (6 to 12 years) continue into adolescence and further into adulthood [2,4]. A few longitudinal studies confirmed the moderate transmission of childhood dietary patterns into young adulthood [5–7]. Nevertheless, results from retrospective studies in adults indicated that selected CFEs may favor future eating behaviors especially in the form of eating styles (ESs) [8–16]. ESs describe psychological aspects of dietary behaviors, such as beliefs, attitudes, motives and feelings towards food and eating [17]. The role of selected ESs, e.g., intuitive eating (IE), restrained eating (ResEat) and external eating (ExtEat), as predictors of the food intake was confirmed in available research [17–20]. IE is a non-dieting approach that promotes eating based on physiological internal signals rather than emotional (EmoEat) or external (ExtEat) ones [21]. Identification of the individual's ES and searching for its origin may be useful in prevention and treatment of diet-related diseases [22].

To date, research has confirmed the following associations: (1) the link between parents using food to control the child's behavior (e.g., food pressuring or food rewarding) and more frequent binge-eating or dietary restraint [8], long-lasting food rejection [13], lower level of intuitive eating and higher level of disordered eating in adulthood [9]; (2) the association between parents applying restrictions or emotional regulation feeding and food preoccupation as well as emotional eating in adulthood [10,12]; (3) the link between positive and negative memories about family's food rules and dieting in adulthood [14]; and (4) the association between having regular family meals as a child and having regular family meals as an adult [15,23]. Moreover, the availability of unhealthy foods at home during childhood was associated with less healthful eating [24] and early life eating environments with the development of the food addiction [25] in young adults.

Despite some evidence that there is a link between CFEs and maladaptive ESs in adulthood, e.g., ResEat or ExtEat, the existing studies have mostly included single or selected PFPs [8–16]. Moreover, the majority of research focused on the PFPs with potential short- and long-term negative impacts, such as food rewarding, pressuring to eat, rigid controlling behaviors, etc. [8–15]. Little is known about the link between diverse CFEs and adaptive ESs in adulthood, such as IE [26]. Adaptive ESs are believed to be characterized by the absence or low levels of maladaptive eating, hence they may be differently related to CFEs [21]. Furthermore, few available studies have indicated that PFPs may be gendered, and thus have different impacts on girls' and boys' eating [27–29]. Therefore, it may be hypothesized that CFEs related to the same PFPs can differently predict ESs among women and men [11,26].

The aim of the study was to examine the association between childhood food experiences and selected eating styles separately in adult women and men. The following hypotheses were tested: 1. Childhood food experiences such as healthy eating guidance, monitoring and child control predispose to a greater level of intuitive eating in adulthood, while experiences related to restrictions, food rewarding or pressuring to eat favor restrained and external eating in adulthood; 2. Gender differentiates the association between childhood food experiences and selected eating styles in adulthood.

2. Materials and Methods

2.1. Study Design and Participants

The data for this cross-sectional study were collected in Poland from October 2022 to January 2023 with the use of a Computer-Assisted Web Interview technique. An invitation to participate in the study with a short description of its purpose and a link to a questionnaire were published on social media. The inclusion criteria were age between 18 and 65, ability to read and understand Polish and informed online consent. The exclusion criteria were as follows: age lower than 18 years old or greater than 65 years old, inability to read and understand Polish and lack of consent. The data anonymity and confidentiality were assured. The final study sample included 477 women and 231 men (708 participants in total), who properly filled out the questionnaire. The study design was approved by the Ethics Committee of the Institute of Human Nutrition Sciences, Warsaw University of Life Sciences, in Poland (Resolution No. 02/2020) and was conducted in compliance with the Declaration of Helsinki.

2.2. Measures

2.2.1. Assessment of the Childhood Food Experiences

Adults' memories of childhood food experiences related to PFPs were assessed with The Adults' Memories of Feeding in Childhood questionnaire (AMoFiC) [2]. The tool had a 5-factor structure: 1. "Restrictions" (13 items), 2. "Healthy Eating Guidance" (9 items), 3. "Pressure and Food Reward" (6 items), 4. "Monitoring" (5 items), 5. "Child Control" (6 items). The items were rated with a 5-point Likert scale, ranging from never/disagree (1) to always/agree (5). The additional answer, i.e., "I don't remember", was scored zero points and was further treated as a missing value. The score for each subscale was obtained by calculating mean values.

2.2.2. Assessment of the Eating Styles

Intuitive eating (IE) was assessed with the Polish version of the Intuitive Eating Scale-2 [30]. It had a 4-factor structure: 1. "Reliance on Hunger and Satiety Cues" (6 items), 2. "Eating For Physical Rather Than Emotional Reasons" (4 items), 3. "Body–Food Choice Congruence" (3 items), 4. "Unconditional Permission to Eat" (3 items). The items were rated with a 5-point Likert scale, ranging from strongly disagree (1) to strongly agree (5).

Restrained and external eating were assessed with the Polish version of the Dutch Eating Questionnaire [17]. "Restrained eating" (ResEat) subscale contains 9 items, whereas "External eating" (ExtEat) is a 7-item subscale. The items were rated with a 5-point Likert scale, ranging from never (1) to very often (5). Scores for each IE subscale as well as for ResEat and ExtEat were presented as mean values.

2.2.3. Sociodemographic Characteristics

The following sociodemographic data were collected: age, gender (female or male), education (primary, lower secondary, upper secondary, or higher) and place of residence (village, town below 20,000 inhabitants, town between 20,000 and 100,000 inhabitants, or city with over 100,000 inhabitants).

2.3. Data Analysis

Sociodemographic characteristics were presented with the descriptive statistics. Two groups of participants were distinguished based on their scores for each subscale from the AMoFiC questionnaire: 1. "lower childhood food experiences (lower CFEs)"—mean score below or equal to 3.00, and 2. "higher childhood food experiences (higher CFEs)"—mean score greater than 3.00. Shapiro–Wilk test was used to test the normality of distribution. Mean scores for the four subscales from the Intuitive Eating Scale-2 as well as for Restrained and External eating subscales were compared between those two groups, i.e., lower and higher CFEs, with the Mann–Whitney U test. Significance level was set at $\alpha = 0.05$. All analyses were performed in IBM SPSS Statistics for Windows, version 28.0 (IBM Corp., Armonk, NY, USA).

3. Results

3.1. Participants

The study included a total of 708 participants. The majority of the study group were women (67.4%), people with higher education (83.2%) and people living in a city (62.6%) (Table 1). The mean age of the participants was 36.9 ± 11.5 years.

Table 1. Sociodemographic characteristics of the study sample.

Variables		Total (n = 708) n (%)	Women (n = 477) n (%)	Men (n = 231) n (%)
Age (years)	18–24	94 (13.3)	65 (13.6)	29 (12.5)
	25–39	349 (49.3)	253 (53.0)	96 (41.6)
	40–54	193 (27.2)	120 (25.2)	73 (31.6)
	55–65	72 (10.2)	39 (8.2)	33 (14.3)
Education	Primary	3 (0.4)	3 (0.6)	0 (0.0)
	Lower secondary	3 (0.4)	2 (0.4)	1 (0.4)
	Upper secondary	113 (16.0)	68 (14.3)	45 (19.5)
	Higher (e.g., BSc and MSc)	589 (83.2)	404 (84.7)	185 (80.1)
Place of Residence	Village	113 (15.9)	78 (16.3)	35 (15.2)
	Town below 20,000 inhabitants	43 (6.1)	31 (6.5)	12 (5.2)
	Town between 20,000 and 100,000 inhabitants	109 (15.4)	69 (14.5)	40 (17.3)
	City with over 100,000 inhabitants	443 (62.6)	299 (62.7)	144 (62.3)

n, number of participants; BSc, Bachelor of Science; MSc, Master of Science.

3.2. Childhood Food Experiences and Intuitive Eating in Adulthood

Participants with lower CFEs related to "Restrictions" had higher scores in three subscales of IE, i.e., "Reliance on Hunger and Satiety Cues", "Eating For Physical Rather Than Emotional Reasons" and "Unconditional Permission to Eat", in comparison to people with higher experiences, which was confirmed in the total sample and among women (Table 2). Among men, those with lower experiences of "Restrictions" scored higher in "Unconditional Permission to Eat" and lower in "Body–Food Choice Congruence". CFEs related to "Healthy Eating Guidance" were linked to higher scores for "Reliance on Hunger and Satiety Cues", "Eating For Physical Rather Than Emotional Reasons" and "Body–Food Choice Congruence" in the total sample as well as among women and men separately. The experience of "Pressure and Food Reward" in childhood was associated with a lower score for "Eating For Physical Rather Than Emotional Reasons" in the total sample and in women and men separately. Higher experience of "Monitoring" of the child's eating behaviors favored higher score in "Body–Food Choice Congruence" in the total sample, as well as in women. The experiences of "Child Control" differentiated the score of "Eating For Physical Rather Than Emotional Reasons" in men only, with the greater score among the group with higher experiences of this PFP (Table 2).

Table 2. Childhood food experiences and intuitive eating in the study sample.

Childhood Food Experiences (CFEs)			**Intuitive Eating—Subscales**			
Subscale	**Groups of Respondents**	*n* (%)	**Reliance on Hunger and Satiety Cues Mean ± SD**	**Eating for Physical Rather than Emotional Reasons Mean ± SD**	**Body–Food Choice Congruence Mean ± SD**	**Unconditional Permission to Eat Mean ± SD**
			Total sample (*n* = 708)			
Restrictions	lower CFEs [a]	666 (94.1)	3.42 ± 0.79 *	3.36 ± 1.15 **	3.42 ± 0.77	3.65 ± 0.81 **
	higher CFEs [b]	42 (5.9)	3.07 ± 1.03 *	2.86 ± 1.10 **	3.60 ± 0.91	3.30 ± 0.81 **
Healthy Eating Guidance	lower CFEs	292 (41.2)	3.20 ± 0.85 ***	3.09 ± 1.19 ***	3.32 ± 0.77 ***	3.58 ± 0.86
	higher CFEs	416 (58.8)	3.53 ± 0.76 ***	3.50 ± 1.09 ***	3.51 ± 0.78 ***	3.66 ± 0.78
Pressure and Food Reward	lower CFEs	485 (68.5)	3.43 ± 0.81	3.45 ± 1.14 ***	3.46 ± 0.74	3.60 ± 0.82
	higher CFEs	223 (31.5)	3.33 ± 0.81	3.08 ± 1.14 ***	3.36 ± 0.85	3.67 ± 0.81
Monitoring	lower CFEs	479 (67.7)	3.38 ± 0.79	3.38 ± 1.14	3.38 ± 0.76 **	3.64 ± 0.79
	higher CFEs	229 (32.3)	3.44 ± 0.86	3.24 ± 1.16	3.53 ± 0.81 **	3.59 ± 0.87
Child Control	lower CFEs	538 (76.0)	3.43 ± 0.78	3.34 ± 1.13	3.45 ± 0.77	3.63 ± 0.80
	higher CFEs	170 (24.0)	3.30 ± 0.89	3.30 ± 1.22	3.38 ± 0.82	3.61 ± 0.86
			Women (*n* = 477)			
Restrictions	lower CFEs	444 (93.1)	3.39 ± 0.83 *	3.16 ± 1.16 *	3.44 ± 0.80	3.62 ± 0.83 *
	higher CFEs	33 (6.9)	2.98 ± 1.05 *	2.73 ± 1.12 *	3.49 ± 0.89	3.34 ± 0.78 *
Healthy Eating Guidance	lower CFEs	196 (41.1)	3.15 ± 0.90 ***	2.85 ± 1.18 ***	3.35 ± 0.79 *	3.53 ± 0.89
	higher CFEs	281 (58.9)	3.51 ± 0.79 ***	3.32 ± 1.12 ***	3.51 ± 0.82 *	3.65 ± 0.78
Pressure and Food Reward	lower CFEs	316 (66.2)	3.40 ± 0.86	3.23 ± 1.15 **	3.48 ± 0.77	3.58 ± 0.84
	higher CFEs	161 (33.8)	3.30 ± 0.84	2.93 ± 1.16 **	3.37 ± 0.88	3.64 ± 0.80
Monitoring	lower CFEs	317 (66.5)	3.35 ± 0.82	3.16 ± 1.15	3.38 ± 0.78 **	3.64 ± 0.79
	higher CFEs	160 (33.5)	3.40 ± 0.93	3.06 ± 1.20	3.57 ± 0.85 **	3.54 ± 0.89
Child Control	lower CFEs	351 (73.6)	3.40 ± 0.83	3.16 ± 1.15	3.48 ± 0.80	3.61 ± 0.81
	higher CFEs	126 (26.4)	3.26 ± 0.92	3.05 ± 1.21	3.35 ± 0.82	3.57 ± 0.87

Table 2. *Cont.*

Childhood Food Experiences (CFEs)			Intuitive Eating—Subscales			
Subscale	Groups of Respondents	n (%)	Reliance on Hunger and Satiety Cues Mean ± SD	Eating for Physical Rather than Emotional Reasons Mean ± SD	Body–Food Choice Congruence Mean ± SD	Unconditional Permission to Eat Mean ± SD
			Men (n = 231)			
Restrictions	lower CFEs	222 (96.1)	3.46 ± 0.70	3.77 ± 0.99	3.39 ± 0.70 *	3.70 ± 0.78 *
	higher CFEs	9 (3.9)	3.41 ± 0.93	3.36 ± 0.94	3.96 ± 0.90 *	3.15 ± 0.91 *
Healthy Eating Guidance	lower CFEs	96 (41.6)	3.31 ± 0.73 **	3.56 ± 1.07 *	3.25 ± 0.72 *	3.68 ± 0.80
	higher CFEs	135 (58.4)	3.57 ± 0.68 **	3.88 ± 0.91 *	3.52 ± 0.69 *	3.67 ± 0.79
Pressure and Food Reward	lower CFEs	169 (73.2)	3.48 ± 0.71	3.85 ± 0.99 **	3.44 ± 0.69	3.64 ± 0.77
	higher CFEs	62 (26.8)	3.42 ± 0.71	3.48 ± 0.97 **	3.33 ± 0.76	3.76 ± 0.86
Monitoring	lower CFEs	162 (70.1)	3.43 ± 0.72	3.79 ± 1.01	3.40 ± 0.71	3.65 ± 0.79
	higher CFEs	69 (29.9)	3.54 ± 0.68	3.65 ± 0.96	3.43 ± 0.73	3.72 ± 0.79
Child Control	lower CFEs	187 (81.0)	3.48 ± 0.69	3.69 ± 1.00 *	3.40 ± 0.69	3.67 ± 0.78
	higher CFEs	44 (19.0)	3.41 ± 0.79	4.01 ± 0.95 *	3.46 ± 0.81	3.70 ± 0.83

n, number of participants; [a] mean score for the subscale below or equal to 3.00, [b] mean score for the subscale above 3.00; SD, standard deviation; significant at * $p < 0.05$, ** $p < 0.01$, *** $p < 0.001$; Mann–Whitney U Test.

3.3. Childhood Food Experiences, Restrained and External Eating in Adulthood

The differences in ResEat were noted only in regard to the "Restrictions" and "Healthy Eating Guidance" subscales (Table 3). Participants who had more experiences of "Restrictions" obtained a higher score for ResEat in comparison to those with lower experiences in the total sample and separately among women and men. Higher experiences of the PFPs related to "Healthy Eating Guidance" were linked to a lower score for ResEat in the total sample, yet no significant differences were noted within the women and within the men. Higher childhood experiences of "Pressure and Food Reward" as well as "Monitoring" were associated with a higher score for ExtEat in the total sample. In the female and male group, only differences resulting from the experiences of the "Pressure and Food Reward" were observed. Both men and women with higher experiences of this PFP obtained a greater score for ExtEat in comparison to the group with lower experiences (Table 3).

Table 3. Childhood food experiences, external and restrained eating in the study sample.

Childhood Food Experiences (CFEs)			Eating Style	
Subscale	Groups of Respondents	n (%)	External Eating Mean ± SD	Restrained Eating Mean ± SD
		Total sample (n = 708)		
Restrictions	lower CFEs [a]	666 (94.1)	2.97 ± 0.71	2.58 ± 0.88 ***
	higher CFEs [b]	42 (5.9)	3.08 ± 0.82	3.12 ± 0.82 ***
Healthy Eating Guidance	lower CFEs	292 (41.2)	3.05 ± 0.76	2.70 ± 0.90 *
	higher CFEs	416 (58.8)	2.92 ± 0.69	2.56 ± 0.87 *
Pressure and Food Reward	lower CFEs	485 (68.5)	2.89 ± 0.71 ***	2.60 ± 0.85
	higher CFEs	223 (31.5)	3.15 ± 0.71 ***	2.66 ± 0.95
Monitoring	lower CFEs	479 (67.7)	2.94 ± 0.73 *	2.58 ± 0.88
	higher CFEs	229 (32.3)	3.04 ± 0.69 *	2.69 ± 0.89
Child Control	lower CFEs	538 (76.0)	2.96 ± 0.69	2.60 ± 0.88
	higher CFEs	170 (24.0)	3.02 ± 0.79	2.67 ± 0.88

Table 3. *Cont.*

Childhood Food Experiences (CFEs)			Eating Style	
Subscale	Groups of Respondents	n (%)	External Eating Mean ± SD	Restrained Eating Mean ± SD
		Women (n = 477)		
Restrictions	lower CFEs	444 (93.1)	3.02 ± 0.72	2.67 ± 0.89 **
	higher CFEs	33 (6.9)	3.18 ± 0.87	3.12 ± 0.74 **
Healthy Eating Guidance	lower CFEs	196 (41.1)	3.16 ± 0.78 **	2.80 ± 0.91
	higher CFEs	281 (58.9)	2.95 ± 0.69 **	2.63 ± 0.86
Pressure and Food Reward	lower CFEs	316 (66.2)	2.96 ± 0.72 ***	2.66 ± 0.85
	higher CFEs	161 (33.8)	3.18 ± 0.73 ***	2.77 ± 0.95
Monitoring	lower CFEs	317 (66.5)	3.02 ± 0.75	2.66 ± 0.88
	higher CFEs	160 (33.5)	3.07 ± 0.70	2.77 ± 0.88
Child Control	lower CFEs	351 (73.6)	3.00 ± 0.70	2.68 ± 0.89
	higher CFEs	126 (26.4)	3.13 ± 0.82	2.76 ± 0.87
		Men (n = 231)		
Restrictions	lower CFEs	222 (96.1)	2.85 ± 0.68	2.42 ± 0.84 *
	higher CFEs	9 (3.9)	2.71 ± 0.47	3.16 ± 1.13 *
Healthy Eating Guidance	lower CFEs	96 (41.6)	2.82 ± 0.66	2.50 ± 0.86
	higher CFEs	135 (58.4)	2.86 ± 0.67	2.41 ± 0.86
Pressure and Food Reward	lower CFEs	169 (73.2)	2.77 ± 0.66 **	2.48 ± 0.85
	higher CFEs	62 (26.8)	3.05 ± 0.65 **	2.37 ± 0.88
Monitoring	lower CFEs	162 (70.1)	2.79 ± 0.66	2.43 ± 0.85
	higher CFEs	69 (29.9)	2.97 ± 0.69	2.50 ± 0.87
Child Control	lower CFEs	187 (81.0)	2.87 ± 0.68	2.45 ± 0.86
	higher CFEs	44 (19.0)	2.73 ± 0.61	2.43 ± 0.88

n, number of participants; [a] mean score for the subscale below or equal to 3.00, [b] mean score for the subscale above 3.00; SD, standard deviation; significant at * $p < 0.05$, ** $p < 0.01$, *** $p < 0.001$; Mann–Whitney U Test.

4. Discussion

The reported differences in the scores for certain eating styles (ESs), i.e., intuitive (IE), restrained (ResEat) and external (ExtEat) eating, in regard to the declared childhood food experiences (CFEs) have confirmed the link between parental feeding practices (PFPs) and dietary behaviors in adulthood. Nevertheless, some results underlined the complexity of this relationship, for example individual IE components were differently associated with CFEs. Moreover, different CFEs explained ResEat and ExtEat in adulthood.

The study results indicate that restrictions in childhood can be linked to lower IE in adulthood. Restrictions, specifically for weight control, may therefore contribute to relying on internal signals less often, eating for reasons unrelated to physical hunger and not allowing oneself to eat whatever is desired [30]. This particular PFP was the least reported one in the study sample; however, it was more common in women. The CFEs of restrictions in women seem to differently modify their ability of IE in comparison to men. Previous research suggests that maternal ESs may differently predict child's ESs, especially in regard to restrained eating [28]. Maternal ResEat may predict daughters' ResEat only [28]. This can be one of the factors explaining different results in women and men in the current study. The sociocultural models that indicate that dietary restrictions are more specific for girls and women in comparison to boys and men [31] seem to explain our findings. We also observed that the results for certain IE components did not differ between men with lower and higher experiences of restrictions in childhood. Moreover, a higher tendency for making food choices that promote better body functioning was observed only in men who have experienced restrictions during childhood. Nevertheless, the role of the childhood restrictions in determining dietary behaviors in men should be further investigated [11,26].

The experiences of parental guidance on healthy eating in childhood favored greater compliance with IE in the total sample as well as in women and men separately, except for giving oneself permission to eat desired foods. Therefore PFPs such as encouraging children in a supportive way to try new foods and eat diversely, modelling healthy eating, involving children in meal planning and preparations seem to favor eating in response to internal cues and possibly promote more healthful diets [2,32,33]. As parental influence is the first factor that may affect a child's eating, the abovementioned practices can promote the inborn ability of IE and prevent the child from eating disturbances later in life [3,34].

The experiences of being pressured to eat or being rewarded with food were linked to more common use of food to deal with unpleasant emotions in the total sample and in both women and men. Such experiences may consequently lead to emotional eating and overeating [28]. This result is contrary to the previous ones that suggested different brain responses to rewarding in women and men [35] and among boys and girls [29,36,37]. It may in turn differently determine diet quality in female and male adults [4]. Perhaps the difference between women's and men's brain processing might be more significant in terms of determining ESs in childhood [29,36,37] rather than in adulthood.

Being monitored by parents in terms of types of foods eaten during childhood favored choosing foods that promote better body functioning in adulthood, in the total sample and in women. Parental control, i.e., being responsive to child's needs and wants, was linked to eating only for physical reasons in men. Previous research has shown that the role of both of these PFPs in determining dietary behaviors in adulthood remains unclear and possibly less significant in comparison to other parenting practices [2,4]. The differences between women and men might result from varying maternal and paternal influences or from different impacts of other caregivers [27,28]; however, it was not measured in this study. Paying attention to the type of foods eaten by the child and being responsive to the child's needs may support healthful long-term outcomes [2,3].

Studies previously conducted on IE have shown several differences between women and men, similarly as this study. The total Intuitive Eating Scale-2 score and subscales for women were significantly lower, except for the one related to the ability of relying on internal signals [38,39]. Women may be more attentive to body signals than men [40]. However, the focus on appearance, weight control behaviors and disordered eating are observed among males as well [41]. A recent meta-analysis found that across a variety of age groups and cultures IE is higher in men in comparison to women [42,43]. This may be the result of an increased societal pressure that women face in terms of body dissatisfaction and internalization of a thin ideal [44]. Evidence suggests that men might also face pressure to conform to ideals [45], yet the one women face is more frequent and severe [44]. Another explanation for the differences in IE scores between men and women may relate to the relationship between personality and IE scores. For example, men with greater global self-esteem (GSE), thus also with narcissistic features, are less likely to give themselves permission to eat what is desired [46]. On the other hand, in women, greater GSE might promote IE [46]. The lower IE in women may also stem from the link between parental warmth and overprotection, which might cause greater parental concern, and in turn decrease eating in response to internal signals [26]. The assumption that different dietary experiences may correlate differently with IE scores in women and men was confirmed in the study group.

Contrary to the intergender differences related to the IE, having experienced restrictions in childhood predicted a greater ResEat score in both female and male adults as well as in the total sample. This association may result from the direct transmission of the behaviors learned during childhood or from the disturbances in the IE later in life [34]. Our observations suggest the complexity of ResEat [47] and the existence of different underlying mechanisms, such as non-food related adverse childhood experiences. For example, childhood abuse or neglect were found to predispose increased concerns about body shape and weight, unhealthy weight control behaviors, overeating or anxiety about food or eating [48,49]. The experience of financial deprivation in childhood was found to predict less favorable food choices in adulthood [50]. On the other hand, in the total sample, parental guidance on healthy eating predisposed to lower level of ResEat in adulthood. It may be concluded that this PFP may favor healthier eating behaviors, yet not in a form of strict, rigid food rules, but rather as a conscious choice, which is in line with the IE principles [19,30].

The practices such as pressuring to eat or food rewarding predisposed to greater ExtEat; however, differences between women and men were observed. Moreover, parental monitoring in terms of types of foods eaten favored greater ExtEat in the total sample, while solely in women parental guidance on healthy eating was linked to a lower ExtEat. Available studies on ExtEat are inconsistent and the role of ExtEat in promoting weight gain has been questioned [17,51–53]. Perhaps selected CFEs may mediate or moderate the relationship between ESs and dietary behaviors, thus further research should focus on explaining those results.

The experiences of restrictions and parental control had no effect on ExtEat while pressuring and food rewarding, parental monitoring and parental control had no effect on ResEat. Thus, the hypotheses related to ResEat and ExtEat were only partially confirmed. On the other hand, hypotheses related to the IE were confirmed. It might be that CFEs are more useful for determining selected adaptive ESs (e.g., IE) rather than the nonadaptive ones (e.g., ResEat, ExtEat). Our findings confirmed a need to conduct more research that would examine the association between CFEs and adaptive ESs [26], also in a representative study sample. Additionally, CFEs seem to differentiate IE among women and men more than they differentiate ExtEat or ResEat, which supports our second hypothesis. The future studies on the link between CFEs and IE or other adaptive ESs, e.g., mindful eating, should include separate analysis of such associations in women and men to confirm these results. Moreover, although some significant results have been noted, differences in ESs between the groups with lower and higher CFEs were quite small. Thus, further research should be carried out to verify these observations. In addition, PFPs may be linked to parenting styles and other non-food related practices that may affect eating behaviors [54]. There is also a need for including those aspects in the longitudinal research for a better understanding of the development of adaptive and maladaptive eating behaviors [54].

The current study contributes to the growing body of literature on the development of eating styles in adulthood. Understanding which factors may contribute to the prevalence of different eating styles in adulthood is crucial, because they can be linked to both successful prevention of disordered eating behaviors and ensuring higher diet quality. The findings of this research indicate that the public health approaches should focus on seeking methods to improve CFEs, most notably by supporting the relationship between parents and children through nutrition education. The latter have the potential to reduce the development of various health-risk behaviors. Furthermore, investing in parenting interventions that target healthful family mealtime has the potential for a long-term impact on their own children's parenting practices [55].

Study Strengths and Limitations

This study is the first to assess the relationships between diverse childhood food experiences and selected eating styles in adulthood in the Polish adults. A relatively large study sample can be pointed out as another study strength. Nevertheless, the study also has a few limitations. Firstly, a cross-sectional character of the study does not allow us to draw any causal associations. Moreover, a non-representative study sample prohibits the generalization of the study results. The possible diverse impact of both parents, thus different use of PFPs and the impact of other caregivers, have not been included in this study. Additionally, only selected eating styles were chosen for this research. Lastly, the childhood food experiences were based on the retrospective reports, which might have been imprecise. Nevertheless, despite the fact that relying on the long-term memories may be subjected to bias, findings from the retrospective studies are worth considering. Even if the participants' food memories are imprecise, the experiences from the past are meaningful and might underlie current beliefs, values or daily activities. Food- or eating-related memories can provide substantial information about people's life and sociocultural environment [56,57], thus they can be used to explain behavior.

5. Conclusions

Findings from the current study suggest that childhood food experiences related to diverse parental feeding practices can differently determine selected eating styles, i.e., intuitive, external and restrained eating, in adulthood. Having experienced "Restrictions" in childhood favored lower intuitive eating ("Reliance on Hunger and Satiety Cues", "Eating for Physical Rather Than Emotional Reasons", "Unconditional Permission to Eat") and higher restrained eating in adulthood. "Healthy Eating Guidance" predisposed to greater intuitive eating ("Eating for Physical Rather Than Emotional Reasons", "Reliance on Hunger and Satiety Cues", "Body-Food Choice Congruence") and lower restrained eating in adulthood. "Pressure and Food Reward" correlated negatively with "Eating for Physical Rather Than Emotional Reasons" (intuitive eating) and positively with external eating. The experience of parental monitoring was linked to greater "Body-Food Choice Congruence" (intuitive eating) and external eating. "Restrictions", "Healthy Eating Guidance", "Monitoring" and "Child Control" were differently linked to intuitive eating components and external eating in women and men. The abovementioned findings suggest that parents' education programs should focus on long-term consequences of feeding practices as well as the existence of the intergender differences among women and men, especially in regard to intuitive eating. Further retrospective studies in the representative samples are needed to confirm these findings. There is also a need for conducting longitudinal studies that would focus on the mechanism linking childhood food experiences and eating behaviors in adulthood.

Author Contributions: Conceptualization, A.M. and M.J.-Z.; methodology, A.M. and M.J.-Z.; formal analysis, A.M. and M.J.-Z.; data curation, A.M. and M.J.-Z.; writing—original draft preparation, A.M.; writing—review and editing, A.M. and M.J.-Z.; visualization, A.M.; supervision, M.J.-Z.; project administration, M.J.-Z. All authors have read and agreed to the published version of the manuscript.

Funding: This research received no external funding.

Institutional Review Board Statement: The study was conducted according to the guidelines of the Declaration of Helsinki and approved by the Ethics Committee of the Institute of Human Nutrition Sciences, Warsaw University of Life Sciences, in Poland (Resolution No. 02/2020).

Informed Consent Statement: Informed consent was obtained from all subjects involved in the study.

Data Availability Statement: The data presented in this study are available on request from the corresponding author.

Conflicts of Interest: The authors declare no conflict of interest.

References

1. Russell, C.G.; Haszard, J.J.; Taylor, R.W.; Heath, A.L.M.; Taylor, B.; Campbell, K.J. Parental feeding practices associated with children's eating and weight: What are parents of toddlers and preschool children doing? *Appetite* **2018**, *128*, 120–128. [CrossRef] [PubMed]
2. Małachowska, A.; Jeżewska-Zychowicz, M. Does Examining the Childhood Food Experiences Help to Better Understand Food Choices in Adulthood? *Nutrients* **2021**, *13*, 983. [CrossRef]
3. Scaglioni, S.; De Cosmi, V.; Ciappolino, V.; Parazzini, F.; Brambilla, P.; Agostoni, C. Factors Influencing Children's Eating Behaviours. *Nutrients* **2018**, *10*, 706. [CrossRef] [PubMed]
4. Małachowska, A.; Gębski, J.; Jeżewska-Zychowicz, M. Childhood Food Experiences and Selected Eating Styles as Determinants of Diet Quality in Adulthood—A Cross-Sectional Study. *Nutrients* **2023**, *15*, 2256. [CrossRef]
5. Movassagh, E.Z.; Baxter-Jones, A.D.G.; Kontulainen, S.; Whiting, S.J.; Vatanparast, H. Tracking Dietary Patterns over 20 Years from Childhood through Adolescence into Young Adulthood: The Saskatchewan Pediatric Bone Mineral Accrual Study. *Nutrients* **2017**, *9*, 990. [CrossRef]

6. Leal, D.B.; de Assis, M.A.A.; Hinnig, P.D.F.; Schmitt, J.; Lobo, A.S.; Bellisle, F.; Di Pietro, P.F.; Kunradi Vieira, F.; De Moura Araujo, P.H.; De Andrade, D.F. Changes in Dietary Patterns from Childhood to Adolescence and Associated Body Adiposity Status. *Nutrients* **2017**, *9*, 1098. [CrossRef]
7. Luque, V.; Escribano, J.; Closa-Monasterolo, R.; Zaragoza-Jordana, M.; Ferré, N.; Grote, V.; Koletzko, B.; Totzauer, M.; Verduci, E.; ReDionigi, A.; et al. Unhealthy Dietary Patterns Established in Infancy Track to Mid-Childhood: The EU Childhood Obesity Project. *J. Nutr.* **2018**, *148*, 752–759. [CrossRef] [PubMed]
8. Puhl, R.M.; Schwartz, M.B. If you are good you can have a cookie: How memories of childhood food rules link to adult eating behaviors. *Eat. Behav.* **2003**, *4*, 283–293. [CrossRef]
9. Ellis, J.M.; Galloway, A.T.; Webb, R.M.; Martz, D.M.; Farrow, C.V. Recollections of pressure to eat during childhood, but not picky eating, predict young adult eating behavior. *Appetite* **2016**, *97*, 58–63. [CrossRef]
10. Tan, C.C.; Ruhl, H.; Chow, C.M.; Ellis, L. Retrospective reports of parental feeding practices and emotional eating in adulthood: The role of food preoccupation. *Appetite* **2016**, *105*, 410–415. [CrossRef]
11. Galloway, A.T.; Farrow, C.V.; Martz, D.M. Retrospective reports of child feeding practices, current eating behaviors, and BMI in college students. *Obesity* **2010**, *18*, 1330–1335. [CrossRef]
12. Williams, N.A.; Dev, D.A.; Hankey, M.; Blitch, K. Role of food preoccupation and current dieting in the associations of parental feeding practices to emotional eating in young adults: A moderated mediation study. *Appetite* **2017**, *111*, 195–202. [CrossRef] [PubMed]
13. Robert Batsell, W.; Brown, A.S.; Ansfield, M.E.; Paschall, G.Y. "You will eat all of that!": A retrospective analysis of forced consumption episodes. *Appetite* **2002**, *38*, 211–219. [CrossRef] [PubMed]
14. Brink, P.J.; Ferguson, K.; Sharma, A. Dieters Project. *J. Child Adolesc. Psychiatr. Nurs.* **1999**, *13*, 17–25. [CrossRef] [PubMed]
15. Branen, L.; Fletcher, J. Comparison of college students' current eating habits and recollections of their childhood food practices. *J. Nutr. Educ. Behav.* **1999**, *31*, 304–310. [CrossRef]
16. Van Tine, M.L.; McNicholas, F.; Safer, D.L.; Agras, W.S. Follow-up of selective eaters from childhood to adulthood. *Eat. Behav.* **2017**, *26*, 61–65. [CrossRef]
17. Małachowska, A.; Jeżewska-Zychowicz, M.; Gębski, J. Polish Adaptation of the Dutch Eating Behaviour Questionnaire (DEBQ): The Role of Eating Style in Explaining Food Intake—A Cross-Sectional Study. *Nutrients* **2021**, *13*, 4486. [CrossRef]
18. Camilleri, G.M.; Méjean, C.; Bellisle, F.; Andreeva, V.A.; Kesse-Guyot, E.; Hercberg, S.; Péneau, S. Intuitive eating dimensions were differently associated with food intake in the general population-based nutrinet-santé study. *J. Nutr.* **2017**, *147*, 61–69. [CrossRef]
19. Małachowska, A.; Jeżewska-Zychowicz, M. Polish Adaptation and Validation of the Intuitive (IES-2) and Mindful (MES) Eating Scales—The Relationship of the Concepts with Healthy and Unhealthy Food Intake (a Cross-Sectional Study). *Nutrients* **2022**, *14*, 1109. [CrossRef]
20. Lluch, A.; Herbeth, B.; Méjean, L.; Siest, G. Dietary intakes, eating style and overweight in the Stanislas Family Study. *Int. J. Obes.* **2000**, *24*, 1493–1499. [CrossRef]
21. Tylka, T.L. Development and psychometric evaluation of a measure of intuitive eating. *J. Couns. Psychol.* **2006**, *53*, 226–240. [CrossRef]
22. Román, N.; Rigó, A.; Gajdos, P.; Tóth-Király, I.; Urbán, R. Intuitive eating in light of other eating styles and motives: Experiences with construct validity and the Hungarian adaptation of the Intuitive Eating Scale-2. *Body Image* **2021**, *39*, 30–39. [CrossRef]
23. Larson, N.I.; Neumark-Sztainer, D.; Hannan, P.J.; Story, M. Family meals during adolescence are associated with higher diet quality and healthful meal patterns during young adulthood. *J. Am. Diet. Assoc.* **2007**, *107*, 1502–1510. [CrossRef]
24. De Backer, C.J.S. Family meal traditions. Comparing reported childhood food habits to current food habits among university students. *Appetite* **2013**, *69*, 64–70. [CrossRef] [PubMed]
25. Wattick, R.A.; Olfert, M.D.; Claydon, E.; Hagedorn-Hatfield, R.L.; Barr, M.L.; Brode, C. Early life influences on the development of food addiction in college attending young adults. *Eat. Weight. Disord. Stud. Anorex. Bulim. Obes.* **2023**, *28*, 14. [CrossRef]
26. Liu, Y.; Cui, T.; Barnhart, W.R.; Wang, Q.; Yu, Y.; He, J. Associations among retrospective parenting styles, retrospective food parenting, and current eating behaviors in Chinese adults. *Appetite* **2023**, *184*, 106512. [CrossRef]
27. Philippe, K.; Chabanet, C.; Issanchou, S.; Monnery-Patris, S. Are food parenting practices gendered? Impact of mothers' and fathers' practices on their child's eating behaviors. *Appetite* **2021**, *166*, 105433. [CrossRef]
28. Zarychta, K.; Kulis, E.; Gan, Y.; Chan, C.K.Y.; Horodyska, K.; Luszczynska, A. Why are you eating, mom? Maternal emotional, restrained, and external eating explaining children's eating styles. *Appetite* **2019**, *141*, 104335. [CrossRef] [PubMed]
29. Loth, K.A.; Maclehose, R.F.; Fulkerson, J.A.; Crow, S.; Neumark-Sztainer, D. Are food restriction and pressure-to-eat parenting practices associated with adolescent disordered eating behaviors? *Int. J. Eat. Disord.* **2014**, *47*, 310. [CrossRef] [PubMed]
30. Tylka, T.L.; Kroon Van Diest, A.M. The Intuitive Eating Scale-2: Item refinement and psychometric evaluation with college women and men. *J. Couns. Psychol.* **2013**, *60*, 137–153. [CrossRef]
31. Weissman, R.S. The Role of Sociocultural Factors in the Etiology of Eating Disorders. *Psychiatr. Clin.* **2019**, *42*, 121–144. [CrossRef] [PubMed]
32. Peters, J.; Dollman, J.; Petkov, J.; Parletta, N. Associations between parenting styles and nutrition knowledge and 2–5-year-old children's fruit, vegetable and non-core food consumption. *Public Health Nutr.* **2013**, *16*, 1979–1987. [CrossRef]

33. Lopez, N.V.; Schembre, S.; Belcher, B.R.; O'Connor, S.; Maher, J.P.; Arbel, R.; Margolin, G.; Dunton, G.F. Parenting styles, food-related parenting practices, and children's healthy eating: A mediation analysis to examine relationships between parenting and child diet. *Appetite* **2018**, *128*, 205–213. [CrossRef] [PubMed]
34. Denny, K.N.; Loth, K.; Eisenberg, M.E.; Neumark-Sztainer, D. Intuitive eating in young adults. Who is doing it, and how is it related to disordered eating behaviors? *Appetite* **2013**, *60*, 13–19. [CrossRef] [PubMed]
35. Del Parigi, A.; Chen, K.; Gautier, J.F.; Salbe, A.D.; Pratley, R.E.; Ravussin, E.; Reiman, E.M.; Antonio Tataranni, P. Sex differences in the human brain's response to hunger and satiation. *Am. J. Clin. Nutr.* **2002**, *75*, 1017–1022. [CrossRef] [PubMed]
36. Harris, H.; Mallan, K.M.; Nambiar, S.; Daniels, L.A. The relationship between controlling feeding practices and boys' and girls' eating in the absence of hunger. *Eat. Behav.* **2014**, *15*, 519–522. [CrossRef] [PubMed]
37. Van Strien, T.; Bazelier, F.G. Perceived parental control of food intake is related to external, restrained and emotional eating in 7–12-year-old boys and girls. *Appetite* **2007**, *49*, 618–625. [CrossRef] [PubMed]
38. Augustus-Horvath, C.L.; Tylka, T.L. The acceptance model of intuitive eating: A comparison of women in emerging adulthood, early adulthood, and middle adulthood. *J. Couns. Psychol.* **2011**, *58*, 110–125. [CrossRef] [PubMed]
39. Muhammad, R.; Ismail, W.N.D.R.A.W.; Firdus, S.; Abdul Hamid, S.B.; Mohd Asmawi, U.M.; Md Nor, N. Intuitive Eating Behaviour among Young Malay Adults in Malaysian Higher Learning Institutions. *Nutrients* **2023**, *15*, 869. [CrossRef]
40. Gan, W.Y.; Yeoh, W.C. Associations between body weight status, psychological well-being and disordered eating with intuitive eating among Malaysian undergraduate university students. *Int. J. Adolesc. Med. Health* **2017**, *32*, 20170095. [CrossRef]
41. Christoph, M.; Järvelä-Reijonen, E.; Hooper, L.; Larson, N.; Mason, S.M.; Neumark-Sztainer, D. Longitudinal associations between intuitive eating and weight-related behaviors in a population-based sample of young adults. *Appetite* **2021**, *160*, 105093. [CrossRef]
42. Linardon, J.; Tylka, T.L.; Fuller-Tyszkiewicz, M. Intuitive eating and its psychological correlates: A meta-analysis. *Int. J. Eat. Disord.* **2021**, *54*, 1073–1098. [CrossRef]
43. Argyrides, M.; Anastasiades, E. Intuitive eating in Greek-Cypriot adults: Influence of gender and body mass. *Front. Psychol.* **2022**, *13*, 1033720. [CrossRef]
44. Grogan, S. *Body Image: Understanding Body Dissatisfaction in Men, Women and Children*, 4th ed.; Routledge: London, UK, 2021; ISBN 9781000475432.
45. Frederick, D.A.; Tylka, T.L.; Rodgers, R.F.; Convertino, L.; Pennesi, J.L.; Parent, M.C.; Brown, T.A.; Compte, E.J.; Cook-Cottone, C.P.; Crerand, C.E.; et al. Pathways from sociocultural and objectification constructs to body satisfaction among men: The U.S. Body Project I. *Body Image* **2022**, *41*, 84–96. [CrossRef]
46. Kozłowska, M.; Izydorczyk, B. Global Self-Esteem and Body Esteem as Predictors of Intuitive Eating among Young Adult Men and Women. 2022. Available online: https://ruj.uj.edu.pl/xmlui/handle/item/300893 (accessed on 3 April 2023). [CrossRef]
47. Polivy, J.; Herman, C.P.; Mills, J.S. What is restrained eating and how do we identify it? *Appetite* **2020**, *155*, 104820. [CrossRef] [PubMed]
48. Russell, S.J.; Hughes, K.; Bellis, M.A. Impact of childhood experience and adult well-being on eating preferences and behaviours. *BMJ Open* **2016**, *6*, e007770. [CrossRef]
49. Yoon, C.Y.; Mason, S.M.; Loth, K.; Jacobs, D.R. Adverse childhood experiences and disordered eating among middle-aged adults: Findings from the coronary artery risk development in young adults study. *Prev. Med.* **2022**, *162*, 107124. [CrossRef] [PubMed]
50. Mesler, R.M.; Simpson, B.; Bates, Z.L.; Hinrichs, Y. Unhealthy food choices in adulthood: The role of childhood financial adversity, situational scarcity, and self-control. *Food Qual. Prefer.* **2022**, *100*, 104433. [CrossRef]
51. Magklis, E.; Howe, L.D.; Johnson, L. Eating Style and the Frequency, Size and Timing of Eating Occasions: A cross-sectional analysis using 7-day weighed dietary records. *Sci. Rep.* **2019**, *9*, 15133. [CrossRef] [PubMed]
52. Van Strien, T.; Peter Herman, C.; Verheijden, M.W. Eating style, overeating and weight gain. A prospective 2-year follow-up study in a representative Dutch sample. *Appetite* **2012**, *59*, 782–789. [CrossRef] [PubMed]
53. Van Strien, T.; Herman, C.P.; Verheijden, M.W. Eating style, overeating, and overweight in a representative Dutch sample. Does external eating play a role? *Appetite* **2009**, *52*, 380–387. [CrossRef] [PubMed]
54. Shloim, N.; Edelson, L.R.; Martin, N.; Hetherington, M.M. Parenting styles, feeding styles, feeding practices, and weight status in 4–12 year-old children: A systematic review of the literature. *Front. Psychol.* **2015**, *6*, 1849. [CrossRef] [PubMed]
55. Watts, A.; Berge, J.M.; Loth, K.; Larson, N.; Neumark-Sztainer, D. The transmission of family food and mealtime practices fromadolescence to adulthood: Longitudinal findings from ProjectEAT-IV. *J. Nutr. Educ. Behav.* **2018**, *50*, 141. [CrossRef]
56. Holtzman, J.D. Food and Memory. *Annu. Rev. Anthropol.* **2006**, *35*, 361–378. [CrossRef]
57. Neuman, N.; Eli, K.; Nowicka, P. Childhood memories of food and eating in lower-income families in the United States: A qualitative study. *BMC Public Health* **2021**, *21*, 586. [CrossRef] [PubMed]

nutrients

MDPI

Article

Eating Behavior and Factors of Metabolic Health in Primary Schoolchildren: A Cross-Sectional Study in Greek Children

Aristea Gioxari [1], Charalampia Amerikanou [2], Sevasti Peraki [1], Andriana C. Kaliora [2,*] and Maria Skouroliakou [2]

[1] Department of Nutritional Science and Dietetics, School of Health Science, University of the Peloponnese, Antikalamos, 24100 Kalamata-Messinia, Greece; a.gioxari@uop.gr (A.G.); nds19117@go.uop.gr (S.P.)

[2] Department of Dietetics and Nutritional Science, School of Health Science and Education, Harokopio University, 70 El. Venizelou Ave., 17671 Athens, Greece; amerikanou@windowslive.com (C.A.); mskour@hua.gr (M.S.)

* Correspondence: akaliora@hua.gr; Tel.: +30-210-95-49-226; Fax: +30-210-95-77-050

Abstract: Childhood obesity has been associated with altered blood lipids and bad eating habits. In this cross-sectional study, we assessed cardiorespiratory fitness and metabolic health markers in regard to weight status and dietary habits in schoolchildren. In 134 children (6–11 years), we conducted: (1) Anthropometry, namely z-score BMI (z-BMI), waist-to-height ratio (WHtR), and body composition analysis. (2) Measurements of handgrip strength (HGS), resting metabolic rate (RMR) and VO_2max. (3) Quantification of blood lipids and antioxidant vitamins A, E, C. (4) Eating breakfast assessment. About 35% of children were overweight/obese. The z-BMI positively correlated with WHtR ($r = 0.637$, $p < 0.001$), and adversely correlated with fat-free mass ($r = -0.728$, $p < 0.001$) and vitamin E ($r = -0.286$, $p < 0.001$). RMR and VO_2max were greater in normal weight children compared to those with overweight/obesity ($p < 0.001$). HGS did not differ between these groups, but was negatively correlated with dyslipidemia as shown by TG/HDL-C ratio ($r = -0.224$, $p = 0.037$). According to regression analysis, eating breakfast routinely at home was positively associated with RMR and adversely associated with z-BMI. Hence, regular breakfast consumption at home may improve RMR in kids. Cardiorespiratory fitness and physical strength are key modulators of metabolic health in Greek children added to a social determinant of health i.e., eating breakfast at home.

Keywords: primary school children; breakfast at home; metabolic health; cardiorespiratory fitness; handgrip strength; antioxidant status

1. Introduction

Childhood obesity has emerged as a global public health concern with its prevalence rising drastically both in developed and developing countries. According to the World Health Organization (WHO), more than 340 million children and adolescents aged 5–19 were overweight or obese in 2016 [1]. It is well confirmed that obesity in adults is highly associated with reduced antioxidant status, as indicated by inadequate circulating antioxidant vitamins i.e., carotenoids (vitamin A), tocopherols (vitamin E) and ascorbic acid (vitamin C) [2]. Recently, this redox state imbalance has been also observed in children and adolescents with overweight/obesity, accompanied by an altered blood lipid profile such as reduced levels of high-density lipoprotein-cholesterol (HDL-C) and high triglyceride (TG) concentration [3]. There is evidence that adiposity during childhood is characterized by subclinical inflammation with elevated secretion of proinflammatory adipokines contributing to increased oxidative stress [4,5]. In turn, systemic inflammation and oxidative stress during childhood are associated with the development of obesity-related metabolic complications such as cardiovascular diseases (CVD) in adult life [5,6]. According to a recent case-control study in 1444 children, metabolically unhealthy participants demonstrated lower ratios of vitamin A/TG and vitamin E/TG in plasma compared to their metabolically healthy counterparts, indicating the pivotal role of these antioxidant vitamins in metabolic health [7].

Low cardiorespiratory fitness (CRF) is directly linked to excess adiposity and is a major risk factor for cardiovascular disease in adults [8]. CRF is assessed by measuring maximal oxygen consumption (VO_2max), which is the maximum capacity of the body to transport and use oxygen during physical activity [8]. Improvement in CRF of adults has been associated with ameliorated body composition i.e., visceral fat and total fat mass, and lower waist and hip circumferences [8–10], but for children, data are limited. Very recently, it has been suggested that CRF is a potent indicator of cardiovascular health in children and adolescents as well [11]. Based on epidemiological data, only 40% of 12–15-year-olds in the US have a healthy CRF [12]. What is more, CRF has been currently associated with handgrip strength (HGS), which in turn affects all-cause mortality and CVD risk in young and older adults [13,14]. There is now evidence that low HGS may be associated with poor cardiometabolic outcomes in children and adolescents too [15]. In a recent observational study in 2256 children and adolescents aged 5–18 years, HGS-to-body mass index (BMI) presented a positive correlation with cardiorespiratory fitness [16].

Eating habits may influence metabolic health. A higher meal frequency seems to be predictive for a lower weight status in children, as indicated by z-scores of body mass index (z-BMI) for age and waist circumference to height ratio (WHtR) [17]. In addition, skipping breakfast has been associated with a 43% higher risk of developing obesity [18,19]. It is not doubtful that eating habits are formed during childhood and are crucial for a child's development [20], while the home food environment plays a fundamental role in attaining a healthy body weight [21].

Nevertheless, data regarding the role of CRF and HGS in overweight/obesity and how these factors correlate to adiposity, antioxidant status, blood lipid profile and eating habits in children in Greece are limited. Therefore, in the present cross-sectional study we aimed to investigate differences between normal weight children and children with overweight/obesity, regarding fitness indicators (CRF, HGS), biochemical markers (antioxidant vitamins, lipid profile), and dietary habits such as breakfast consumption at home or snacking at school.

2. Methods and Materials

2.1. Ethics Approval

The research protocol was submitted to the Scientific and Ethical Committee of "IASO Maternity Hospital, Obstetrics—Gynecology (Attica, Greece)" and was authorized with an approval code #J-31052019. Throughout the study, the principles of Helsinki Declaration 1964 were adhered, and the General Data protection Regulation (EU) 2016/679 was assured. To this end, a written informed consent was delivered to all parents (or legal guardians) of recruited children, and a copy of the signed consent was handed to each parent.

2.2. Study Design

The present work is a cross-sectional study, in which community children from Attica (Greece) were enrolled during June and July 2019. Parents or legal guardians were invited to take part in the study through written announcements (posters), electronic invitations and social media posts by the collaborating primary schools. Those who agreed to participate were provided with a detailed information leaflet describing the aims, methods, benefits, and potential hazards of the study.

Participants' inclusion criteria were set as follows:

(a) community children, aged 6 to 11 years, living in Attica (Greece);
(b) apparently healthy children without seasonal infection, chronic or life threatening diseases (as described below);
(c) parental consent.

Exclusion criteria were:

(a) children with infections (e.g., seasonal influenza), chronic diseases (e.g., celiac disease, inflammatory bowel diseases, kidney disease, malabsorption, parathyroid diseases), pediatric metabolism disorders (e.g., type 1 diabetes) or life threating diseases (e.g., cancer, congenital disorders);
(b) children with cognitive disorders (e.g., autism, attention-deficit/hyperactivity disorder);
(c) children under medication treatment that could affect the outcomes of the study;
(d) children following a vegetarian or a vegan diet;
(e) children receiving nutritional supplements including vitamins and minerals;
(f) parental refusal to consent.

2.3. *Clinical, Laboratory and Nutritional Data*

All measurements and data collection were conducted at IASO Maternity Hospital (Attica, Greece) under the supervision of the appointed physician and the collaborating researchers. Parents (or guardians) visited along with their child hospital's facilities in three separate days within two weeks for: (1) medical history record, anthropometric measurements and blood analysis; (2) CRF and HGS assessments; and (3) eating behavior evaluation, respectively. Prior to visiting the clinical site, parents (or guardians) were instructed to ensure that their child was healthy, fully rested, joyful and well hydrated. Throughout each test parents (or guardians) were present, while children were advised to express themselves if they would feel discomfort during measurements. All children were verbally encouraged by the researchers to do their best during the tests providing positive feedback.

2.3.1. Day 1: Anthropometry and Blood Analysis

Medical history: The appointed pediatrician recorded children's medical history from parents (or guardians) including general information, as well as disease specific data (i.e., allergies, medical condition, drug treatment, nutrient supplementation).

Anthropometry: Experienced dieticians performed measurements of body weight (BW), height (Ht), waist circumference (WC), as well as body composition and resting metabolic rate (RMR).

More specifically, Ht was measured on a standard stadiometer without shoes to the nearest millimeter (Seca Mode 220, Hamburg, Germany), and BW on a flat scale with light clothing to the nearest 0.1 kg. BMI was calculated as the ratio of BW (kg) to the square of Ht (m^2). To assess growth and weight status, z-scores of Ht-for-age, BW-for-age and BMI-for-age were calculated according to WHO growth reference data for boys and girls aged 5 to 19 years [22]. WC was measured with a non-stretch but flexible tape on minimal clothing. For defining abdominal adiposity, the WHtR was used with a cut-off $\geq$0.50 [23].

Body composition i.e., fat mass (FM), fat-free mass (FFM) and total body water (TBW), was analyzed with air displacement plethysmography (Bodpod® Body Composition Tracking Systems, Life Measurement, Inc., Rome, Italy) following the manufacturer's instructions. Measurement was performed on minimal clothing. Preparation for the Bodpod test included overnight fasting and abstaining from rigorous activities at the day before the examination [24]. Body composition indicators, FM, FFM and TBW were expressed as kg or % BW.

An open-circuit indirect calorimetry of computerized metabolic system with ventilated canopy (Quark RMR, Cosmed, Rome, Italy) was applied to measure RMR (kcal/day) based on measurements of gas exchange, namely oxygen consumption (VO_2) and carbon dioxide production (CO_2) [25]. The oxygen sensor was calibrated before each measurement with the use of mixed reference gases of known composition. Measurements were conducted after overnight fasting and prior to the measurement children were asked to rest in the recumbent position for 10 min in a thermoneutral environment. Then, the canopy was placed over their head, and they were asked to breathe normally for 25 min avoiding hyperventilation or falling asleep during the test. RMR output was also expressed in relation to BW, namely, kcal/kg of BW/day.

Blood analysis: Blood withdrawal (8 mL) from each child was performed after overnight fasting. To isolate serum, whole blood was allowed to clot at room temperature for 20 min followed by centrifugation at 3000 rpm for 10 min (4 °C). For plasma isolation, whole blood was collected in ethylenediaminetetraacetic acid (EDTA)-filled tubes prior to centrifugation.

Total cholesterol (TC), low-density lipoprotein-cholesterol (LDL-C), HDL-C and TG were quantified in sera with an automatic biochemical analyzer using manufacturer's reagents (Cobas 8000 modular analyzer, Roche Diagnostics GmbH, Mannheim, Germany). A reversed-phase high performance liquid chromatography (HPLC) system (model 1050, Agilent Technologies, Waldbronn, Germany) coupled with ultraviolet (UV) and fluorescence (FL) detectors, quaternary pump, auto-sampler and data analysis software, was used to quantify antioxidant vitamins A (retinol), E (alpha-tocopherol) and C (ascorbic acid) in plasma samples, according to previously published methods [26,27]. All blood analyses were performed in freshly drawn blood samples.

2.3.2. Day 2: CRF and HGS

CRF: The appointed pediatrician was responsible for conducting the maximal oxygen consumption (VO_2max) examination test. Measurement of VO_2max was performed on a treadmill (Woodway ELG 55, Waukesha, Germany) according to a modified Balke protocol for children [28]. Initially, children were asked to warm up on the treadmill at a self-selected speed for 10 min. Next, children performed an exercise test to fatigue at a constant speed of 5.0 mph consisting of 2 min stages of progressively increasing the incline of the treadmill by 2.5%. VO_2max was determined as the highest oxygen consumption attained during the test, upon fulfillment of three out of four criteria: (a) VO_2 reached a plateau; (b) respiratory exchange ratio (RER) was greater than 1.2; (c) rating of perceived exertion (RPE) was greater than 17; heart rate (HR) approached the maximum age-predicted heart rate ($\pm$10 beats/min) [29]. Output of VO_2max was expressed as mL O_2 per kg of BW per min (mL O_2/kg/min).

HGS: The appointed dieticians conducted two HGS measurements of the dominant hand, each on a separate day. The average of both measurements was calculated and HGS output was expressed as kg. To this scope, the Jamar Plus+ Digital Hand Dynamometer (Patterson Medical, Warrenville, IL, USA) was used. Before HGS test, children were asked to familiarize themselves with the dynamometer by grasping the handle, adjusting grip to the handle and performing 2–3 tests. Then, measurements were preformed according to the standard procedures recommended by the American Society of Hand Therapists (ASHT) [30]. More specifically, children were asked to sit upright on a chair with their feet supported on the ground and to place their tested hand on the table in front, maintaining the arm position during the test. Shoulders had to be slightly abducted and neutrally rotated, the elbow in 90° of flexion, the forearm in 0° between pronation and supination, and the wrist in neutral resting position [31,32]. Children were then asked to squeeze the grip continuously for 3 sec. Children were not aware of the HGS test outcome as the display of the dynamometer always faced the researcher. The second HGS measurement was performed on the third visit, before nutritional data collection.

2.3.3. Day 3: Nutritional Behavior Assessment

Children's behavior regarding breakfast and snacking at school during the last month was assessed by applying the KIDMED questionnaire via face-to-face interviews with the parents (or guardians) and children [33]. Questions denoting a negative connotation with respect to the Mediterranean diet were assigned a value of −1 and those with a positive aspect +1 [33].

All children invited to participate were attending public schools that have food canteens. Children who positively responded of eating breakfast daily (or most of the days) were further asked if they consumed breakfast at home or not. Children who consumed breakfast on a regular basis but apart from home were also recorded.

3. Statistical Analysis

Statistical analysis was performed using the SPSS software for Windows (Version 26, Armork, NY, USA, IBM Corporation). Significance level was set at p-value ≤ 0.05. The Kolmogorov–Smirnov test was used to assess normality of variable distribution. Dichotomous variables were presented as counts (N) or relative frequencies (N %) and quantitative variables as mean and standard deviation of the mean (SD).

Children were categorized according to z-BMI, as underweight (z-BMI < −2), normal weight (z-BMI −2 to 0.99) or overweight/obese (z-BMI ≥ 1) [34]. Only two children were scored as underweight, and were excluded from further statistical analysis. The independent-samples t-test was conducted to compare variable means between the normal weight and the overweight/obesity group. To compare eating behavior frequencies between groups, the chi-square test was used.

Children were also categorized according to the frequency of having breakfast. All children who reported eating breakfast daily (or most of the days) consumed this meal exclusively at home. Conversely, those reporting not having breakfast at home, all skipped this meal in the morning. Therefore, two categories of breakfast frequency were used: "daily/most of the days" or "sometimes/no". The independent-samples t-test was performed for the comparison of means between the two groups.

Pearson's correlation was used to examine the relations between quantitative variables of the population. The stronger the association of the two variables, the closer the Pearson correlation coefficient, r, was to either +1 or −1, depending on whether the relationship was positive or negative, respectively.

Linear regression models, unadjusted and adjusted for confounders (adjusted model 1: age, sex; adjusted model 2: age, sex, WC) were then performed to quantify associations showing significant correlations. The z-BMI, VO_2max, HGS and RMR were used as the dependent variables. Parameters of metabolic health and eating behavior were used as predictor variables. Regression beta coefficients, b, were assessed explaining the degree of change in the outcome variable for every 1-unit of change (increase or decrease depending on whether the relationship is positive or negative) in the predictor variable.

4. Results

4.1. Children's General Characteristics

As shown in Figure 1, a total of 175 children were assessed to participate in the study. When study criteria were applied, 20 children were excluded due to seasonal influenza and 4 children due to the presence of chronic diseases (3 with diabetes type 1 and one child with celiac disease). Additionally, 17 children withdrew from the study as their parents (or guardians) did not respond to our communication efforts or were willing to discontinue for personal reasons. Consequently, 134 children completed the study. All children were Greek, lived in urban area of Attica and belonged to a middle-class socio-economic status.

Descriptive characteristics regarding anthropometry, CRF, physical strength, biochemical markers and eating habits in the whole sample (n = 134) are shown in Table 1. The mean age of participants was 8.8 years and 57.5% were boys. Based on z-BMI, 81.7% of children had a normal weight, while 35.1% had overweight/obesity. Only two children (1.9%) belonged to the category of underweight (z-BMI < −2). Using the WHtR ≥ 0.5 cut-off [23], abdominal adiposity was found in 36.2% of children with overweight/obesity and 2.4% in normal weight children. Most children consumed breakfast (75.4%) and snacked during school time (73.1%).

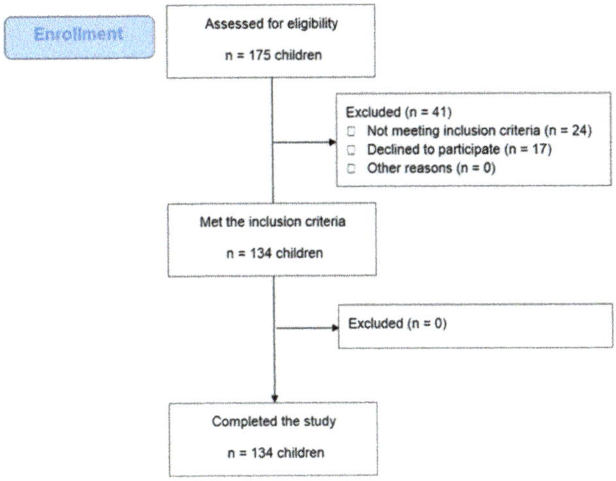

Figure 1. Study flow chart.

Table 1. Children characteristics in the whole sample and on different sexes.

Parameters	Enrolled (N = 134)	Boys (N = 77)	Girls (N = 57)	*p*-Value
Anthropometry				
Age (years); mean (SD)	8.8 (1.8)	8.8 (1.7)	8.9 (1.8)	0.709
Height (m); mean (SD)	1.4 (0.1)	1.4 (0.1)	1.4 (0.1)	0.577
Weight (kg); mean (SD)	33.6 (10.0)	34.4 (10.9)	32.6 (8.7)	0.326
BMI (kg/m^2); mean (SD)	17.8 (3.1)	18.1 (3.4)	17.5 (2.5)	0.301
Z-score weight; mean (SD)	0.9 (1.2)	1.0 (1.2)	0.6 (1.0)	**0.042**
Z-score height; mean (SD)	0.8 (1.1)	0.9 (1.1)	0.6 (1.0)	0.064
Z-score BMI; mean (SD)	0.6 (1.2)	0.7 (1.3)	0.4 (1.1)	0.156
Weight status based on z-score BMI; N (%)				
<−2, underweight	2 (1.9)	1 (1.3)	1 (1.8)	-
−2 to +0.99, normal weight	85 (81.7)	48 (62.3)	37 (64.9)	0.531
≥1, overweight/obese	47 (35.1)	28 (36.4)	19 (33.3)	0.393
WC (cm); mean (SD)	61.1 (8.7)	62.0 (9.5)	59.8 (7.4)	0.149
WHtR; mean (SD)	0.4 (0.6)	0.4 (0.7)	0.4 (0.0)	0.564
FM (%); mean (SD)	23.7 (9.5)	22.4 (10.4)	25.4 (7.9)	0.070
FM (kg); mean (SD)	8.6 (5.8)	8.5 (6.7)	8.8 (4.3)	0.777
FFM (%); mean (SD)	76.3 (9.6)	77.5 (10.6)	74.6 (7.9)	0.082
FFM (kg); mean (SD)	25.0 (5.7)	25.8 (5.5)	24.0 (5.8)	0.064
TBW (%); mean (SD)	63.7 (9.2)	64.6 (9.9)	62.4 (8.0)	0.169
Cardiorespiratory fitness and strength				
RMR (kcal/day); mean (SD)	1565.5 (278.9)	1628.0 (276.2)	1479.8 (261.4)	**0.003**
RMR (kcal/kg/day); mean (SD)	49.0 (10.0)	49.6 (9.8)	48.1 (10.3)	**0.414**

Table 1. *Cont.*

Parameters	Enrolled (N = 134)	Boys (N = 77)	Girls (N = 57)	*p*-Value
VO_2max (mL/kg/min); mean (SD)	49.9 (9.5)	52.5 (10.2)	47.0 (7.6)	**0.003**
HRmax (bpm); mean (SD)	202.9 (11.3)	201.9 (10.5)	204.2 (12.3)	0.297
HGS (kg); mean (SD)	15.2 (5.2)	16.3 (5.4)	13.2 (4.7)	**0.018**
Blood indices				
Vit A (mg/L); mean (SD)	0.3 (0.2)	0.3 (0.1)	0.3 (0.2)	0.852
Vit E (mg/L); mean (SD)	10.9 (2.6)	10.9 (2.8)	10.8 (2.4)	0.859
Vit C (mg/L); mean (SD)	5.6 (1.3)	5.6 (1.0)	5.6 (1.7)	0.826
Total cholesterol (mg/dL); mean (SD)	164.3 (26.8)	166.1 (25.1)	161.8 (29.1)	0.366
HDL-C (mg/dL); mean (SD)	53.2 (12.2)	53.5 (11.1)	52.7 (12.6)	0.729
LDL-C (mg/dL); mean (SD)	99.6 (23.6)	101.5 (22.4)	97.1 (26.2)	0.288
TG (mg/dL); mean (SD)	57.4 (19.1)	55.5 (16.5)	59.9 (22.0)	0.196
TG/HDL-C ratio; mean (SD)	1.2 (0.7)	1.1 (0.5)	1.3 (0.8)	0.268
Meals				
Daily breakfast (YES/NO); N (%)	101 (75.4)/23 (17.2)	58 (75.3)/13 (16.9)	43 (75.4)/10 (17.5)	0.937
Daily snacking at school (YES/NO); N (%)	98 (73.1)/22 (16.4)	52 (67.5)/15 (19.5)	46 (80.7)/7 (12.3)	0.197

Data are presented as counts (%) or means (standard deviation) (SD). For continuous values, the independent-samples *t*-test was conducted to compare means between sexes. For categorical variables, the chi-square test was used. Level of statistical significance was set at $p \leq 0.05$. Bold *p*-values represent statistically significant differences between groups. BMI, body mass index; WC, waist circumference; WHtR, waist to height ratio; FM, fat mass; FFM, fat-free mass; TBW, total body water; RMR, resting metabolic rate; HRmax, maximal heart rate; HGS, handgrip strength; HDL-C, high-density lipoprotein-cholesterol; LDL-C, low-density lipoprotein-cholesterol; TG, triglycerides.

Table 1 also presents mean levels for all tested variables between sexes. Concerning anthropometry, boys showed significantly higher z-scores of weight ($p = 0.042$) than girls. Additionally, boys demonstrated higher CRF and physical strength compared to girls, as indicated by VO_2max ($p = 0.003$) and HGS ($p = 0.018$) respectively. Biochemical markers and eating habits did not differ between sexes.

4.2. Differences of Tested Variables According to Body Weight Status

Table 2 presents mean differences for all tested variables between normal weight children and children with overweight/obesity. In regard to anthropometry, children with overweight/obesity demonstrated higher z-BW for age ($p < 0.001$), WC ($p < 0.001$), WHtR ($p < 0.001$) and FM % ($p < 0.001$) compared to their normal weight counterparts. On the contrary, FFM % ($p < 0.001$) and TBW % ($p < 0.001$) were significantly lower in children with overweight/obesity. Additionally, correlation analysis showed that z-BMI was strongly and positively correlated with WC (r = 0.722, $p < 0.001$), WHtR (r = 0.637, $p < 0.001$), FM % (r = 0.725, $p < 0.001$), while a strong and inverse correlation with FFM % (r = −0.728, $p < 0.001$) and TBW % (r = −0.623, $p < 0.001$) was detected. A negative correlation with plasma alpha-tocopherol was also recorded (r = −0.286, $p < 0.001$).

Mean value of RMR (kcal/kg/day) was lower in participants with overweight/obesity compared to those with normal weight ($p < 0.001$). At the same time RMR was positively correlated with FFM % (r = 0.650, $p <$ 001) and negatively correlated with FM % (r = −0.642, $p < 0.001$) and z-BMI (r = −0.575, $p < 0.001$).

Table 2. Differences in tested variables based on body weight status.

Parameters: Mean (SD)	Normal Weight (N = 85)	Overweight/Obese (N = 47)	p-Value
Anthropometry			
z-score BMI	−0.05 (0.7)	1.9 (0.8)	**<0.001**
z-score height	0.6 (1.0)	1.1 (1.1)	**0.002**
z-score weight	0.3 (0.8)	2.0 (0.9)	**<0.001**
Age (years)	8.8 (1.8)	8.8 (1.7)	0.897
Height (m)	1.3 (0.1)	1.4 (0.1)	0.076
Weight (kg)	29.9 (7.3)	40.7 (10.8)	**<0.001**
BMI (kg/m^2)	16.2 (1.5)	20.9 (2.8)	**<0.001**
WC (cm)	57.4 (5.8)	68.1 (8.9)	**<0.001**
WHtR	0.4 (0.1)	0.5 (0.05)	**<0.001**
FM (%)	18.9 (6.4)	32.4 (8.2)	**<0.001**
FM (kg)	5.6 (2.7)	13.7 (6.5)	**<0.001**
FFM (%)	81.1 (6.4)	67.5 (8.3)	**<0.001**
FFM (kg)	24.0 (5.6)	27.0 (5.5)	**0.004**
TBW (%)	67.5 (7.7)	56.4 (7.0)	**<0.001**
Cardiorespiratory fitness and strength			
RMR (kcal/kg/day)	52.9 (9.0)	42.3 (8.1)	**<0.001**
VO_2max (mL/kg/min)	52.4 (8.4)	46.1 (10.1)	**<0.001**
HRmax (bpm)	202.8 (11.7)	203.0 (10.7)	0.932
HGS (kg)	14.8 (4.8)	15.8 (5.9)	0.371
Blood indices			
Vit A (mg/L)	0.3 (0.1)	0.3 (0.2)	0.582
Vit E (mg/L)	10.9 (2.4)	10.5 (2.9)	0.435
Vit C (mg/L)	5.5 (1.1)	5.7 (1.7)	0.591
Total cholesterol (mg/dL)	165.0 (27.5)	163.3 (26.0)	0.736
HDL-C (mg/dL)	53.2 (11.9)	53.3 (12.8)	0.968
LDL-C (mg/dL)	100.2 (21.5)	98.6 (22.4)	0.719
TG (mg/dL)	57.9 (20.0)	56.9 (17.5)	0.764
TG/HDL C ratio	1.2 (0.7)	1.2 (0.6)	0.859
Meals			
Daily breakfast (YES/NO); N (%)	68 (80.0)/9 (10.6)	31 (66.0)/14 (29.8)	**0.009**
Daily snacking at school (YES/NO); N (%)	62 (72.9)/15 (17.6)	34 (72.3)/7 (14.9)	0.478

Data are presented as means (standard deviation) (SD) or counts (%). The independent-samples t-test was conducted to compare variable means between children of overweight/obesity and normal weight. To compare eating behavior frequencies between groups, the chi-square test was used. Level of statistical significance was set at $p \leq 0.05$. Bold p-values represent statistically significant differences between groups. BMI, body mass index; WC, waist circumference; WHtR, waist to height ratio; FM, fat mass; FFM, fat-free mass; TBW, total body water; RMR, resting metabolic rate; HRmax, maximal heart rate; HGS, handgrip strength; HDL-C, high-density lipoprotein-cholesterol; LDL-C, low-density lipoprotein-cholesterol; TG, triglycerides.

With respect to CRF, VO_2max was lower in children with overweight/obesity than those of normal weight ($p < 0.001$). VO_2max was positively correlated with FFM %

(r = 0.326, $p < 0.001$) and negatively correlated with FM % (r = −0.349, $p < 0.001$) and z-BMI (r = −0.195, $p = 0.029$).

HGS did not differ between the normal weight and the overweight/obesity group ($p = 0.371$), but was strongly and positively correlated with FFM (r = 0.869, $p < 0.001$) and RMR (r = 0.567, $p < 0.001$). HGS tended to correlate significantly with HDL-C (r = 0.207, $p = 0.055$) and showed a significantly negative correlation with TG/HDL-C ratio (r = −0.224, $p = 0.037$).

Blood lipid profile and antioxidant vitamin levels did not differ between groups. However, a negative correlation of z-BMI with plasma vitamin E was identified (r = −0.286, $p = 0.001$).

4.3. *Differences between Tested Variables According to Breakfast Eating Behavior*

As regards breakfast, this was consumed exclusively at home. Children who reported not having breakfast at home, all skipped this meal in the morning. According to Table 2, the proportion of children having breakfast regurarly was greater in normal weight children than that of the overweight/obesity group ($p = 0.009$). The proportion of children who snacked during school did not differ between normal weight and overweight/obesity groups.

Lower mean values of z-BMI, WC, WHtR and FM %, and higher FFM % were found in children who had breakfast daily or most of the days, than those who skipped this meal (Table 3). It is noteworthy that RMR was found to be greater in children having breakfast than those who did not ($p = 0.035$). Mean values of HGS and VO_2max did not differ between these two groups.

Table 3. Differences in tested variables based on eating behavior.

Parameters: Mean Values (SD)	Consuming Breakfast		p-Value
	Daily or Most of the Days (N = 101)	Sometimes/No (N = 23)	
z-score BMI	0.5 (1.3)	1.2 (1.2)	**0.012**
z-score height	0.8 (1.1)	0.6 (1.2)	0.393
z-score weight	0.8 (1.2)	1.2 (1.3)	0.175
Age (years)	8.6 (1.8)	9.4 (1.3)	**0.042**
Height (m)	1.3 (0.1)	1.4 (0.1)	0.165
Weight (kg)	32.3 (9.4)	37.9 (10.0)	**0.012**
BMI (kg/m^2)	17.4 (3.0)	19.5 (3.3)	**0.002**
WC (cm)	60.0 (8.3)	65.5 (9.6)	**0.006**
WHtR	0.4 (0.1)	0.5 (0.1)	**0.025**
FM (%)	23.1 (9.5)	27.7 (9.2)	**0.041**
FM (kg)	8.2 (5.5)	11.1 (6.5)	**0.029**
FFM (%)	76.9 (9.5)	72.4 (9.2)	**0.044**
FFM (kg)	24.2 (5.3)	26.8 (5.0)	**0.035**
TBW (%)	64.0 (9.4)	60.2 (7.9)	0.082
RMR (kcal/kg/day)	49.6 (9.9)	44.6 (7.3)	**0.035**
VO_2 max (mL/kg/min)	49.7 (10.1)	48.6 (6.3)	0.642
HRmax (bpm)	202.2 (12.0)	205.2 (8.5)	0.304
HGS (kg)	14.5 (5.0)	16.2 (3.8)	0.159

Table 3. *Cont.*

Parameters: Mean Values (SD)	Consuming Breakfast		
	Daily or Most of the Days (N = 101)	Sometimes/No (N = 23)	*p*-Value
Vit A (mg/L)	0.3 (0.2)	0.3 (0.1)	0.531
Vit E (mg/L)	10.9 (2.8)	10.7 (2.3)	0.769
Vit C (mg/L)	5.5 (1.4)	5.7 (1.1)	0.733
Total cholesterol (mg/dL)	163.8 (27.7)	163.0 (23.5)	0.895
HDL (mg/dL)	52.8 (12.1)	54.9 (11.8)	0.460
LDL (mg/dL)	99.5 (24.1)	96.9 (22.1)	0.629
TG (mg/dL)	57.2 (19.8)	56.1 (15.6)	0.814
TG/HDL-C ratio	1.2 (0.7)	1.1 (0.4)	0.524

Data are presented as counts (%) or means (standard deviation) (SD). Independent-samples *t*-test was conducted to compare variable means between groups. Level of statistical significance was set at $p \leq 0.05$. Bold *p*-values represent statistically significant differences between groups. BMI, body mass index; WC, waist circumference; WHtR, waist to height ratio; FM, fat mass; FFM, fat-free mass; TBW, total body water; RMR, resting metabolic rate; HRmax, maximal heart rate; HGS, handgrip strength; HDL-C, high-density lipoprotein-cholesterol; LDL-C, low-density lipoprotein-cholesterol; TG, triglycerides.

4.4. Linear Regression Analyis

Table 4 presents outcomes of linear regression models (unadjusted model, adjusted model 1, and adjusted model 2), regarding the associations of z-BMI, RMR, CRF and HGS with eating behavior and parameters of metabolic health. In agreement with correlation analysis, z-BMI was significantly associated with body composition (FM and FFM), even when controlling for age, sex, and WC. An inverse association with antioxidant plasma vitamin E (alpha-tocopherol) was also evident in both adjusted regression models. With regard to eating behavior, z-BMI was negatively associated with having breakfast regularly at home ($p = 0.016$), even when adjusted to age and sex ($p = 0.010$).

Table 4. Regression analysis addressing the associations between metabolic health factors and eating behavior.

Tested Associations	Unadjusted Model		Adjusted Model 1		Adjusted Model 2	
	Beta	*p*-Value	Beta	*p*-Value	Beta	*p*-Value
z-BMI						
FFM (kg)	0.414	**<0.001**	0.823	**<0.001**	0.258	**0.009**
FM (kg)	0.709	**<0.001**	0.845	**<0.001**	0.461	**<0.001**
Plasma vitamin E (mg/L)	−0.286	**0.001**	−0.293	**0.001**	−0.161	**0.004**
Eating breakfast regularly	−0.218	**0.016**	−0.237	**0.010**	−0.082	0.173
VO2max (mL/kg/min)						
FFM (kg)	0.135	0.143	0.122	0.367	0.092	0.560
FM (kg)	−0.258	**0.005**	−0.425	**<0.001**	−0.602	**<0.001**
HGS (kg)						
FFM (kg)	0.869	**<0.001**	0.658	**<0.001**	0.627	**<0.001**
FM (kg)	0.450	**<0.001**	0.248	**<0.001**	0.066	0.520
HDL-C (mg/dL)	0.207	0.055	0.118	0.094	0.063	0.343

Table 4. *Cont.*

Tested Associations	Unadjusted Model		Adjusted Model 1		Adjusted Model 2	
	Beta	*p*-Value	Beta	*p*-Value	Beta	*p*-Value
TG/HDL-C	−0.224	**0.037**	−0.103	0.142	−0.075	0.247
RMR (kcal/day)						
FFM (kg)	0.704	**<0.001**	0.638	**<0.001**	0.464	**<0.001**
FM (kg)	0.504	**<0.001**	0.335	**<0.001**	0.028	0.812
Eating breakfast regularly	0.212	**0.020**	0.213	**0.005**	0.196	**0.050**

Level of statistical significance was set at $p \leq 0.05$. Bold *p*-values represent statistically significant associations between variables. Model 1: adjusted for age and sex. Model 2: adjusted for age, sex and WC. BMI, body mass index; WC, waist circumference; FM, fat mass; FFM, fat-free mass; RMR, resting metabolic rate; HGS, handgrip strength; HDL-C, high-density lipoprotein-cholesterol; TG, triglycerides.

Similarly, RMR and HGS were significantly associated with FFM in all tested regression models, while CRF, as indicated by VO_2max was negatively associated with FM even after controlling for age, sex and WC. RMR was positively associated with eating breakfast on a regular basis ($p = 0.020$), and after adjusting for sex, age and WC, this association persisted ($p = 0.05$). Furthermore, HGS was inversely associated with TG/HDL-C ($p = 0.037$), but this association discontinued in both adjusted regression models.

5. Discussion

In the present study, we explored the role of CRF, physical strength and dietary habits in different food environments, either breakfast exclusively at home or snacking exclusively at school, in metabolic health of primary children in Greece. To the best of our knowledge, this is the first study aiming at investigating VO_2max, HGS and RMR, and how these factors simultaneously correlate to adiposity, antioxidant status, blood lipid profile and eating habits of Greek children. For this purpose, 134 children, aged 6 to 11 years old, visited our clinical site along with their parents to get a full screening regarding anthropometry (i.e., BMI, RMR, body circumferences, bod composition), cardiorespiratory fitness (i.e., VO_2max), physical strength (i.e., HGS), blood analysis (i.e., blood lipids and antioxidant vitamins A, E, C) and assessment of particular eating behavior.

In the European region childhood obesity is a major health concern. Outcomes of the WHO European Childhood Obesity Surveillance Initiative (COSI) recording obesity trends in children aged 6–9 years during 2015–2017 have revealed that overall, 28.7% of boys and 26.5% of girls had overweight/obesity [35]. In fact, children of Southern Europe were characterized as the heaviest, while the mean z-score BW-for-age of Greek children was among the highest [35]. Additionally, Greece was found to possess the highest z-BMI-for-age for boys [35]. In the same study, sex affected obesity prevalence. Based on the WHO growth reference data, Greek boys had a prevalence of overweight/obesity of 42% [95% Confidence Interval (CI) 38.5–45.5] compared to girls, who had a prevalence of 37.8% [95% CI 34.5–41.1] [35]. Similar to the previous study, we found that almost 35% of participants were classified as overweight or obese, with the z-score BW-for-age being substantially higher in boys than in girls.

With regard to abdominal adiposity prevalence, data from a large cohort study in Greece during 2015 showed a prevalence of about 95% in children with obesity, 66% in children with overweight and 12% in normal weight children [36]. For the prediction of abdominal adiposity, authors used the established cut-off point of WHtR ≥ 0.5 [36]. In the current study, we found that abdominal adiposity was less common, occurring at a rate of 36.2% in children who were overweight or obese and 2.4% in children who were of normal weight. These variations may be attributed to differences in sample sizes, geographic regions, as well as the declining prevalence of childhood obesity since 2010, as many preventive interventions targeting primary schoolchildren in Greece have taken place [37].

According to some research, abdominal adiposity in children and adolescents can predict the likelihood of developing cardiometabolic abnormalities such as dyslipidemia, type 2 diabetes, hypertension, and coronary artery disease more accurately than BMI alone [38]. For instance, abdominal adiposity has been linked to childhood dyslipidaemia, regardless of BMI [39]. Abdominal adiposity in children is determined by several indexes, mainly WC and WHtR [38]. Compared to WC, the WHtR is considered more useful, since the 0.5 cut-off value is universal and would help standardize clinical practice independently of age, sex, height and race [40,41]. Additionally, the role of WHtR for the prediction of cardiometabolic risk factors in children has been well established [41]. Results from an observational study in Italian primary schoolchildren showed that WHtR was positively correlated with BMI [42]. In line with this, our results indicated that z-BMI was strongly and positively correlated with WC and WHtR. This observation was confirmed by body composition analysis, as children with overweight/obesity demonstrated higher mean values of FM % and lower values of FFM % compared to their normal weight counterparts. In fact, z-BMI was strongly and positively correlated with FM % and negatively correlated with FFM % and TBW %, highlighting the vital role of assessing body composition in children [43,44].

Additionally, we recorded an inverse correlation of z-BMI with plasma vitamin E, probably indicating the negative impact of overweight/obesity on redox balance and metabolic health [45]. To assess vitamin E, we quantified plasma alpha-tocopherol, the main form of vitamin E in the human body and the most metabolically active [46]. Vitamin E is mostly accumulated in the adipose tissue (~90%), as well as in the liver and the adrenal glands [46]. There is evidence that vitamin E supplementation significantly increases alpha-tocopherol in plasma, reaching a maximum concentration at 8 h post-ingestion followed by substantial decline [47]. This observation could explain the non-detectable differences for vitamin E between the normal weight and overweight/obesity group in our study. Metabolic abnormalities, however, seem to affect vitamin's bioavailability. According to a randomized controlled study, alpha-tocopherol concentration in plasma was lower in adults with metabolic syndrome compared to healthy individuals. It is suggested that the presence of systemic inflammation and oxidative stress affects intestinal absorption of the vitamin and impairs hepatic alpha-tocopherol trafficking [48]. The role of vitamin E in childhood obesity has been investigated in randomized clinical trials. For instance, it has been shown that oral vitamin E administration in children with obesity-related liver disease normalized or stabilized serum aminotransferase and alkaline phosphatase levels [49,50]. Therefore, the observed negative association between z-BMI and vitamin E in our study, even after controlling for age, sex and adiposity (WC), could imply the pivotal role of vitamin E dietary intake in child overweight/obesity.

It is well documented that absolute RMR (kJ/day) is higher in children with obesity than in lean ones [51–53], an outcome also evident in the present study. However, RMR is directly related to body weight, which in turn accounts for about 70 to 80% of the variance in RMR [51]. To this end, we also presented RMR output as kcal/kg of BW/day, and results showed that the mean value was greater in normal weight participants compared to those with overweight/obesity, verifying the indisputable role of body size in child's resting energy metabolism. Furthermore, body composition is considered a main determinant of RMR. Zwiauer et al. showed a strong correlation of RMR with FFM in children [52], which was also the case in the present study. We also recorded a negative correlation of RMR with FM, while absolute RMR (kcal/day) was greater in boys than in girls, an observation conforming that FM and sex are additional determinants of RMR [53].

Nevertheless, little is known regarding the association of overweight/obesity with CRF, namely VO_2max. In 2021, Grzyb et al. have shown that children and adolescents with obesity demonstrated similar VO_2max values compared to those with overweight, but significantly greater than children of normal weight [54]. There is evidence that augmentation of VO_2max in adults is related to lower FM and WC [8–10], but in the case of children, data are still limited. Morinder et al. have demonstrated that VO_2max was a stronger marker for insulin sensitivity compared to FM in severely obese children and adolescents, an outcome that may implies the imperative role of CRF measurement for predicting metabolic syndrome in children [55]. Likewise, in the present study the mean VO_2max was higher in the group with overweight/obesity than in lean children, also showing a negative association with FM, even after adjusting for age, sex and WC.

VO_2max is directly correlated with HGS, a strong predictor of cardiovascular health in both young adults and children [13,14,16]. Recently, children with overweight/obesity showed higher HGS and lower CRF compared to their normal weight counterparts [16,56]. In the present study, HGS did not differ between the two groups, but was strongly and positively correlated with % FFM and RMR, verifying that HGS can be used as a metabolic health indicator in children [57]. We also reported that HGS was negatively associated with TG/HDL-C ratio, a well-known marker of cardiometabolic health [58]. When adjusted to adiposity (WC), HGS showed no association with TG/HDL-C. This is also confirmed by previous studies, as the negative impact of overweight and obesity on cardiometabolic health in both children and adults is well established [56].

It has been suggested that certain meals are important for children's weight status. Breakfast consumption has been linked to a healthier BMI, according to observational studies in the Greek child population [59,60]. Similarly, the present study indicated that children who ate breakfast had lower z-BMI, WHtR and FM than those who did not. Moreover, RMR was positively associated with having breakfast adjusting for age, sex and adiposity, an observation that has been reported by Tambalis for Greek children [61]. Breakfast intake in the current survey was restricted to eating at home. There is evidence that increasing breakfast consumption at home may limit the amount of unhealthful snack foods children consume later in the day, especially for those children on greater socioeconomic disadvantage [62]. Breakfast at home environment is considered more nutritious and access to nutritious meals is a fundamental determinant of health. To this end, it is suggested that parents should be advised to provide their children a healthful breakfast at home in order to attain a healthy body weight [62].

The present study also had some limitations. We are aware that the sample size is relatively small. To overcome this, we applied strict inclusion and exclusion criteria, while all appointed researchers were well trained to avoid measurement errors. Additionally, measurements and interview sessions for each child were conducted by the same researchers to omit bias. Furthermore, we did not evaluate levels of physical activity. In addition, we did not assess nutrient composition of breakfast meals. In the future, large case-control studies are needed to investigate the implication of nutrients and non-nutrients obtained from breakfast in children's CRF and metabolic health.

6. Conclusions

In the present study, we explored the role of cardiorespiratory fitness, physical strength and particular meal consumption in metabolic health of 134 primary children in Greece. Results indicated that z-BMI had a positive correlation with WC, WHtR, and fat mass but a negative correlation with CRF, antioxidant status (as measured by blood vitamin E levels), and frequent breakfast consumption. According to the TG/HDL-C ratio, HGS had a negative correlation with dyslipidemia but a positive correlation with FFM. A positive association of RMR with eating breakfast at home on a regular basis was also found, even after adjusting of sex, age and adiposity. Therefore, CRF, physical strength and breakfast intake before school are promising key modulators of cardiometabolic health in Greek children.

Author Contributions: Conceptualization, M.S.; Methodology, M.S., A.C.K., A.G. and C.A.; Validation, A.G., C.A., A.C.K. and M.S.; Formal analysis, A.G., C.A. and S.P.; Writing—original draft preparation, A.G., C.A. and S.P.; Writing—review and editing, A.G., C.A., A.C.K. and M.S.; Supervision, A.C.K. and M.S. All authors have read and agreed to the published version of the manuscript.

Funding: This research received no external funding.

Institutional Review Board Statement: The study was conducted according to the guidelines of the Declaration of Helsinki and approved by the Ethics Committee of IASO HOSPITAL in Athens-Greece (Approval Code #J-31052019).

Informed Consent Statement: Informed consent was obtained from all subjects involved in the study. Written informed consent has been obtained from the parents publish this paper.

Data Availability Statement: Data is unavailable due to privacy or ethical restrictions.

Acknowledgments: The authors would like to express their gratitude to all volunteers who participated in the study.

Conflicts of Interest: The authors declare no conflict of interest.

References

1. World Health Organization. Obesity and Overweight: Key Facts. 2020. Available online: https://www.who.int/news-room/fact-sheets/detail/obesity-and-overweight (accessed on 9 June 2021).
2. Hosseini, B.; Saedisomeolia, A.; Allman-Farinelli, M. Association between antioxidant intake/status and obesity: A systematic review of observational studies. *Biol. Trace Elem. Res.* **2016**, *175*, 287–297. [CrossRef] [PubMed]
3. Barbosa, P.; Melnyk, S.; Bennuri, S.C.; Delhey, L.; Reis, A.; Moura, G.R.; Børsheim, E.; Rose, S.; Carvalho, E. Redox Imbalance and Methylation Disturbances in Early Childhood Obesity. *Oxidative Med. Cell. Longev.* **2021**, *2021*, 2207125. [CrossRef]
4. Paltoglou, G.; Schoina, M.; Valsamakis, G.; Salakos, N.; Avloniti, A.; Chatzinikolaou, A.; Margeli, A.; Skevaki, C.; Papagianni, M.; Kanaka-Gantenbein, C.; et al. Interrelations among the adipocytokines leptin and adiponectin, oxidative stress and aseptic inflammation markers in pre- and early-pubertal normal-weight and obese boys. *Endocrine* **2017**, *55*, 925–933. [CrossRef] [PubMed]
5. Hertiš Petek, T.; Petek, T.; Močnik, M.; Marčun Varda, N. Systemic Inflammation, Oxidative stress and cardiovascular health in children and adolescents: A systematic review. *Antioxidants* **2022**, *11*, 894. [CrossRef] [PubMed]
6. Kilic, E.; Özer, Ö.F.; Erek Toprak, A.; Erman, H.; Torun, E.; Kesgin Ayhan, S.; Caglar, H.G.; Selek, S.; Kocyigit, A. Oxidative stress status in childhood obesity: A potential risk predictor. *Med. Sci. Monit.* **2016**, *22*, 3673–3679. [CrossRef]
7. Rupérez, A.I.; Mesa, M.D.; Anguita-Ruiz, A.; González-Gil, E.M.; Vázquez-Cobela, R.; Moreno, L.A.; Gil, Á.; Gil-Campos, M.; Leis, R.; Bueno, G.; et al. Antioxidants and oxidative stress in children: Influence of puberty and metabolically unhealthy status. *Antioxidants* **2020**, *9*, 618. [CrossRef]
8. Berge, J.; Støren, Ø.; Hertel, J.K.; Gjevestad, E.; Småstuen, M.C.; Hjelmesæth, J. Associations between cardiorespiratory fitness and weight loss in patients with severe obesity undergoing an intensive lifestyle intervention program: Retrospective cohort study. *BMC Endocr. Disord.* **2019**, *19*, 69. [CrossRef]
9. Rosenkilde, M.; Nordby, P.; Stallknecht, B. Maintenance of improvements in fitness and fatness 1 year after a 3-month lifestyle intervention in overweight men. *Eur. J. Clin. Nutr.* **2016**, *70*, 1212–1214. [CrossRef]
10. Nicklas, B.J.; Wang, X.; You, T.; Lyles, M.F.; Demons, J.; Easter, L.; Berry, M.J.; Lenchik, L.; Carr, J.J. Effect of exercise intensity on abdominal fat loss during calorie restriction in overweight and obese postmenopausal women: A randomized, controlled trial. *Am. J. Clin. Nutr.* **2009**, *89*, 1043–1052. [CrossRef]
11. Raghuveer, G.; Hartz, J.; Lubans, D.R.; Takken, T.; Wiltz, J.L.; Mietus-Snyder, M.; Perak, A.M.; Baker-Smith, C.; Pietris, N.; Edwards, N.M. Cardiorespiratory fitness in youth: An important marker of health: A scientific statement from the American Heart Association. *Circulation* **2020**, *142*, e101–e118. [CrossRef] [PubMed]
12. Gahche, J.; Fakhouri, T.; Carroll, D.D.; Burt, V.L.; Wang, C.Y.; Fulton, J.E. Cardiorespiratory fitness levels among U.S. youth aged 12–15 years: United States, 1999–2004 and 2012. *NCHS Data Brief* **2014**, *153*, 1–8.
13. Zhou, M.; Zha, F.; Chen, Y.; Liu, F.; Zhou, J.; Long, J.; Luo, W.; Huang, M.; Zhang, S.; Luo, D.; et al. Handgrip strength-related factors affecting health outcomes in young adults: Association with cardiorespiratory fitness. *BioMed Res. Int.* **2021**, *2021*, 6645252. [CrossRef] [PubMed]
14. Wu, Y.; Wang, W.; Liu, T.; Zhang, D. Association of Grip Strength with Risk of All-Cause Mortality, Cardiovascular Diseases, and Cancer in Community-Dwelling Populations: A Meta-analysis of Prospective Cohort Studies. *J. Am. Med. Dir. Assoc.* **2017**, *18*, 551.e17–551.e35. [CrossRef]
15. Abe, T.; Thiebaud, R.S.; Ozaki, H.; Yamasaki, S.; Loenneke, J.P. Children with Low Handgrip Strength: A Narrative Review of Possible Exercise Strategies to Improve Its Development. *Children* **2022**, *9*, 1616. [CrossRef]
16. Manzano-Carrasco, S.; Garcia-Unanue, J.; Haapala, E.A.; Felipe, J.L.; Gallardo, L.; Lopez-Fernandez, J. Relationships of BMI, muscle-to-fat ratio, and handgrip strength-to-BMI ratio to physical fitness in Spanish children and adolescents. *Eur. J. Pediatr.* **2023**, *182*, 2345–2357. [CrossRef]
17. Juton, C.; Berruezo, P.; Torres, S.; Castañer, O.; Según, G.; Fitó, M.; Homs, C.; Gómez, S.F.; Schröder, H. Association between meal frequency and weight status in spanish children: A prospective cohort study. *Nutrients* **2023**, *15*, 870. [CrossRef] [PubMed]
18. Ardeshirlarijani, E.; Namazi, N.; Jabbari, M.; Zeinali, M.; Gerami, H.; Jalili, R.B.; Larijani, B.; Azadbakht, L. The link between breakfast skipping and overweigh/obesity in children and adolescents: A meta-analysis of observational studies. *J. Diabetes Metab. Disord.* **2019**, *18*, 657–664. [CrossRef]

19. Monzani, A.; Ricotti, R.; Caputo, M.; Solito, A.; Archero, F.; Bellone, S.; Prodam, F. A Systematic Review of the Association of Skipping Breakfast with Weight and Cardiometabolic Risk Factors in Children and Adolescents. What Should We Better Investigate in the Future? *Nutrients* **2019**, *11*, 387. [CrossRef] [PubMed]
20. Kuźbicka, K.; Rachoń, D. Bad eating habits as the main cause of obesity among children. *Pediatr. Endocrinol. Diabetes Metab.* **2013**, *19*, 106–110.
21. Nowicka, P.; Keres, J.; Ek, A.; Nordin, K.; Sandvik, P. Changing the home food environment: Parents' perspectives four years after starting obesity treatment for their preschool aged child. *Int. J. Environ. Res. Public Health* **2021**, *18*, 11293. [CrossRef]
22. World Health Organization (WHO). Growth Reference Data for 5–19 Years—Indicators. Available online: https://www.who.int/tools/growth-reference-data-for-5to19-years/indicators (accessed on 28 June 2023).
23. Eslami, M.; Pourghazi, F.; Khazdouz, M.; Tian, J.; Pourrostami, K.; Esmaeili-Abdar, Z.; Ejtahed, H.S.; Qorbani, M. Optimal cut-off value of waist circumference-to-height ratio to predict central obesity in children and adolescents: A systematic review and meta-analysis of diagnostic studies. *Front. Nutr.* **2023**, *9*, 985319. [CrossRef]
24. Nuñez, C.; Kovera, A.J.; Pietrobelli, A.; Heshka, S.; Horlick, M.; Kehayias, J.J.; Wang, Z.; Heymsfield, S.B. Body composition in children and adults by air displacement plethysmography. *Eur. J. Clin. Nutr.* **1999**, *53*, 382–387. [CrossRef] [PubMed]
25. Ashcraft, C.M.; Frankenfield, D.C. Validity test of a new open-circuit indirect calorimeter. *JPEN J. Parenter. Enter. Nutr.* **2015**, *39*, 738–742. [CrossRef]
26. Nierenberg, D.W.; Lester, D.C. Determination of vitamins A and E in serum and plasma using a simplified clarification method and high-performance liquid chromatography. *J. Chromatogr.* **1985**, *345*, 275–284. [CrossRef]
27. Liau, L.S.; Lee, B.L.; New, A.L.; Ong, C.N. Determination of plasma ascorbic acid by high-performance liquid chromatography with ultraviolet and electrochemical detection. *J. Chromatogr.* **1993**, *612*, 63–70. [CrossRef]
28. Marinov, B.; Kostianev, S.; Turnovska, T. Modified treadmill protocol for evaluation of physical fitness in pediatric age group—Comparison with Bruce and Balke protocols. *Acta Physiol. Pharmacol. Bulg.* **2003**, *27*, 47–51.
29. Beltz, N.M.; Gibson, A.L.; Janot, J.M.; Kravitz, L.; Mermier, C.M.; Dalleck, L.C. Graded exercise testing protocols for the determination of VO2max: Historical perspectives, progress, and future considerations. *J. Sports Med. (Hindawi Publ. Corp.)* **2016**, *2016*, 3968393. [CrossRef]
30. Fess, E.E. Grip Strength. In *Clinical Assessment Recommendations*, 2nd ed.; Casanova, J.S., Ed.; American Society of Hand Therapists: Chicago, IL, USA, 1992; pp. 41–45, 163–177.
31. Gąsior, J.S.; Pawłowski, M.; Jeleń, P.J.; Rameckers, E.A.; Williams, C.A.; Makuch, R.; Werner, B. Test-retest reliability of handgrip strength measurement in children and preadolescents. *Int. J. Environ. Res. Public Health* **2020**, *17*, 8026. [CrossRef]
32. Gąsior, J.S.; Pawłowski, M.; Williams, C.A.; Dąbrowski, M.J.; Rameckers, E.A. Assessment of maximal isometric hand grip strength in school-aged children. *Open Med.* **2018**, *13*, 22–28. [CrossRef] [PubMed]
33. Serra-Majem, L.; Ribas, L.; Ngo, J.; Ortega, R.M.; García, A.; Pérez-Rodrigo, C.; Aranceta, J. Food, youth and the Mediterranean diet in Spain. Development of KIDMED, Mediterranean diet quality index in children and adolescents. *Public Health Nutr.* **2004**, *7*, 931–935. [CrossRef] [PubMed]
34. Anderson, L.N.; Carsley, S.; Lebovic, G.; Borkhoff, C.M.; Maguire, J.L.; Parkin, P.C.; Birken, C.S. Misclassification of child body mass index from cut-points defined by rounded percentiles instead of z-scores. *BMC Res. Notes* **2017**, *10*, 639. [CrossRef]
35. Spinelli, A.; Buoncristiano, M.; Nardone, P.; Starc, G.; Hejgaard, T.; Júlíusson, P.B.; Fismen, A.-S.; Weghuber, D.; Musić Milanović, S.; García-Solano, M.; et al. Thinness, overweight, and obesity in 6- to 9-year-old children from 36 countries: The World Health Organization European Childhood Obesity Surveillance Initiative-COSI 2015–2017. *Obes. Rev.* **2021**, *22* (Suppl. S6), e13214. [CrossRef] [PubMed]
36. Tambalis, K.D.; Panagiotakos, D.B.; Psarra, G.; Sidossis, L.S. Current data in Greek children indicate decreasing trends of obesity in the transition from childhood to adolescence; results from the National Action for Children's Health (EYZHN) Program. *J. Prev. Med. Hyg.* **2018**, *59*, e36–e47. [CrossRef] [PubMed]
37. Hassapidou, M. Prevalence of childhood obesity in Greece: Results from WHO Childhood Obesity Surveillance Initiative 2010–2020. *Public Health Toxicol.* **2022**, *2*, A45. [CrossRef]
38. Kelishadi, R.; Mirmoghtadaee, P.; Najafi, H.; Keikha, M. Systematic review on the association of abdominal obesity in children and adolescents with cardio-metabolic risk factors. *J. Res. Med. Sci.* **2015**, *20*, 294–307.
39. Calcaterra, V.; Larizza, D.; De Silvestri, A.; Albertini, R.; Vinci, F.; Regalbuto, C.; Dobbiani, G.; Montalbano, C.; Pelizzo, G.; Cena, H. Gender-based differences in the clustering of metabolic syndrome factors in children and adolescents. *J. Pediatr. Endocrinol. Metab.* **2020**, *33*, 279–288. [CrossRef]
40. Muñoz-Hernando, J.; Escribano, J.; Ferré, N.; Closa-Monasterolo, R.; Grote, V.; Koletzko, B.; Gruszfeld, D.; ReDionigi, A.; Verduci, E.; Xhonneux, A.; et al. Usefulness of the waist-to-height ratio for predicting cardiometabolic risk in children and its suggested boundary values. *Clin. Nutr.* **2022**, *41*, 508–516. [CrossRef]
41. Li, W.-C.; Chen, I.-C.; Chang, Y.-C.; Loke, S.-S.; Wang, S.-H.; Hsiao, K.-Y. Waist-to-height ratio, waist circumference, and body mass index as indices of cardiometabolic risk among 36,642 Taiwanese adults. *Eur. J. Nutr.* **2013**, *52*, 57–65. [CrossRef] [PubMed]
42. Santomauro, F.; Lorini, C.; Pieralli, F.; Niccolai, G.; Picciolli, P.; Vezzosi, S.; Bonaccorsi, G. Waist-to-height ratio and its associations with body mass index in a sample of Tuscan children in primary school. *Ital. J. Pediatr.* **2017**, *43*, 53. [CrossRef]
43. Rusek, W.; Baran, J.; Leszczak, J.; Adamczyk, M.; Baran, R.; Weres, A.; Inglot, G.; Czenczek-Lewandowska, E.; Pop, T. Changes in children's body composition and posture during puberty growth. *Children* **2021**, *8*, 288. [CrossRef]

44. Ofenheimer, A.; Breyer-Kohansal, R.; Hartl, S.; Burghuber, O.C.; Krach, F.; Franssen, F.M.E.; Wouters, E.F.M.; Breyer, M.-K. Using body composition groups to identify children and adolescents at risk of dyslipidemia. *Children* **2021**, *8*, 1047. [CrossRef]
45. Barzegar-Amini, M.; Khorramruz, F.; Ghazizadeh, H.; Sahebi, R.; Mohammadi-Bajgyran, M.; Mohaddes Ardabili, H.; Tayefi, M.; Darroudi, S.; Moohebati, M.; Heidari-Bakavoli, A.; et al. Association between serum vitamin E concentrations and the presence of metabolic syndrome: A population-based cohort study. *Acta Biomed.* **2021**, *92*, e2021047. [CrossRef]
46. Szewczyk, K.; Chojnacka, A.; Górnicka, M. Tocopherols and tocotrienols-bioactive dietary compounds; what is certain, what is doubt? *Int. J. Mol. Sci.* **2021**, *22*, 6222. [CrossRef]
47. Jaafar, F.; Abdullah, A.; Makpol, S. Cellular uptake and bioavailability of tocotrienol-rich fraction in SIRT1-inhibited human diploid fibroblasts. *Sci. Rep.* **2018**, *8*, 10471. [CrossRef] [PubMed]
48. Mah, E.; Sapper, T.N.; Chitchumroonchokchai, C.; Failla, M.L.; Schill, K.E.; Clinton, S.K.; Bobe, G.; Traber, M.G.; Bruno, R.S. α-Tocopherol bioavailability is lower in adults with metabolic syndrome regardless of dairy fat co-ingestion: A randomized, double-blind, crossover trial. *Am. J. Clin. Nutr.* **2015**, *102*, 1070–1080. [CrossRef] [PubMed]
49. Vajro, P.; Mandato, C.; Franzese, A.; Ciccimarra, E.; Lucariello, S.; Savoia, M.; Capuano, G.; Migliaro, F. Vitamin E treatment in pediatric obesity-related liver disease: A randomized study. *J. Pediatr. Gastroenterol. Nutr.* **2004**, *38*, 48–55. [CrossRef]
50. Lavine, J.E. Vitamin E treatment of nonalcoholic steatohepatitis in children: A pilot study. *J. Pediatr.* **2000**, *136*, 734–738. [CrossRef]
51. Epstein, L.H.; Wing, R.R.; Cluss, P.; Fernstrom, M.H.; Penner, B.; Perkins, K.A.; Nudelman, S.; Marks, B.; Valoski, A. Resting metabolic rate in lean and obese children: Relationship to child and parent weight and percent-overweight change. *Am. J. Clin. Nutr.* **1989**, *49*, 331–336. [CrossRef]
52. Zwiauer, K.F.; Mueller, T.; Widhalm, K. Resting metabolic rate in obese children before, during and after weight loss. *Int. J. Obes. Relat. Metab. Disord.* **1992**, *16*, 11–16.
53. Molnár, D.; Schutz, Y. The effect of obesity, age, puberty and gender on resting metabolic rate in children and adolescents. *Eur. J. Pediatr.* **1997**, *156*, 376–381. [CrossRef] [PubMed]
54. Grzyb, A.; Domagalska-Szopa, M.; Siwiec, A.; Kwiecień-Czerwieniec, I.; Szopa, A. Cardiopulmonary capacity in overweight and obese children and adolescents: A cross-sectional study. *Front. Physiol.* **2021**, *12*, 671827. [CrossRef]
55. Morinder, G.; Larsson, U.E.; Norgren, S.; Marcus, C. Insulin sensitivity, VO2max and body composition in severely obese Swedish children and adolescents. *Acta Paediatr.* **2009**, *98*, 132–138. [CrossRef] [PubMed]
56. Blakeley, C.E.; Van Rompay, M.I.; Schultz, N.S.; Sacheck, J.M. Relationship between muscle strength and dyslipidemia, serum 25(OH)D, and weight status among diverse schoolchildren: A cross-sectional analysis. *BMC Pediatr.* **2018**, *18*, 23. [CrossRef] [PubMed]
57. Steffl, M.; Chrudimsky, J.; Tufano, J.J. Using relative handgrip strength to identify children at risk of sarcopenic obesity. *PLoS ONE* **2017**, *12*, e0177006. [CrossRef]
58. Nur Zati Iwani, A.K.; Jalaludin, M.Y.; Wan Mohd Zin, R.M.; Fuziah, M.Z.; Hong, J.Y.H.; Abqariyah, Y.; Mokhtar, A.H.; Wan Mohamud, W.N. TG: HDL-C ratio is a good marker to identify children affected by obesity with increased cardiometabolic risk and insulin resistance. *Int. J. Endocrinol.* **2019**, *2019*, 8586167. [CrossRef]
59. Tambalis, K.D.; Panagiotakos, D.B.; Psarra, G.; Sidossis, L.S. Breakfast skipping in Greek schoolchildren connected to an unhealthy lifestyle profile. Results from the National Action for Children's Health Program: Breakfast Skipping and Lifestyle Factors. *Nutr Diet.* **2019**, *76*, 328–335. [CrossRef]
60. Kyriazis, I.; Rekleiti, M.; Saridi, M.; Beliotis, E.; Toska, A.; Souliotis, K.; Wozniak, G. Prevalence of obesity in children aged 6–12 years in Greece: Nutritional behaviour and physical activity. *Arch. Med. Sci.* **2012**, *8*, 859–864. [CrossRef]
61. Tambalis, K.D.; Panagiotakos, D.B.; Psarra, G.; Sidossis, L.S. Association of cardiorespiratory fitness levels with dietary habits and lifestyle factors in schoolchildren. *Appl. Physiol. Nutr. Metab.* **2019**, *44*, 539–545. [CrossRef] [PubMed]
62. Utter, J.; Scragg, R.; Mhurchu, C.N.; Schaaf, D. At-home breakfast consumption among New Zealand children: Associations with body mass index and related nutrition behaviors. *J. Am. Diet. Assoc.* **2007**, *107*, 570–576. [CrossRef]

nutrients

MDPI

Article

Women's Autonomy and Anemia in Children under Five Years of Age: A Peruvian Population-Based Survey

Rosa Campos-Guerrero, Xiomara Genoveva Diaz-Molina, Rodrigo Vargas-Fernández and Diego Azañedo *

Faculty of Health Sciences, Universidad Científica del Sur, Lima 15067, Peru; 100032454@cientifica.edu.pe (R.C.-G.); 100033619@cientifica.edu.pe (X.G.D.-M.); jvargasf@cientifica.edu.pe (R.V.-F.)

* Correspondence: dazanedo@cientifica.edu.pe

Abstract: To determine the association between women's autonomy and the presence of childhood anemia in children under five years of age in Peru, a cross-sectional study utilizing data from the 2019 Demographic and Family Health Survey was carried out. The study employed generalized linear models with a Poisson distribution and log link function. Crude and adjusted prevalence ratios (aPR) were calculated, along with their corresponding 95% confidence intervals (CI), to assess the association of interest. A total of 15,815 women and their children under five years of age were analyzed. The prevalence of childhood anemia was 30.4% (95%CI: 29.5–31.3%), while the proportions of low, moderate and high autonomy of the mothers were 44.5%, 38.4% and 17.1%, respectively. Children under five years of age of women with a low level of autonomy were more likely to have anemia (aPR: 1.10; 95%CI: 1.00–1.21). Three out of ten children under five years of age suffer from anemia, and four out of ten mothers have a low level of autonomy. A low level of women's autonomy was associated with a higher probability of anemia in children under 5 years of age.

Keywords: child nutrition disorders; personal autonomy; decision making; health surveys; Peru

1. Introduction

Target 2.2 of the Sustainable Development Goals aims to eradicate all forms of malnutrition by 2030, and to achieve international targets on stunting and wasting in children under 5 years of age [1]. Despite this, according to the World Health Organization, it is currently estimated that 40% of children under five years of age worldwide suffer from anemia [2]. Likewise, developing countries alone present a burden of 89% of global disability related to anemia in the general population [3]. Meanwhile, in India 2017, it was estimated that 8.3 million disability-adjusted life years were lost due to anemia in children under 5 years of age [4]. In Latin America and the Caribbean (LAC) in 2019, the prevalence of anemia in children under five was 21%, similar to the prevalence in Europe and Central Asia (20%), although much higher than in North America (7%) [5]. Likewise, in that same year in LAC, the highest prevalences were reported in Bolivia (37%) and Peru (30%), while the lowest were found in Costa Rica (19%), Argentina (19%), Cuba (18%) and Brazil (12%) [5]. This condition has a great impact on children, since it is associated with alterations in the gastrointestinal tract, immune system, thermoregulation, cognitive and motor function and physical performance, which in adulthood lead to a greater burden of disease and loss of work productivity [6–8].

Childhood anemia is associated with the presence of various factors [9–13], which can be grouped into health and hygiene factors, sociodemographic and economic factors and those related to food security, which involve adequate nutrition and nutritional supplementation. In the household, women play a fundamental role in the nutrition and care of children; therefore, within the framework of women's human rights, women's autonomy is the fundamental basis for making decisions related to food, finances and family health [14–16]. Women's autonomy is a construct that has three dimensions that include the capacity to make decisions, control over finances, and degree of freedom of movement. Greater autonomy allows mothers to make decisions regarding the feeding and hygiene of their children and the distribution of resources for household care, thus influencing child health [16–18]. However, a study using data from low- and middle-income countries between 2000 and 2015 reported that only 19.9% of women had autonomy to make household decisions and 61.6% to make decisions about their health [19]. In this regard, low autonomy in decision-making by women could be related to anemia in children, through mechanisms such as low access to health services, as well as inadequate nutrition and nutritional supplementation in children [16,20].

To date, most studies have focused on assessing the association between women's autonomy and child health status by focusing on anthropometric indicators, mortality, and the prevalence of diarrhea [21]. However, evidence regarding the association between women's autonomy and anemia in children is scarce. The only study identified used data from the Sub-Saharan Africa Demographic and Family Health Survey (DHS) for the years 2006 to 2019, and reported that the odds of anemia decrease as women's autonomy increases [22]. Although low female autonomy and a high prevalence of anemia are important social and public health problems in low- and middle-income countries such as in Latin America, their association has not been studied in this context.

Peru is one of the Latin American countries with the lowest female autonomy (only 19% with high autonomy) and the highest prevalence of anemia [5,23–26]. We hypothesize that women's autonomy can be a crucial factor affecting the presence of anemia in children under 5 years of age. Therefore, the present study aimed to determine the association between women's autonomy and the presence of childhood anemia in children under five years of age using the Demographic and Family Health Survey (ENDES—acronym in Spanish) 2019 conducted in Peru.

2. Materials and Methods

2.1. Study Design and Data Source

This cross-sectional study was based on ENDES data collected in 2019. ENDES 2019 is a survey conducted between January and December 2019 by the National Institute of Statistics and Informatics (an institution that regulates, controls and manages the statistical information of Peru) under the framework of the DHS Program, which is the format of many surveys conducted in low- and middle-income countries. Likewise, the ENDES aims to provide updated information on demographic dynamics, the health status of mothers and children under five and other health determinants such as communicable and non-communicable diseases [27]. In fact, the ENDES is composed of three questionnaires: (i) a household questionnaire, which collects information on housing characteristics (water source, sanitation, household equipment, etc.); (ii) an individual woman's questionnaire, which collects information on sociodemographic characteristics, reproductive history, pregnancy of women aged 15 to 49 years and information on health characteristics of their children under five years; and (iii) a health questionnaire, which collects information on communicable and non-communicable diseases and their risk factors in people aged 15 years and older, and mental, oral and eye health in children under 12 years of age. In addition, the level of inference of the ENDES is at the national level, by urban/rural area and in the 25 departments of Peru [27]. The data presented in this study are openly available: https://proyectos.inei.gob.pe/microdatos/ (accessed on 18 May 2023).

2.2. Sampling and Data Collection

The sampling framework for the selection of the ENDES sample consists of information from the National Population Census XI and Housing Census VI of 2007 and the Household Targeting System Update 2012–2013 and updated cartographic material. The ENDES has a complex sampling method characterized by being two-stage, probabilistic, balanced, stratified and independent, at the departmental level and by urban and rural area. The primary and secondary sampling units are divided by area of residence: (i) clusters and private households in urban areas and (ii) rural census area and private households in rural areas [27]. The ENDES research unit is made up of the usual residents and the people who spent the previous night in the dwelling. For the year 2019, the collection of information was carried out through direct interviews by previously evaluated and trained staff, and the answers of the respondents were recorded on an electronic device (tablet). Further details on the ENDES methodology can be found in the technical report [27].

2.3. *Inclusion/Exclusion Criteria*

For the purposes of the present study, all children under five years whose mothers had complete information on the sociodemographic and economic characteristics that determined their level of autonomy and children who had a recorded hemoglobin value were included. Children whose mother had not spent the previous night at home and children aged six months or younger were excluded. Thus, a total of 15,815 mothers and children under five years of age were included in the present study.

2.4. *Variables*

2.4.1. Outcome Measures

The dependent variable was the presence of anemia in children under five years of age. The cut-off point for the diagnosis of anemia was <11 g/dL. The definition of anemia in a child under five years of age was considered to be a hemoglobin value less than 11.0 g/dL based on the Technical Standard for the preventive management of anemia in children, adolescents, pregnant and puerperal women from 2017 [28]. Thus, the dependent variable was recoded as 1 (yes) when the hemoglobin value was less than 11 g/dL and 0 (no) when the hemoglobin value was greater than or equal to 11 g/dL. It should be noted that the value used in the present study was hemoglobin adjusted for the level of altitude of the child's residence [29].

The determination of hemoglobin levels in the ENDES was performed under universal standards with a HemoCue® hemoglobinometer model Hb 201+ previously calibrated by a trained anthropometrist on the same day as the interview [29]. To perform the procedure, the sample collection process first had to be explained to the mother of the child under five years of age and informed consent had to be obtained [29]. Sample collection in children aged 12 to 71 months was performed with the child on the mother's or caregiver's lap, with the anthropometrist holding the lateral area of the child's hand and extending the arm diagonally downward. The middle finger was then punctured with a lancet to obtain a drop of sufficient quantity (10 microliters) to fill a microwell. For children under 12 months of age, the puncture was made in the heel area without squeezing or pressing, to obtain the appropriate amount of blood (10 microliters) for hemoglobin measurement in a microwell. The filled cuvette was then checked for air bubbles and placed parallel to the cuvette holder [29]. Finally, the anthropometrist recorded the result that appeared on the digital display of the hemoglobinometer on the collection card. Further details on sample collection can be found in the anemia measurement methodology report [29].

2.4.2. Exposure

The variable of women's autonomy was constructed based on four dimensions. Each of these dimensions was composed of different characteristics of the woman and were based on specific questions from the ENDES, as follows: (i) Related to decision-making, which includes economic characteristics: Who has the last word in deciding what to do with the money the husband earns [V743F], Who has the last word in large household purchases [V743B], Who has the last word in buying basic necessities [V743C]; health: Who has the last word in health care? [V743A]); and free transit: Who has the last word in visiting family or relatives? [V743D]) (ii) Attitudes towards violence that consider the reasons for justifying the violence experienced by the woman (based on battered wife explains that she leaves without telling him [V744A], battered wife explains that she neglects the children [V744B], battered wife explains that she argues with him [V744C], battered wife explains that she refuses to have sex with him [V744D], and battered wife explains that she burns food [V744E]); (iii) Socioeconomic aspects, which include characteristics such as employment (based on work in the last 12 months [V731]), and head of household (based on sex of the head of household [V151]); and (iv) Socio-cultural aspects such as educational level (based on highest level of education [V106]) and access to television, radio and newspapers (based on frequency of watching television [V159], frequency of listening to radio [V158], and frequency of reading newspaper or magazine [V157]).

After identifying the variables that make up women's autonomy, the following recoding was carried out: (i) variables that make up the decision-making dimension were recoded as 1 when the woman had the last word in decision-making, and 0 when she did not; (ii) variables related to the justification for violence were recoded as 1 when the woman gave an affirmative answer and 0 when it was negative; (iii) economic aspects were recoded as 1 when the woman had worked in the last 12 months, and when the head of the household was a woman, and 0 when a negative answer was given about work and when the head of the household was a man; and (iv) for socio-cultural aspects, the following categorizations were made: educational level was coded as 0 = no education or only primary education, 1 = secondary education and 2 = higher education, while the variables on access to media were coded as 1 when the woman had access to television, radio and newspapers at least once a week or every day and 0 when she did not. After recoding the variables, an index was constructed with the sum of the final scores of each of the variables included, with the highest scores determining the highest level of autonomy. Finally, the constructed index was classified into tertiles to determine low, moderate and high levels of autonomy. The inclusion and recoding of the variables, the creation of an index and its division into tertiles were based on previous studies [25,30–34].

It should be noted that the mother's information and the child's hemoglobin determination were collected in a single interview conducted on the same day.

2.4.3. Covariables

The inclusion of covariables was made on the basis of previous studies that had evaluated the association of interest [16,35–37]. Thus, the following variables were included: age of child (6–23, 24–35, 36–59), sex of child (male, female), age of mother (15–24, 25–34, 35–49), ethnicity (native, non-native), marital status (married, cohabiting), health insurance (yes, no), number of children (0, 1–3, 4–7), number of people in the household (0–4, 5 or more), area of residence (urban, rural), wealth quintile (poorest [Q1], poorer, middle, richer, richest [Q5]), natural region (Coast, Highlands, Jungle).

2.5. Statistical Analysis

The statistical program Stata version 17.0 (StataCorp, College Station, TX, USA) was used to merge the databases of mothers and their children and perform the analyses. In addition, the svy command was used to consider complex sampling and the ENDES weighting factor in all analyses. Population characteristics were reported with absolute and relative frequencies. In addition, a bivariate analysis was performed using the chi-square test to evaluate differences between the proportions of the variables and the dependent and independent variables. The association between the level of autonomy of the woman and the presence of anemia in children under the age of five years was evaluated using generalized linear models of the Poisson family, and log link functions and crude (PR) and adjusted prevalence ratios (aPR), along with their corresponding 95% confidence intervals (CI), were reported for covariates that had a value of $p < 0.05$ in the bivariate analysis of the dependent variable. Models were fitted for the following variables: child's sex and age, mother's age, mother's ethnicity, mother's marital status, number of children, number of people in the household, place of residence, wealth quintile, and natural region. Finally, the multicollinearity of the variables included in the adjusted model was evaluated, and this event was not found. Statistical significance was determined with a p value <0.05 in all analyses.

2.6. Ethical Considerations

The data used in this study were obtained from the secondary database of ENDES 2019, and each participant had previously signed an informed consent form. It should be noted that the ENDES databases are anonymized, thereby preventing the identification of participants. For the measurement of hemoglobin in the child, the surveyor asked the mother for informed consent, which had to be accepted by the mother in order to obtain the blood sample.

3. Results

3.1. Characteristics of the Study Population

A total of 15,815 mother–child pairs were included in the analysis. Most of the children were between 36 and 59 months old (45.2%) and were male (50.9%). Regarding the mothers of these children, 47.9% were between 25 and 34 years old, 9.2% were of native ethnicity, and 72.1% had between one and three children. Further information on the characteristics of the population included is shown in Table 1.

Table 1. Characteristics of the population included in this study.

Characteristics	*n*	Weighted Proportion *
Age of child (in months)		
6–23	5228	32.9
24–35	3450	21.9
36–59	7137	45.2
Sex of child		
Male	8048	50.9
Female	7767	49.1
Age of mother (in years)		
15–24	3421	21.2
25–34	7640	47.9
35–49	4754	30.9
Ethnicity		
Native	1461	9.2
Non-native	14,354	90.8
Marital status		
Married	4225	27.8
Cohabitant	11,590	72.2
Health insurance		
Yes	14,426	91.2
No	1389	8.8
Number of children		
0	4010	25.4
1–3	11,397	72.1
4–7	408	2.5
Number of people in the household		
0–4	7190	45.5
5 or more	8625	54.5
Area of residence		
Urban	11,083	70.1
Rural	4732	29.9

Table 1. *Cont.*

Characteristics	*n*	Weighted Proportion *
Wealth quintile		
Poorest (Q1)	4471	26.3
Poorer	4335	24.8
Middle	3129	19.6
Richer	2296	16.3
Richest (Q5)	1584	13.0
Natural region		
Coast	6569	52.8
Highlands	5260	28.8
Jungle	3986	18.4

* The weighting factor and sample specifications of ENDES were included.

3.2. Anemia in Children under Five Years of Age

The prevalence of anemia in children under five years of age was 30.4% (CI: 29.5–31.3%) in 2019. The highest proportions of anemia were found in children who were aged 0–23 months (50.0%) and were male (32.5%). In addition, these higher proportions were found in children whose mothers were aged between 15 and 24 years (37.6%), belonged to a native ethnicity (45.8%), were cohabiting (32.3%), and had between four and seven children (39.9%). Additionally, the highest proportions of childhood anemia were found in children whose mothers had a low (35.1%) and moderate (27.5%) level of autonomy (Table 2).

Table 2. Characteristics of the population included according to the presence of anemia in the child, ENDES 2019.

Characteristics	Presence of Anemia		*p*-Value **
	No (*n* = 10,684) % * (95% CI)	Yes (*n* = 5131) % * (95% CI)	
Total	69.6 (68.7–70.5)	30.4 (29.5–31.3)	
Age of child (in months)			
6–23	49.9 (48.3–51.6)	50.0 (48.4–51.7)	<0.001
24–35	73.4 (71.7–75.2)	26.5 (24.8–28.3)	
36–59	82.1 (81.0–83.2)	17.9 (16.8–19.0)	
Sex of child			
Male	67.5 (66.2–68.8)	32.5 (31.2–33.8)	<0.001
Female	71.8 (70.5–73.0)	28.2 (27.0–29.5)	
Age of mother (in years)			
15–24	62.4 (60.4–64.3)	37.6 (35.7–39.6)	<0.001
25–34	69.7 (68.4–71.0)	30.3 (29.0–31.6)	
35–49	74.4 (72.9–76.0)	25.6 (24.0–27.2)	
Ethnicity			
Native	54.2 (50.9–57.6)	45.8 (42.4–49.1)	<0.001
Non-native	70.8 (69.8–71.7)	29.2 (28.3–30.2)	
Marital status			
Married	74.6 (72.9–76.1)	25.4 (23.9–27.1)	<0.001
Cohabitant	67.7 (66.6–68.8)	32.3 (31.2–33.4)	
Health insurance			
Yes	69.7 (68.7–70.6)	30.3 (29.4–31.3)	0.800
No	69.3 (66.2–72.2)	30.7 (27.8–33.8)	
Number of children			
0	72.7 (71.0–74.4)	27.3 (25.6–29.0)	<0.001
1–3	68.8 (67.8–69.9)	31.2 (30.1–32.2)	
4–7	60.1 (53.9–66.0)	39.9 (34.1–46.1)	

Table 2. *Cont.*

Characteristics	Presence of Anemia		p-Value **
	No (n = 10,684) % * (95% CI)	Yes (n = 5131) % * (95% CI)	
Number of people in the household			
0–4	71.0 (69.7–72.3)	29.0 (27.7–30.3)	0.007
5 or more	68.5 (67.2–69.8)	31.5 (30.2–32.8)	
Area of residence			
Urban	72.9 (71.8–73.9)	27.1 (26.1–28.2)	<0.001
Rural	61.4 (59.6–63.3)	38.6 (36.7–40.4)	
Wealth quintile			
Poorest (Q1)	60.0 (58.2–61.9)	40.0 (38.1–41.8)	<0.001
Poorer	67.4 (65.6–69.1)	32.6 (30.9–34.4)	
Middle	72.2 (70.2–74.2)	27.8 (25.8–29.8)	
Richer	75.1 (72.7–77.3)	24.9 (22.8–27.3)	
Richest (Q5)	82.4 (80.1–84.6)	17.6 (15.4–19.9)	
Natural region			
Coast	75.9 (74.6–77.2)	24.1 (22.8–25.4)	<0.001
Highlands	61.4 (59.6–63.2)	38.6 (36.8–40.4)	
Jungle	64.4 (62.5–66.3)	35.6 (33.7–37.5)	
Women's Autonomy			
Low	64.9 (63.5–66.3)	35.1 (33.7–36.5)	<0.001
Moderate	72.5 (71.0–73.8)	27.5 (26.2–29.0)	
High	75.6 (73.5–77.6)	24.4 (22.4–26.5)	

CI: confidence interval. * The weighting factor and sample specifications of ENDES were included. ** Estimated *p*-value using the Chi-square test.

3.3. Level of Mothers' Autonomy

The proportions of low, moderate and high levels of autonomy were 44.5%, 38.4% and 17.1%, respectively. Regarding a low level of autonomy, the highest proportions were found in mothers aged 15 to 24 years (50.6%) who belonged to a native ethnicity (74.7%), were cohabiting (46.7%), had health insurance (45.1%) and had between four and seven children (71.8). More information about the characteristics according to the level of autonomy is presented in Table 3.

Table 3. Characteristics of the population included by level of maternal autonomy, ENDES 2019.

Characteristics	Women's Autonomy			p-Value **
	High (n = 2567) % * (95% CI)	Moderate (n = 6021) % * (95% CI)	Low (n = 7227) % * (95% CI)	
Total	17.1 (16.3–18.0)	38.4 (37.3–39.5)	44.5 (43.3–45.7)	
Age of child (in months)				
6–23	16.9 (15.8–18.1)	38.9 (37.5–40.4)	44.2 (42.6–45.7)	0.617
24–35	17.5 (15.9–19.3)	38.7 (36.6–40.9)	43.8 (41.6–46.0)	
36–59	17.1 (15.8–18.6)	37.4 (35.8–39.1)	45.5 (43.7–47.2)	
Sex of child				
Male	17.0 (15.9–18.2)	39.0 (37.5–40.5)	44.0 (42.5–45.5)	0.467
Female	17.2 (16.0–18.5)	37.8 (36.3–39.2)	45.0 (43.5–46.6)	
Age of mother (in years)				
15–24	12.9 (11.3–14.7)	36.5 (34.4–38.7)	50.6 (48.3–52.9)	<0.001
25–34	17.8 (16.6–19.1)	40.6 (39.0–42.3)	41.6 (30.0–43.3)	
35–49	19.0 (17.4–20.7)	36.2 (34.2–38.2)	44.8 (42.8–46.9)	
Ethnicity				
Native	5.0 (3.6–6.9)	20.3 (17.4–23.7)	74.7 (71.0–78.0)	<0.001
Non-native	18.1 (17.1–19.0)	39.7 (38.6–40.9)	42.2 (41.0–43.5)	

Table 3. *Cont.*

Characteristics	Women's Autonomy			*p*-Value **
	High (n = 2567) % * (95% CI)	Moderate (n = 6021) % * (95% CI)	Low (n = 7227) % * (95% CI)	
Marital status				
Married	21.9 (20.0–23.9)	39.4 (37.3–41.6)	38.7 (36.6–40.9)	<0.001
Cohabitant	15.3 (14.4–16.3)	38.0 (36.7–39.3)	46.7 (45.4–48.1)	
Health insurance				
Yes	16.9 (16.0–17.9)	38.0 (36.8–39.1)	45.1 (43.9–46.4)	<0.001
No	18.8 (16.0–21.9)	42.2 (38.6–45.8)	39.0 (35.5–42.8)	
Number of children				
0	21.4 (19.5–23.5)	40.1 (38.0–42.2)	38.5 (36.4–40.6)	<0.001
1–3	16.1 (15.1–17.0)	38.2 (37.0–39.5)	45.7 (44.4–47.1)	
4–7	3.4 (1.1–10.2)	24.8 (18.9–31.7)	71.8 (64.4–78.2)	
Number of people in the household				
0–4	19.7 (18.4–21.1)	40.6 (39.0–42.2)	39.7 (38.1–41.3)	<0.001
5 or more	15.0 (13.9–16.2)	36.6 (35.1–38.1)	48.4 (46.8–50.0)	
Area of residence				
Urban	22.1 (20.9–23.3)	44.5 (43.2–45.8)	33.4 (32.1–34.8)	<0.001
Rural	4.6 (3.8–5.6)	22.9 (21.1–24.9)	72.5 (70.3–74.6)	
Wealth quintile				
Poorest (Q1)	2.9 (2.3–3.7)	19.6 (17.8–21.4)	77.5 (75.6–79.4)	<0.001
Poorer	10.6 (9.4–11.9)	40.8 (38.8–42.9)	48.6 (46.4–50.7)	
Middle	18.8 (17.1–20.7)	48.8 (46.3–51.3)	32.4 (30.1–34.8)	
Richer	28.6 (26.0–31.4)	47.5 (44.7–50.5)	23.9 (21.5–26.4)	
Richest (Q5)	41.1 (37.6–44.8)	44.6 (41.1–48.1)	14.3 (12.1–16.8)	
Natural region				
Coast	21.1 (19.7–22.6)	44.3 (42.6–46.1)	34.6 (32.8–36.4)	<0.001
Highlands	14.4 (13.1–15.8)	33.7 (31.9–35.5)	51.9 (49.8–54.1)	
Jungle	10.0 (8.9–11.3)	28.8 (26.7–30.9)	61.2 (58.8–63.6)	

CI: confidence interval. * The weighting factor and sample specifications of ENDES were included. ** Estimated *p*-value using the Chi-square test.

3.4. Association between the Level of Mother's Autonomy and the Presence of Anemia in Children under Five Years of Age

In the crude analysis, it was found that low (PR: 1.44; 95%CI: 1.31–1.58) and moderate (PR: 1.13; 95%CI: 1.02–1.25) autonomy were associated with the presence of anemia in children under five years of age, while in the analysis adjusted for the child's, mother's and household characteristics, only women with a low level of autonomy had a higher probability of their children under five years of age having anemia (aPR: 1.10; 95% CI: 1.00–1.21; p = 0.047) (Table 4).

Table 4. Association between mothers' level of autonomy and the presence of childhood anemia.

Variable	Crude		Adjusted *	
	PR (95% CI)	*p*-Value	aPR (95% CI)	*p*-Value
Autonomy				
High	Reference		Reference	
Moderate	1.13 (1.02–1.25)	0.015	1.03 (0.93–1.13)	0.567
Low	1.44 (1.31–1.58)	<0.001	1.10 (1.00–1.21)	0.047

PR: prevalence ratio. aPR: adjusted prevalence ratio. CI: confidence interval. Weighting factors and sample specifications of ENDES were included for all analysis. * Model adjusted for the following variables: sex and age of the child, age of the mother, ethnicity of the mother, marital status of the mother, number of children, number of people in the household, place of residence, wealth quintile and natural region.

4. Discussion

The present study aimed to determine the association between women's autonomy and the presence of anemia in children under five years of age in the Peruvian population in 2019. In this regard, it was found that three out of ten Peruvian children under five years of age had anemia at the time of the study. Likewise, in relation to women's autonomy, it was determined that eight out of ten Peruvian women had low to moderate autonomy. In addition, children under five years of age of women with low autonomy were more likely to have anemia.

Children under five years of age have high nutritional demands and constitute a high-risk group for anemia, which is the main cause of years lived with disability in this age group [4,12,38]. In Peru, it is estimated that around 30% of children under five years of age suffered from anemia in 2019, a figure higher than the LAC average (21%) [5]. Although the figures are still high, a decreasing trend has been observed in the country in the last decade [5], with the prevalence of childhood anemia having reached 40% in 2010. This reduction is consistent with that reported by a study that identified absolute and relative reductions in the prevalence of anemia in children under 5 years of age in 29 low- and middle-income countries in the period 2000–2018 [39]. In this regard, the presence of low income is common in a large proportion of households in these countries, limiting the purchase of quality food and favoring the consumption of foods with high caloric content but low in micronutrients [40]. In Peru, characteristics related to a low socioeconomic level, as well as inadequate housing conditions and access to basic services, are associated with a greater probability of presenting childhood anemia [41–43]. Likewise, limited access to prenatal checkups, nutritional supplementation and anemia screening may increase the frequency of anemia in Peruvian children [41]. The absence of this type of care could hinder access to preventive anemia messages, as well as timely control and treatment of this condition, further contributing to its high frequency. On the other hand, although various strategies for the prevention of anemia have been implemented at the national level [44], it appears that they have not achieved the desired impact, probably due to the scarce monitoring and strengthening of these strategies, especially in vulnerable populations [45,46]. Furthermore, the design of these interventions does not account for the articulation of the plans of the different ministries involved, making their implementation inefficient [47], in addition to the fact that the multisectoral plan to combat anemia was intended to be valid until 2021, and to date no report has been published [44]. Therefore, there is a need to reevaluate the national anemia reduction strategies so that they are directed at the population at greatest risk and their incidence can be reduced; likewise, their continuity must be guaranteed.

The level of autonomy of the women assessed was found to be worryingly low, with 40% of women presenting low autonomy, while only 10% demonstrated a high level of autonomy. This finding is consistent with that reported in a previous study conducted in Africa in 2020, in which 47% of the women assessed showed low autonomy on a scale that combined four dimensions of autonomy: general, maternal and child health, financial, and social [16]. In addition, the same study showed that only half of the participants had autonomy in the care of their own health and that of their children [16]. A systematic review of studies conducted in low- and middle-income countries also showed that only 55% of women had the autonomy to decide about their own maternal health [48]. These similarities could be largely attributed to the gender roles established in these countries, which reduce women's educational and work opportunities, diminishing their capacity to make decisions in the home [49]. Likewise, characteristics such as older age, higher educational level, urban residence and household income level have been identified as factors associated with women's autonomy in low and middle-income contexts [48]. In Peru, with the support of various national institutions, the Ministry of Women and Vulnerable Populations has implemented policies and programs to promote gender equality and women's empowerment in line with the sustainable development objectives of the United

Nations [50]. It is essential that the progress of these policies be monitored at the national level to assess their impact on women's autonomy.

As a main finding, it was found that women with a lower level of autonomy had a higher probability of having a child with anemia, which coincides with the results of studies carried out in Africa and Asia [22,51]. In contrast, evidence shows that women with a higher level of autonomy and financial stability tend to invest more in household nutrition, which translates into improved nutritional status and growth in children [16,35–37]. In addition, it has been observed that the dimension of autonomy in health-related decisions is a key factor in obtaining positive nutritional outcomes in children [16,36]. This is because mothers with greater autonomy have more access, understanding and awareness of information on child health and nutrition, allowing improved food security in the home [52]. On the other hand, a woman with greater autonomy in health care tends to seek timely and adequate care to prevent, detect and manage her own or her child's health problems [14], which could represent greater probabilities of preventing childhood anemia through hemoglobin screening tests, and the adequate administration of iron and micronutrient supplements. We must acknowledge that the association reported in our study is on the borderline, which prevents us from drawing categorical conclusions about the relationship of interest. Consequently, we recommend further investigation of this association in different populations to ensure the consistency of results.

The public health implications of this research are diverse and require concrete actions. First, it is necessary to strengthen the supervisory bodies responsible for ensuring compliance with national strategies aimed at the prevention and timely, sustained and prolonged treatment of childhood anemia, mainly the Multisectoral Plan to Combat Anemia, the completion date of which was in 2021, and which, at present, has not shown the results of its evaluation [44]. In addition, the Ministry of Health should strengthen its role and provide constant epidemiological surveillance of childhood anemia, with the aim of directing strategies and raising awareness among authorities and the population about the impact of this public health problem on children [53]. Likewise, it is crucial that government entities in our country commit to the fulfillment of Sustainable Development Goals 2, "Zero Hunger", 3, "Health and Well-Being, and 5, "Gender Equality and Women's Empowerment". These goals seek to guarantee food security and access to food for vulnerable populations, ensure the adequate provision of health services, and finally provide the necessary tools to achieve women's autonomy in all areas and defend their rights [54].

The present study has limitations that should be considered when interpreting its results. In the first place, there may be the possibility of information bias, because the women surveyed may have provided erroneous information on the dimensions of women's autonomy for fear of being listened to by their partners or family members, or to fit within socially acceptable standards. On the other hand, enumerators may have made recording errors or omissions when recording information on any of the variables of interest. However, the team that collected the data was trained to perform this task appropriately, minimizing this type of bias. On the other hand, the cross-sectional nature of the study prevents the establishment of cause-and-effect relationships Additionally, there are characteristics of the child (nutritional status, health, or birth characteristics) that have not been included as confounding variables due to their lack of availability and presence of missing values. Despite the limitations identified, there are strengths of the study that should be reported. First, internationally accepted measurement instruments were used to measure the exposure and outcome of interest. Similarly, the ENDES is supported by the DHS, which provides guidance for the application of population-based surveys worldwide. Likewise, the present study provides important evidence on the role of women's autonomy in the anemia status of their children under 5 years of age, with information that allows inferences to be made at the population level.

5. Conclusions

A low level of women's autonomy was associated with a higher probability of anemia in children under 5 years of age. It is necessary to strengthen the promotion of Peruvian women's autonomy in order to empower them to make decisions regarding their children's health care, and thus contribute to the reduction of anemia levels in children. It is also essential to evaluate the impact of anemia prevention and treatment interventions in the country in order to improve their effectiveness and ensure their continuity. The implementation of these strategies can contribute to the fulfillment of the Sustainable Development Goals related to Peruvian women and children.

Author Contributions: R.V.-F. initiated the research idea, designed the study and analyzed the data. All authors participated in the interpretation of the data and the drafting of the manuscript and approved the final version. All authors have read and agreed to the published version of the manuscript.

Funding: This research did not receive any specific grant from funding agencies in the public, commercial or not-for-profit sectors.

Institutional Review Board Statement: Not applicable.

Informed Consent Statement: Not applicable.

Data Availability Statement: Not applicable.

Acknowledgments: We express our gratitude to the Universidad Científica del Sur for their invaluable support in proofreading the manuscript in English and covering the Article Processing Charges.

Conflicts of Interest: The authors declare no conflict of interest.

References

1. Organización de las Naciones Unidas. Objetivo 2: Poner Fin al Hambre—Hambre Cero. Objetivos de DEsarrollo Sostenible. 2022. Available online: https://www.un.org/sustainabledevelopment/es/hunger/ (accessed on 30 January 2023).
2. World Health Organization. Anaemia in Women and Children. The Global Health Observatory. 2021. Available online: https://www.who.int/data/gho/data/themes/topics/anaemia_in_women_and_children (accessed on 30 January 2023).
3. Kassebaum, N.J. The Global Burden of Anemia. *Hematol. Oncol. Clin. N. Am.* **2016**, *30*, 247–308. [CrossRef] [PubMed]
4. Plessow, R.; Arora, N.K.; Brunner, B.; Tzogiou, C.; Eichler, K.; Brügger, U.; Wieser, S. Social Costs of Iron Deficiency Anemia in 6–59-Month-Old Children in India. *PLoS ONE* **2015**, *10*, e0136581. [CrossRef] [PubMed]
5. Banco Mundial. Prevalencia de Anemia en la Infancia (% de Menores de 5 Años). 2019. Available online: https://datos.bancomundial.org/indicador/SH.ANM.CHLD.ZS?end=2019&name_desc=true&start=2000&view=chart (accessed on 30 January 2023).
6. Zavaleta, N.; Astete-Robilliard, L. Effect of anemia on child development: Long-term consequences. *Rev. Peru. Med. Exp. Salud Pública* **2017**, *34*, 716–722. [CrossRef] [PubMed]
7. Safiri, S.; Kolahi, A.-A.; Noori, M.; Nejadghaderi, S.A.; Karamzad, N.; Bragazzi, N.L.; Sullman, M.J.M.; Abdollahi, M.; Collins, G.S.; Kaufman, J.S.; et al. Burden of anemia and its underlying causes in 204 countries and territories, 1990–2019: Results from the Global Burden of Disease Study 2019. *J. Hematol. Oncol.* **2021**, *14*, 185. [CrossRef]
8. World Health Organization (WHO). Nutritional Anaemias: Tools for Effective Prevention. 2017. Available online: https://apps.who.int/iris/bitstream/handle/10665/259425/?sequence=1 (accessed on 18 May 2023).
9. da Silva, L.L.S.; Fawzi, W.W.; Cardoso, M.A. Factors associated with anemia in young children in Brazil. *PLoS ONE* **2018**, *13*, e0204504. [CrossRef]
10. Endris, B.S.; Dinant, G.J.; Gebreyesus, S.H.; Spigt, M. Risk factors of anemia among preschool children in Ethiopia: A Bayesian geo-statistical model. *BMC Nutr.* **2022**, *8*, 2. [CrossRef]
11. Pasqualino, M.M.; Thorne-Lyman, A.L.; Manohar, S.; Kc, A.; Shrestha, B.; Adhikari, R.; Klemm, R.D.; West, K.P. The Risk Factors for Child Anemia Are Consistent across 3 National Surveys in Nepal. *Curr. Dev. Nutr.* **2021**, *5*, nzab079. [CrossRef]
12. Gedfie, S.; Getawa, S.; Melku, M. Prevalence and Associated Factors of Iron Deficiency and Iron Deficiency Anemia Among Under-5 Children: A Systematic Review and Meta-Analysis. *Glob. Pediatr. Health* **2022**, *9*, 2333794X221110860. [CrossRef]
13. Belachew, A.; Tewabe, T. Under-five anemia and its associated factors with dietary diversity, food security, stunted, and deworming in Ethiopia: Systematic review and meta-analysis. *Syst. Rev.* **2020**, *9*, 31. [CrossRef]
14. Osamor, P.E.; Grady, C. Women's autonomy in health care decision-making in developing countries: A synthesis of the literature. *Int. J. Womens Health* **2016**, *8*, 191–202. [CrossRef]
15. Rahman, M.M.; Mostofa, M.G.; Hoque, M.A. Women's household decision-making autonomy and contraceptive behavior among Bangladeshi women. *Sex. Reprod. Healthc.* **2014**, *5*, 9–15. [CrossRef] [PubMed]

16. Saaka, M. Women's decision-making autonomy and its relationship with child feeding practices and postnatal growth. *J. Nutr. Sci.* **2020**, *9*, e38. [CrossRef] [PubMed]
17. Nigatu, D.; Gebremariam, A.; Abera, M.; Setegn, T.; Deribe, K. Factors associated with women's autonomy regarding maternal and child health care utilization in Bale Zone: A community based cross-sectional study. *BMC Womens Health* **2014**, *14*, 79. [CrossRef] [PubMed]
18. Bloom, S.S.; Wypij, D.; Das Gupta, M. Dimensions of women's autonomy and the influence on maternal health care utilization in a north Indian city. *Demography* **2001**, *38*, 67–78. [CrossRef]
19. Doku, D.T.; Bhutta, Z.A.; Neupane, S. Associations of women's empowerment with neonatal, infant and under-5 mortality in low- and /middle-income countries: Meta-analysis of individual participant data from 59 countries. *BMJ Glob. Health* **2020**, *5*, e001558. [CrossRef]
20. Castillo-Guerra, S. Efecto del empoderamiento femenino sobre la nutrición infantil en Colombia. *Soc. Y Econ.* **2019**, *36*, 106–122. [CrossRef]
21. Abreha, S.K.; Zereyesus, Y.A. Women's Empowerment and Infant and Child Health Status in Sub-Saharan Africa: A Systematic Review. *Matern. Child Health J.* **2021**, *25*, 95–106. [CrossRef]
22. Wilunda, C.; Wanjohi, M.; Takahashi, R.; Kimani-Murage, E.; Mutoro, A. Association of women's empowerment with anaemia and haemoglobin concentration in children in sub-Saharan Africa: A multilevel analysis. *Matern. Child Nutr.* **2023**, *19*, e13426. [CrossRef]
23. CEPAL. La Autonomía Económica de las Mujeres en la Recuperación Sostenible Y Con Igualdad. 2021. Available online: https://repositorio.cepal.org/bitstream/handle/11362/46633/S2000740_es.pdf?sequence=5&isAllowed=y (accessed on 18 May 2023).
24. Fondo de Población de Naciones Unidas. Estado de Población Mundial. Estado la Población Mund 2021 Mi Cuerpo Me Perten. 2021. Available online: https://drive.google.com/file/d/1ndu3RByuCsawOwVYLeCcLxexTvpCdgpe/view (accessed on 18 May 2023).
25. Barón-Lozada, F.A.; Basualdo-Meléndez, G.W.; Vargas-Fernández, R.; Hernández-Vásquez, A.; Bendezu-Quispe, G. Women's Autonomy and Intimate Partner Violence in Peru: Analysis of a National Health Survey. *Int. J. Environ. Res. Public Health* **2022**, *19*, 14373. [CrossRef]
26. The World Bank. Prevalence of Anemia Among Children (% of Children Ages 6–59 Months)—Peru. 2019. Available online: https://data.worldbank.org/indicator/SH.ANM.CHLD.ZS?locations=PE (accessed on 18 May 2023).
27. INEI. Encuesta Demográfica y de Salud Familiar-ENDES 2019. 2019. Available online: https://www.inei.gob.pe/media/MenuRecursivo/publicaciones_digitales/Est/Endes2019/ (accessed on 18 May 2023).
28. Ministerio de Salud. Norma Técnica-Manejo Terapéutico Y Preventivo De La Anemia. 2017. Available online: http://www.minsa.gob.pe/ (accessed on 18 May 2023).
29. Instituto Nacional de Estadística e Informática. Metodología de La Medición de La Anemia. 2018. Available online: https://proyectos.inei.gob.pe/endes/2018/documentos_2018/METODOLOGIA_DE_LA_MEDICION_DE_LA_ANEMIA.pdf (accessed on 18 May 2023).
30. Bengesai, A.V.; Khan, H.T.A. Female autonomy and intimate partner violence: Findings from the Zimbabwe demographic and health survey, 2015. *Cult. Health Sex.* **2021**, *23*, 927–944. [CrossRef]
31. Mganga, A.E.; Renju, J.; Todd, J.; Mahande, M.J.; Vyas, S. Development of a women's empowerment index for Tanzania from the demographic and health surveys of 2004–05, 2010, and 2015–16. *Emerg. Themes Epidemiol.* **2021**, *18*, 13. [CrossRef] [PubMed]
32. Rettig, E.M.; Fick, S.E.; Hijmans, R.J. The Female Empowerment Index (FEMI): Spatial and temporal variation in women's empowerment in Nigeria. *Heliyon* **2020**, *6*, e03829. [CrossRef]
33. Asaolu, I.O.; Alaofè, H.; Gunn, J.K.L.; Adu, A.K.; Monroy, A.J.; Ehiri, J.E.; Hayden, M.H.; Ernst, K.C. Measuring Women's Empowerment in Sub-Saharan Africa: Exploratory and Confirmatory Factor Analyses of the Demographic and Health Surveys. *Front. Psychol.* **2018**, *9*, 994. [CrossRef]
34. Wado, Y.D. Women's autonomy and reproductive health-care-seeking behavior in Ethiopia. *Women Health* **2018**, *58*, 729–743. [CrossRef] [PubMed]
35. Wemakor, A.; Awuni, V.; Issah, S. Maternal autonomy but not social support is a predictor of child feeding indicators in the Northern Region, Ghana. *BMC Nutr.* **2022**, *8*, 135. [CrossRef] [PubMed]
36. Komakech, J.J.; Walters, C.N.; Rakotomanana, H.; Hildebrand, D.A.; Stoecker, B.J. The associations between women's empowerment measures, child growth and dietary diversity: Findings from an analysis of demographic and health surveys of seven countries in Eastern Africa. *Matern. Child Nutr.* **2022**, *18*, e13421. [CrossRef] [PubMed]
37. Jones, R.; Haardörfer, R.; Ramakrishnan, U.; Yount, K.M.; Miedema, S.; Girard, A.W. Women's empowerment and child nutrition: The role of intrinsic agency. *SSM—Popul. Health* **2019**, *9*, 100475. [CrossRef]
38. Hernández-Vásquez, A.; Peñares-Peñaloza, M.; Rebatta-Acuña, A.; Farfan, C.A.C.; Bordón-Luján, C.; Santero, M.; Bendezu-Quispe, G. Is anemia a public health problem among children under five years ago in peru? Findings from a national healthcare administrative database (2012 and 2016) using geographic information systems. *Rev. Chil. Nutr.* **2019**, *46*, 718–726. [CrossRef]
39. Sun, J.; Wu, H.; Zhao, M.; Magnussen, C.G.; Xi, B. Prevalence and changes of anemia among young children and women in 47 low- and middle-income countries, 2000–2018. *EClinicalMedicine* **2021**, *41*, 101136. [CrossRef]

40. Kovalskys, I.; Rigotti, A.; Koletzko, B.; Fisberg, M.; Gómez, G.; Herrera-Cuenca, M.; Sanabria, L.Y.C.; García, M.C.Y.; Pareja, R.G.; Zimberg, I.Z.; et al. Latin American consumption of major food groups: Results from the ELANS study. *PLoS ONE* **2019**, *14*, e0225101. [CrossRef]
41. Velásquez-Hurtado, J.E.; Rodríguez, Y.; Gonzáles, M.; Astete-Robilliard, L.; Loyola-Romaní, J.; Vigo, W.E.; Rosas-Aguirre, M. Factors associated with anemia in children under three years of age in Perú: Analysis of the Encuesta Demográfica y de Salud Familiar, ENDES, 2007–2013. *Biomedica* **2016**, *36*, 220–229. [CrossRef]
42. Morocho-Alburqueque, N.; Quincho-Lopez, A.; Nesemann, J.M.; Cañari-Casaño, J.L.; Elorreaga, O.A.; Muñoz, M.; Talero, S.; Harding-Esch, E.M.; Saboyá-Díaz, M.I.; Honorio-Morales, H.A.; et al. Prevalence of and factors associated with childhood anaemia in remote villages of the Peruvian Amazon: A cross-sectional study and geospatial analysis. *Trans. R. Soc. Trop. Med. Hyg.* **2023**, trad018. [CrossRef] [PubMed]
43. Westgard, C.M.; Orrego-Ferreyros, L.A.; Calderón, L.F.; Rogers, A.M. Dietary intake, intestinal infection, and safe drinking water among children with anemia in Peru: A cross-sectional analysis. *BMC Nutr.* **2021**, *7*, 11. [CrossRef] [PubMed]
44. Gobierno del Perú. Plan Multisectorial de Lucha Contra la Anemia 2018–2021. 2018. Available online: https://sdv.midis.gob.pe/Sis_Anemia/Quehacemos/PlanesSectoriales (accessed on 19 April 2023).
45. Berky, A.J.; Robie, E.; Ortiz, E.J.; Meyer, J.N.; Hsu-Kim, H.; Pan, W.K. Evaluation of Peruvian Government Interventions to Reduce Childhood Anemia. *Ann. Glob. Health* **2020**, *86*, 98. [CrossRef]
46. Louzado-Feliciano, P.; Vargas, B.; Dandu, M.; Fuller, S.; Santos, N.; Quiñones, Á.; Martin, H.M.; Caban-Martinez, A.J. A Qualitative Assessment of Mothers' Experience With Pediatric Anemia Care in Arequipa, Peru. *Front. Public Health* **2020**, *8*, 598136. [CrossRef]
47. Informes, S. Intervención del Estado Para la Reducción de la Anemia Infantil: Resultados de la Supervisión Nacional. 2018.
48. Gebeyehu, N.A.; Gelaw, K.A.; Lake, E.A.; Adela, G.A.; Tegegne, K.D.; Shewangashaw, N.E. Women decision-making autonomy on maternal health service and associated factors in low- and middle-income countries: Systematic review and meta-analysis. *Women's Health* **2022**, *18*, 17455057221122618. [CrossRef]
49. ECLAC. Women's Autonomy in Changing Economic Scenarios. January 2020. Available online: https://repositorio.cepal.org/bitstream/handle/11362/45037/S1900722_en.pdf?sequence=4&isAllowed=y (accessed on 18 May 2023).
50. Ministerio de la Mujer y Poblaciones Vulnerables. Política Nacional de Igualdad de Género. 2022.
51. Ray, R. Mother's autonomy and child anemia: A case study from India. *Child. Youth Serv. Rev.* **2020**, *112*, 104537. [CrossRef]
52. Pratley, P. Associations between quantitative measures of women's empowerment and access to care and health status for mothers and their children: A systematic review of evidence from the developing world. *Soc. Sci. Med.* **2016**, *169*, 119–131. [CrossRef]
53. Zavaleta, N. Anemia infantil: Retos y oportunidades al 2021. *Rev. Peru. Med. Exp. Salud Publica* **2017**, *34*, 588–589. [CrossRef]
54. Organizacion de las Naciones Unidas. Objetivos de Desarrollo Sostenible. 2022. Available online: https://www.un.org/sustainabledevelopment/es/objetivos-de-desarrollo-sostenible/ (accessed on 14 April 2023).

nutrients

MDPI

Article

Differences in Nutrient Intake and Diet Quality among Non-Hispanic Black Adults by Place of Birth and Length of Time in the United States

Oluwafikayo S. Adeyemi-Benson [1,*], Alexandra M. Roehll [1], Edson Flores [2] and Chelsea R. Singleton [3]

1 Department of Kinesiology & Community Health, College of Applied Health Sciences, University of Illinois at Urbana-Champaign, Champaign, IL 61820, USA; aroehll2@illinois.edu
2 Department of Kinesiology and Nutrition, University of Illinois at Chicago, Chicago, IL 60612, USA; flore836@umn.edu
3 Department of Social, Behavioral, and Population Sciences, Tulane School of Public Health and Tropical Medicine, New Orleans, LA 70112, USA; csingle1@tulane.edu
* Correspondence: oadey2@illinois.edu; Tel.: +1-(516)-603-0424

Abstract: Prior research suggests that migrating to the United States (US) can negatively affect the diets and health of immigrants. There is limited information on how relocating to the US affects the diets of Black-identifying immigrants. To address this gap, this study examined differences in nutrient intake and diet quality among non-Hispanic Black adults by place of birth and length of time in the US. Cross-sectional data from the National Health and Nutrition Examination Survey (2005–2016) were analyzed. Approximately 6508 non-Hispanic Black adults were categorized into three groups: foreign-born (FB) living in the US <10 years (n = 167), FB living in the US ≥ 10 years (n = 493), and US-born (n = 5848). Multivariable-adjusted logistic and linear regression models were evaluated to identify differences in nutrient intake and diet quality (as measured by the Healthy Eating Index (HEI) of 2015) across the three groups when controlling for socio-demographics. Compared to US-born adults, both FB groups had significantly higher HEI-2015 scores and higher odds of meeting dietary recommendations for several nutrients: saturated fat, sodium, and cholesterol. There were no differences in nutrient intake between the two FB groups; however, FB (<10 years) adults had better diet quality than FB (≥10 years) ones. Place of birth and length of time in the US were associated with dietary intake among non-Hispanic Black adults. More research is needed to improve understanding of dietary acculturation among Black identifying immigrants in the US.

Keywords: acculturation; diet quality; nutrient intake; disparities; non-Hispanic Black; NHANES

1. Introduction

A healthy diet and lifestyle are essential to chronic disease prevention [1]. While dietary preferences and habits can vary substantially between people with different cultural backgrounds, most Americans' diets exceed the recommended intake for saturated fats, sodium, added sugars, and refined grains [2]. Poor diet is a known risk factor for several chronic diseases, including obesity, cardiovascular disease (CVD), strokes, cancer, and type 2 diabetes [3]. Recognizing how poor diet quality and nutrient intake affect the health status of racial/ethnic minorities is an important public health priority in the United States (US) [4]. Despite recently documented improvements to the quality of Americans' diets, not every subpopulation has benefitted [5]. Non-Hispanic Black adults have experienced the least improvement among all racial/ethnic groups [5]. Furthermore, previous studies found that Black adults have less-favorable nutrient intakes, lower adherence to dietary guidelines, and poorer dietary quality compared to their White counterparts [5,6]. These nutritional inequities have great potential to further exacerbate disparities in chronic disease risk by race/ethnicity in the US [4].

Unfortunately, the field's understanding of the diets of Black-identifying populations in the US is limited in scope. Currently, there is limited understanding of differences in dietary practices and preferences among Black adults given their culture and lived experiences. The recent immigration wave of people who self-identify as non-Hispanic Black (i.e., people from African, Caribbean, Central American, or South American nations) underscores the need to expand understanding of the diets of Black adults and children in the US [7,8]. Between 2000 and 2013, the number of Black immigrants in the US increased by 56%, with migration from Africa increasing by 137% [7]. In 2017, there were an estimated four million Caribbean immigrants living in the US [8].

Moving to the US can result in dietary acculturation, which entails changes to an individual's traditional diet that result in alignment with the typical American diet [9]. In general, dietary acculturation has been found to have detrimental effects on the diets of immigrants, which consequently can increase the risk of diet-related chronic diseases among immigrant populations [9]. For example, a prior study found that adapting to the US lifestyle was associated with the loss of cultural culinary preferences and increased the consumption of unhealthy foods among immigrants despite improvements in their socioeconomic status [10]. Several studies have linked acculturation measures to changes in dietary intake in several immigrant populations, including Puerto Rican, South Asian, and Filipino adults [11–13]. Overall, findings from the literature support the hypothesis that relocating to the US can result in significant declines in diet quality.

Given the scarcity of scientific research on the diets of Black-identifying immigrant populations and the growing number of Black immigrants in the US, there is a need to study the differences in nutrient intake and diet quality by place of birth and length of time in the US among Black adults. A prior study reported disparities in diet quality between US-born and foreign-born Black adults, with the former having poorer diet quality [14]. However, the study did not examine diet in relation to the 2015–2020 Dietary Guidelines for Americans (DGAs). Thus, this study aimed to examine differences in nutrient intake and diet quality between US-born and foreign-born (henceforth, FB) non-Hispanic Black adults who participated in the National Health and Nutrition Examination Survey (NHANES). In addition, this study evaluated the role of length of time in the US by examining differences between FB Black adults who migrated to the US fewer than 10 years ago and those who migrated more than 10 years ago. It was hypothesized that FB Black adults (<10 years) would have better diet quality than US-born Black adults; however, FB Black adults (≥10 years) would have diet profiles similar to US-born Black adults. When comparing the FB groups, FB Black adults (<10 years) were expected to have better diet quality than FB Black adults (≥10 years).

2. Materials and Methods

2.1. Data Source

Cross-sectional data collected from participants of the Centers for Disease Control and Prevention's National Health and Nutrition Examination Survey (NHANES) cycles in 2005–2016 were obtained and analyzed. NHANES collects data from a multistage, stratified probability-cluster sample of the non-institutionalized U.S. population [15]. Data on nutrition and health are collected from participants by conducting a series of interviewer-administered questionnaires and physical examinations [15]. A total of 60,936 adults and children participated in the six selected cycles. Individuals who did not self-identify as non-Hispanic Black and were less than <20 years of age (n = 53,863) were excluded from this study, which left 7073 non-Hispanic Black adults. Participants with missing day one 24 h recall data were also excluded (n = 565). Thus, the analytical sample for this study comprised 6508 non-Hispanic Black adults.

Measures representing place of birth (US vs. other) and length of time in the U.S. were used to categorize participants into three distinct groups: FB Black adults who migrated fewer than 10 years ago (n = 167; 3.0%), FB Black adults who migrated more than 10 years ago (n = 493; 7.2%), and US-born Black adults (n = 5848; 89.8%). NHANES collects self-reported information about place of birth and length of time in the US [15]. These two measures are often used as proxy measures of acculturation in studies on the health and health behaviors of immigrant populations in the US [11–14]. Since NHANES does provide separate race and ethnicity data, Black-identifying Hispanics could not be separated from other Hispanic adults. Therefore, the current study only included non-Hispanic Black adults. The National Center for Health Statistics Institutional Review Board (IRB) approved NHANES, and all participants provided written informed consent [15]. The IRB at the University of Illinois at Urbana-Champaign deemed this research exempt.

2.2. Nutrient Intake

Nutrient intake data were examined for all participants included in the analytical sample. The dietary intake interview of NHANES, titled "What We Eat in America", was conducted in partnership with the U.S. Department of Agriculture using a computerized data collection instrument [16]. Each participant was eligible for two days of 24 h recall; the first day was conducted in-person during the initial NHANES interview, while the second day was conducted over the telephone approximately 3–10 days later [16]. As stated above, 6508 non-Hispanic Black adults participating in NHANES 2005–2016 had complete dietary data for the first day; 4867 (69%) had complete data for the second day. Only data from the first day were analyzed since 31% of the sample did not complete the second 24 h dietary recall.

Measures examined included total energy (kcal per day), protein (grams per day), carbohydrates (grams per day), total sugar (grams per day), dietary fiber (grams per day), total fat (grams per day), saturated fat (grams per day), cholesterol (milligrams per day), and sodium (milligrams per day). To identify participants who met recommendations for nutrient intake, participants' consumption levels for each nutrient were compared to the recommended level of intake mentioned in the 2015–2020 Dietary Guidelines for Americans (DGAs) [17]. According to the DGAs, the following are the recommended intake range(s): 20–35% of energy from total fat, 10–35% of energy from protein, 45–65% of energy from carbohydrates, 14 g/1000 kcal/day from fiber, <10% of energy from saturated fat, and <2300 mg/day of sodium [17]. The 2015–2020 DGAs do not have a recommended consumption amount for total sugars and cholesterol. However, the World Health Organization (WHO) recommends that <5% of energy intake should come from added sugar. Thus, total sugar intake was compared to this recommendation to identify the proportion of FB Black adults and U.S.-born Black adults who had a total sugar intake amount of <5% of energy intake [18]. As for the daily recommendation for cholesterol intake, the goal of <300 mg/day was utilized. This goal was included in the prior iteration of the DGAs (2010–2015) [17].

2.3. Diet Quality

The Healthy Eating Index (HEI) is a diet quality index that measures an individual or population's dietary alignment with the DGAs [19,20]. It can be used to assess the conformance of any meal or group of foods to the diet recommendations outlined in the DGAs [19,20]. For the current study, study participants' (n = 6508) day one 24 h recall data were analyzed using the simple HEI scoring algorithm to generate HEI-2015 total and component scores [21]. Since the simple HEI scoring algorithm was used, the HEI-2015 scores presented in this study do not represent usual intake (i.e., long-term intake). Rather, they represent an estimation of how each participant's consumption on day one of the dietary interview aligned with the DGAs.

The HEI-2015 total score ranges from 0 to 100, with 100 indicating perfect alignment. It consists of 13 components, including total fruits, whole fruits, total vegetables, greens and beans, total protein foods, seafood and plant proteins, whole grains, dairy, fatty acids, refined grains, sodium, added sugars, and saturated fats. Total fruits, whole fruits, total protein foods, total vegetables, seafood and plant proteins, and greens and beans all contribute five points each to the total score. The other dietary components all contribute ten points to the total score [19]. Refined grains, sodium, added sugars, and saturated fats are considered measures of moderation; higher consumption of these foods will lower the HEI total score. All others are considered measures of adequacy, so higher consumption of these items will increase HEI total score.

2.4. Other Measures

In addition to nutrient intake and diet quality, the following measures were examined: current age (years), sex (male vs. female), education level (<high school diploma, high school diploma or equivalent, some college, or ≥college degree), marital status (married vs. other), number of people living in the household, poverty-to-income ratio (PIR), and day of the week the 24 h recall interview was completed. These socio-demographic measures were obtained via the interviewer-administered questionnaires. NHANES investigators estimated each participant's PIR from their self-reported annual income. The PIR represents the ratio of an individual's annual household income to the federal poverty level for their household size the year the NHANES interview was conducted [22]. Days of the week for the recall interview were categorized to compare participants who had their interviews on the weekend (Friday–Sunday) to participants who had interviews on a weekday (Monday–Thursday).

2.5. Statistical Analysis

To examine the characteristics of the analytical sample, descriptive statistics were calculated (i.e., weighted means and frequencies). Analysis of variance (ANOVA) and chi-square tests were used to identify differences in socio-demographic measures across the three groups representing acculturation: FB Black adults (<10 years), FB Black adults (≥10 years), and U.S.-born Black adults. The weighted mean intake of each nutrient among the three groups and the weighted percentage of participants in the groups who met the dietary recommendations for each nutrient were calculated. Logistic regression was used to determine if the odds of meeting dietary recommendations for nutrient intake were significantly different among the three acculturation groups. Models were run to compare (1) both groups of FB Black adults to US-born Black adults and (2) FB Black adults (<10 years) to FB Black adults (≥10 years).

Linear regressions were used to examine the association differences in HEI-2015 total scores between the three acculturation groups and both groups of FB Black adults. The unadjusted model included only the variables representing the three groups. The adjusted model also included the variables of age, sex, education level, marital status, PIR, number of household members, and day of the week of the 24 h recall interview. These socio-demographic variables were included because prior research has shown they are associated with dietary intake [23]. Confidence intervals that did not include the null value of 1.0 and had p values < 0.05 were considered statistically significant. All analyses were conducted by using SAS version 9.4 [24]. Since NHANES employs a complex sampling scheme, appropriate sampling weights were applied to the descriptive statistics and regression analyses.

3. Results

Descriptive statistics stratified by the three groups are presented in Table 1. Among the 6508 non-Hispanic Black adults, the mean age was 44.6, 44.3% were male, and 17.6% had ≥college degree. Most of the study participants (65.8%) reported a marital status other than "married". Participants had three household members on average and a poverty-to-income ratio of 2.3. Significant demographic differences were observed across the three groups for every measure of interest except the PIRs. A higher percentage of FB Black adults (≥10 years) had ≥college degree compared to the FB Black adults (<10 years) and US-born Black adults, and a higher percentage of FB Black adults (<10 years) reported being married compared to the other two groups.

Table 1. Demographic characteristics of study participants stratified by foreign-born status and length of time in the US, *n* (%) or mean (±SE) [a,b,c].

Characteristic:	All Participants $n = 6508$ [d,e]	Foreign-Born (<10 years) 167 (3.0%)	Foreign-Born (≥10 years) 493 (7.23%)	US-Born 5848 (89.76%)	*p* Value [f]
Age, years	44.6 (0.3)	36.5(1.1)	47.4 (0.7)	44.6 (0.4)	0.0006
Sex:					0.002
Male	3123 (44.3)	96 (56.9)	249 (46.6)	2778 (43.7)	
Female	3385 (55.7)	71 (43.1)	244 (53.4)	3070 (56.3)	
Education Level:					0.0001
<High School	1569 (21.6)	33 (19.2)	98 (16.2)	1438 (22.1)	
HS or Equivalent	1687 (25.8)	34 (22.5)	92 (18.1)	1561 (26.5)	
Some College	2159 (35.0)	53 (30.9)	167 (36.1)	1939 (35.0)	
≥College Degree	1087 (17.6)	47 (27.5)	134 (29.6)	906 (16.3)	
Marital Status:					0.0001
Married	2350 (34.2)	89 (51.8)	250 (48.8)	2011 (32.5)	
Other	4154 (65.8)	78 (48.2)	243 (51.2)	3833 (67.5)	
Number of Household Members	3.1 (0.0)	3.6 (0.2)	3.2 (0.1)	3.1 (0.0)	0.0001
Poverty-to-Income Ratio	2.3 (0.1)	2.1 (0.1)	2.7 (0.1)	2.3 (0.1)	0.11

[a] NHANES, National Health and Nutrition Examination Survey. [b] SE, Standard Error. [c] Data Source: National Health and Nutrition Examination Survey. [d] Cell counts may not total to sample size because of missing data. [e] Percentages may not total to 100 because of rounding. [f] *p* values determined by χ^2 test or analysis of variance (ANOVA), with $p < 0.05$ considered statistically significant.

Descriptive information on nutrient intake is displayed in Table 2. Less than 3% of participants in all three groups met the intake recommendations for dietary fiber, and less than 4% met recommendations for total sugar intake. Less than 16% of participants in all three groups met the intake recommendation for sodium. While ≥60% of foreign-born adults met intake recommendations for saturated fat, only 43% of US-born adults met the saturated fat recommendation.

Results from the logistic regression models examining associations between foreign-born status, length of time in the US, and odds of meeting recommendations for nutrient intake are displayed in Table 3. The unadjusted logistic regression models indicated that FB Black adults (<10 years) had greater odds of meeting the dietary recommendations for saturated fat and carbohydrates than US-born Black adults. FB Black adults (≥10 years) had greater odds of meeting the dietary recommendations for total fat, saturated fat, protein, and cholesterol compared to US-born Black adults. After adjusting for age, sex, education level, marital status, PIR, number of household members, and day of the week, FB Black adults (<10 years) had significantly higher odds of meeting the dietary recommendations for saturated fat (odds ratio (OR), 2.74; 95% CI, 1.62–4.63), protein (OR, 1.84; 95% CI, 1.01–3.34), carbohydrates (OR, 1.71; 95% CI, 1.17–2.49), cholesterol (OR, 1.71; 95% CI, 1.16–2.52), and sodium (OR, 2.19, 95% CI = 1.16–4.14) than US-born Black adults. FB Black adults (≥10 years) had significantly higher odds of meeting dietary recommendations for total fat (OR, 1.65; 95% CI, 1.34–2.04), saturated fat (OR, 2.24; 95% CI, 1.77–2.83), cholesterol (OR, 1.56, 95% CI, 1.22–1.99), and sodium (OR, 1.57; 95% CI, 1.11–2.20) than US-born Black adults. When comparing the two groups of FB Black adults, no significant differences in the odds of meeting nutrient intake recommendations were detected, except for carbohydrates. After adjusting for covariates, FB Black adults (<10 years) had higher odds of meeting the carbohydrate recommendation (OR, 1.63; 95% CI, 1.24–2.13).

Table 2. Descriptive information on nutrient intake by foreign-born status and length of time in the US [a].

Nutrient:	Mean Intake (SE) [b]	Recommended Intake	% Meeting Guideline
Total Energy Intake, kcal			
Foreign Born (<10 years)	1883 (65)	—	—
Foreign Born (≥10 years)	1876 (63)		
US Born	2164 (21)		
Total Fat, g [c]			
Foreign Born (<10 years)	61.9 (3.4)	20–35% of energy	51.1
Foreign Born (≥10 years)	64.7 (2.7)		56.3
US Born	84.4 (0.1)		44.7
Saturated Fat, g			
Foreign Born (<10 years)	20.0 (1.2)	<10% of energy	66.4
Foreign Born (≥10 years)	20.3 (1.0)		64.1
US Born	26.6 (0.3)		43.2
Protein, g			
Foreign Born (<10 years)	77.9 (2.8)	10–35% of energy	91.4
Foreign Born (≥10 years)	77.1 (2.2)		90.3
US Born	80.0 (0.8)		85.9
Dietary Fiber, g			
Foreign Born (<10 years)	15.8 (0.9)	14 g/1000 kcal	1.8
Foreign Born (≥10 years)	16.8 (0.5)		2.9
US Born	13.8 (0.2)		2.3
Carbohydrates, g			
Foreign Born (<10 years)	252.2 (9.2)	45–65% of energy	65.9
Foreign Born (≥10 years)	241.9 (8.7)		60.3
US Born	257.5 (2.6)		55.4
Total Sugars, g			
Foreign Born (<10 years)	96.2 (4.6)	<5% of energy [d]	3.4
Foreign Born (≥10 years)	101.4 (4.2)		3.1
US Born	123.0 (1.7)		3.6
Cholesterol, mg			
Foreign Born (<10 years)	254.6 (16.0)	<300 mg [e]	68.3
Foreign Born (≥10 years)	259.4 (13.6)		70.9
US Born	314.4 (3.7)		60.1
Sodium, mg			
Foreign Born (<10 years)	3011.9 (140.0)	<2300 mg [e]	15.2
Foreign Born (≥10 years)	2975.0 (107.6)		13.6
US Born	3444.5 (33.0)		10.5

[a] NHANES, National Health and Nutrition Examination Survey. [b] SE, standard error. [c] g, grams. [d] Recommended intake of added sugars from the World Health Organization. [e] mg, milligrams.

Table 3. Results from logistic regression models examining associations between foreign-born status, length of time in the U.S., and odds of meeting national recommendations for nutrient intake [a].

Nutrient:	Odds Ratio (95% CI) [b]		Odds Ratio (95% CI)	
	Unadjusted [c]	Adjusted [d]	Unadjusted [c]	Adjusted [d]
Total Energy Intake				
Foreign Born (<10 years)				
Foreign Born (≥10 years)	—	—	—	—
US Born				
Total Fat				
Foreign Born (<10 years)	1.29 (0.87–1.92)	1.49 (0.93–2.38)	0.81 (0.57–1.16)	1.11 (0.74–1.67)
Foreign Born (≥10 years)	1.60 (1.33–1.91)	1.65 (1.34–2.04)	REF	REF
US Born	REF [e]	REF	-	-
Saturated Fat				
Foreign Born (<10 years)	2.60 (1.58–4.26)	2.74 (1.62–4.63)	1.10 (0.73–1.66)	1.33(0.93–1.89)
Foreign Born (≥10 years)	2.35 (1.88–2.94)	2.24 (1.77–2.83)	REF	REF
US Born	REF	REF	-	-
Protein				
Foreign Born (<10 years)	1.76 (0.97–3.19)	1.84 (1.01–3.34)	1.14 (0.66–1.99)	1.14 (0.73–1.77)
Foreign Born (≥10 years)	1.54 (1.08–2.20)	1.36 (0.94–1.96)	REF	REF
US Born	REF	REF	-	-
Dietary Fiber				
Foreign Born (<10 years)	0.79 (0.29–2.17)	0.93 (0.32–2.71)	0.62 (0.19–2.01)	0.78 (0.17–3.53)
Foreign Born (≥10 years)	1.27 (0.63–2.55)	1.27 (0.60–2.74)	REF	REF
US Born	REF	REF	-	-
Carbohydrates				
Foreign Born (<10 years)	1.56 (1.10–2.19)	1.71 (1.17–2.49)	1.27 (0.94–1.73)	1.63 (1.24–2.13)
Foreign Born (≥10 years)	1.22 (0.98–1.53)	1.19 (0.95–1.50)	REF	REF
US Born	REF	REF	-	-
Total Sugars				
Foreign Born (<10 years)	0.95 (0.31–2.92)	1.10 (0.33–3.66)	1.09 (0.35–3.37)	0.90 (0.27–3.09)
Foreign Born (≥10 years)	0.88 (0.44–1.76)	1.07 (0.54–2.14)	REF	REF
US Born	REF	REF	-	-
Cholesterol				
Foreign Born (<10 years)	1.43 (0.96–2.13)	1.71 (1.16–2.52)	0.89 (0.59–1.32)	0.95 (0.68–1.32)
Foreign Born (≥10 years)	1.62 (1.29–2.03)	1.56 (1.22–1.99)	REF	REF
US Born	REF	REF	-	-
Sodium				
Foreign Born (<10 years)	1.52 (0.92–2.51)	2.19 (1.16–4.14)	1.14 (0.68–1.92)	1.32 (0.77–2.27)
Foreign Born (≥10 years)	1.33 (0.96–1.84)	1.57 (1.11–2.20)	REF	REF
US Born	REF	REF	-	-

[a] NHANES, National Health and Nutrition Examination Survey. [b] CI, confidence interval. [c] The unadjusted model with only the variable(s) representing foreign-born status and/or length of time in the US. [d] Model adjusted for age, sex, education level, marital status, poverty level, number of household members, and day of the week. [e] REF, reference group.

Table 4 presents results from linear regression models assessing associations between foreign-born status, length of time in the US, and HEI-2015 total score. The mean HEI-2015 total scores were 54.6 for FB Black adults (<10 years), 56.3 for FB Black adults (≥10 years), and 47.8 for US-born Black adults. Compared to US-born Black adults, FB Black adults (≥10 years) [β = 8.5; standard error [SE] = 0.7; p = 0.0001] and FB Black adults (<10 years) [β = 6.8; SE = 1.2; p = 0.0001] had higher HEI-2015 total scores. The significance was retained after adjusting for age, sex, education level, marital status, PIR, number of household members, and day of the week. When comparing the groups of FB Black adults, the unadjusted model yielded no significant results. However, the adjusted model indicated that FB adults (<10 years) had a higher HEI-2015 total scores than FB (≥10 years) after adjusting for all covariates [β = 2.6; SE = 0.7; p = 0.0004].

Table 4. Results from linear regression models examining the association between foreign-born status, length of time in the US, and HEI-2015 total score [a,b].

Group:	Mean Score (SE)	β (SE) [*p* Value] [c,d]		β (SE) [*p* Value]	
		Unadjusted [e]	Adjusted [f]	Unadjusted [e]	Adjusted [f]
Foreign Born (<10 years)	54.6 (1.2)	6.8 (1.2) [<0.0001]	8.9 (1.3) [<0.0001]	−1.7 (1.4) [0.23]	2.6 (0.7) [0.004]
Foreign Born (≥10 years)	56.3 (0.7)	8.5 (0.7) [<0.0001]	7.3 (0.7) [<0.0001]	REF	REF
US Born	47.8 (0.2)	REF [g]	REF	-	-

[a] HEI, Healthy Eating Index. [b] NHANES, National Health and Nutrition Examination Survey. [c] Coefficient estimate. [d] SE, standard error. [e] The unadjusted model with only the variable(s) representing foreign-born status and/or length of time in the US. [f] Model adjusted for age, sex, education level, marital status, poverty level, number of household members, and day of the week. [g] REF, reference group.

4. Discussion

This study aimed to determine if acculturation, place of birth, and length of time in the US are associated with nutrient intake and diet quality among non-Hispanic Black adults who participated in NHANES. It was hypothesized that FB Black adults who migrated to America fewer than 10 years ago would have better diet quality than US-born Black adults and FB Black adults who migrated 10 years ago or more. Overall, the findings from this study supported the hypothesis that FB Black adults (<10 years) had better diet quality than US-born Black adults. However, FB Black adults who migrated more than 10 years ago also had better diet quality than US-born Black adults. This finding does not align with the hypothesis that FB Black adults who have been in the US for more than 10 years would have diets similar to US-born Black adults. It appears that FB Black adults, regardless of their length of time in the US, had better diets than US-born Black adults. When comparing the FB groups, the odds of meeting nutrient recommendations were similar between the groups; however, the estimates from the linear regression model revealed that FB Black adults (<10 years) had slightly higher diet quality scores than FB Black adults (≥10 years).

Unlike studies that focused on Latino and Asian immigrants [11–13,25–27], FB Black adults had better diet quality than US-born ones, regardless of the year they migrated to America. This finding aligns with results from a study by Brown et al., which reported that being foreign-born is associated with significantly higher diet quality scores (as measured by the Alternative HEI-2010 and DASH scores) and greater intake of healthier foods (e.g., fruits, vegetables) among Black adults in the US [14]. Brown et al. also concluded that diet quality did vary significantly by length of time in the US among FB Black adults. Thus, it is possible that length of time in the US is not associated with dietary intake among foreign-born adults who self-identify as non-Hispanic Black in the same manner as immigrants from other regions of the world.

Evidence from qualitative studies provides more in-depth information on the relationship between the measures that represent acculturation and dietary intake among immigrants of African descent. Paxton et al. found that West-African immigrants living in New York, NY, reported strong efforts to maintain their traditional diets over time, which typically comprised fruits, vegetables, and grains [28]. However, they found it difficult to maintain this diet in their new environment. The participants did see evidence of dietary acculturation among their children [28], which aligns with findings from a study by Jakub et al. [29]. Jakub et al. discovered that the children of African immigrants had diets closer in profile to American youth and were more influenced by their peers and environment [29]. It is possible that Black adults who migrate to the US try hard to maintain their traditional diets over time, and the effects of dietary acculturation are more evident in their children. Given the limited number of quantitative studies on this topic, additional research is needed to confirm these findings and connect behavioral factors (e.g., cooking practices, food-purchasing habits, food preferences, etc.) to dietary outcomes among FB Black adults and their children.

As previously mentioned, prior studies have linked measures that represent acculturation, such as length of time in the US, to poorer dietary quality among immigrant populations [11–13,25–27]. A study by Thomson et al. reported that acculturation was associated with poorer dietary quality and higher body mass indexes among Mexican immigrants in the US [25]. It is likely that acculturation influences diet and health differently across immigrant populations in the US. Greater emphasis and study should be devoted to assessing these differences and their connection to racial/ethnic disparities in dietary behavior and chronic disease risk.

Overall, it is important to note that all three groups had large proportions of individuals who were not meeting national nutrient recommendations. For example, a small percentage of participants in all three groups met recommendations for intake of dietary fiber, total sugars, and sodium. These findings align with evidence from population-based studies of nutrient intake and adherence to dietary recommendations that focused on non-Hispanic Black adults [5,6,23,30]. A study by Thompson et al., which examined differences in nutrient intake between non-Hispanic White and Black men living in the U.S., found that less than 5% of men met the recommendations for dietary fiber and total sugar intake [30]. Furthermore, a recent "What We Eat in America" assessment of usual intake among non-Hispanic Black adults reported that most Black adults in the US surpass national recommendations for sodium intake [31]. Meeting national recommendations for nutrient intake is important, as scientific evidence indicates strong associations between saturated fat, dietary cholesterol, sodium, and CVD [32]. Since Black Americans experience high prevalence rates of many CVD risk factors (e.g., obesity, metabolic syndrome, type 2 diabetes, and high blood pressure), it is important that the field identifies factors that influence dietary intake, such as acculturation [7,33–35].

Strengths and Limitations

This study has strengths and limitations. Use of the nationwide NHANES dataset was a strength because it included a large, diverse sample of non-Hispanic Black adults. In addition, use of HEI-2015 was a strength because it directly measured how an individual's diet aligned with the DGAs. Key limitations included the low sample size for FB Black adults (<10 years), which might have affected ability to observe statistically significant findings for some dietary measures. This study employed a cross-sectional design, so causal associations could not be studied. Because a significant number of study participants had missing data for the second 24 h recall interview, only data from the first recall interview were analyzed. Thus, HEI-2015 scores reflecting usual intake were not calculated. All findings on nutrient intake and diet quality solely reflect the consumption reported by participants on the first day of the dietary interview. As previously mentioned, the inability to examine Black-identifying Hispanic adults was a limitation. Individuals included in the analytical sample solely reflect non-Hispanic Black adults living in the US. Future studies should include Black Hispanic adults, which likely includes individuals from Latin America and the Caribbean with diverse cultural backgrounds.

The primary independent variables (i.e., foreign-born status and length of time in the US) were a major limitation of this study for two key reasons. First, these variables are only proxy measures of acculturation. Although used in prior research, they do not capture the full extent and experience of acculturation among immigrant populations [14]. Future studies should use a validated acculturation scale tailored to the target population of interest. Second, these variables only permit a simplistic comparison of foreign-born to US-born Black-identifying adults, which does not capture the generational effects associated with immigration. Studies have found intergenerational differences in dietary change among West-African immigrants, with first-generation West-African adults exhibiting more dietary acculturation compared to their immigrant parents [36]. NHANES data do not provide data to determine their generational status. In addition, the data source does not have information on ancestry, cultural beliefs, family dynamics (e.g., gender roles, cooking behaviors), or relevant environmental factors (e.g., urban/rural status, access to healthy food retailers, etc.). Having this information would have facilitated a more in-depth analysis of dietary differences between foreign-born and US-born Black adults that accounted for the complexity of these associations and the historical diversity of these groups. Future studies should consider these limitations and conduct qualitative and quantitative research that addresses these gaps in knowledge.

5. Conclusions

In summary, FB Black adults had higher odds of meeting several nutrient recommendations and had better diet quality compared to US-born Black adults, regardless of their length of time in the US. Understanding the similarities and differences among these groups is valuable for developing tailored dietary and lifestyle interventions and decreasing the risk of diet-related chronic diseases among non-Hispanic Black adults in the US. The lived experience of Black-identifying adults that migrate to US should be studied in relation to dietary intake. Although length of time in the US appears to not be a salient factor, there may be other factors that may be relevant the dietary behaviors of foreign-born Black adults: stress, underemployment, racial discrimination, economic expectations from family/community back home. Overall, this study contributes to the bodies of knowledge about the diets of immigrant populations and differences in the diets of adult immigrants who self-identify as Black in the US. This study provides valuable knowledge to the field on diet quality and nutrient intake among non-Hispanic Black immigrants. The results may be useful to nutrition educators and practitioners working to improve the health of this minority population. Additional studies are needed to explore the importance of factors contributing to changes in diet due to acculturation and their overall impact on the health and health behaviors of immigrants who self-identify as non-Hispanic Black in the US.

Author Contributions: Conceptualization, O.S.A.-B. and C.R.S.; methodology, O.S.A.-B. and C.R.S.; formal analysis, O.S.A.-B.; writing—original draft preparation, O.S.A.-B.; writing—review and editing, O.S.A.-B., E.F., A.M.R. and C.R.S. All authors have read and agreed to the published version of the manuscript.

Funding: This research received no external funding.

Institutional Review Board Statement: The Institutional Review Board at the University of Illinois at Urbana-Champaign deemed this research exempt.

Informed Consent Statement: Not applicable.

Data Availability Statement: The data used for this research project are publicly available on the website for the National Health and Nutrition Examination Survey (NHANES): https://www.cdc.gov/nchs/nhanes/index.htm. The data were accessed on 15 December 2019.

Conflicts of Interest: The authors declare no conflict of interest.

References

1. Lagström, H.; Stenholm, S.; Akbaraly, T.; Pentti, J.; Vahtera, J.; Kivimäki, M.; Head, J. Diet quality as a predictor of cardiometabolic disease–free life expectancy: The Whitehall II cohort study. *Am. J. Clin. Nutr.* **2020**, *111*, 787–794. [CrossRef] [PubMed]
2. U.S. Department of Agriculture; U.S. Department of Health and Human Services. Dietary Guidelines for Americans, 2020–2025. Available online: https://www.dietaryguidelines.gov/sites/default/files/2020-12/Dietary_Guidelines_for_Americans_2020-2025.pdf (accessed on 11 February 2022).
3. Fanelli, S.M.; Jonnalagadda, S.S.; Pisegna, J.L.; Kelly, O.J.; Krok-Schoen, J.L.; Taylor, C.A. Poorer Diet Quality Observed among US Adults with a Greater Number of Clinical Chronic Disease Risk Factors. *J. Prim. Care Community Health* **2020**, *11*, 2150132720945898. [CrossRef]
4. Kris-Etherton, P.M.; Petersen, K.S.; Velarde, G.; Barnard, N.D.; Miller, M.; Ros, E.; O'Keefe, J.H.; Williams, K., Sr.; Van Horn, L.; Na, M.; et al. Barriers, Opportunities, and Challenges in Addressing Disparities in Diet-Related Cardiovascular Disease in the United States. *J. Am. Heart Assoc.* **2020**, *9*, e014433. [CrossRef] [PubMed]
5. McCullough, M.L.; Chantaprasopsuk, S.; Islami, F.; Rees-Punia, E.; Um, C.Y.; Wang, Y.; Leach, C.R.; Sullivan, K.R.; Patel, A.V. Association of socioeconomic and geographic factors with diet quality in US adults. *JAMA Netw. Open* **2022**, *5*, e2216406. [CrossRef] [PubMed]
6. Liu, J.; Steele, E.M.; Li, Y.; Karageorgou, D.; Micha, R.; Monteiro, C.A.; Mozaffarian, D. Consumption of ultraprocessed foods and diet quality among US children and adults. *Am. J. Prev. Med.* **2022**, *62*, 252–264. [CrossRef]
7. Anderson, M. A Rising Share of the US Black Population is Foreign Born. Pew Research Center's Social Demographic Trends Project. Available online: https://www.pewresearch.org/social-trends/2015/04/09/a-rising-share-of-the-u-s-black-population-is-foreign-born/ (accessed on 5 September 2020).
8. Zong, J.; Batalova, J. Carribean Immigrants in the United States. Available online: https://www.migrationpolicy.org/article/caribbean-immigrants-united-states-2017 (accessed on 17 October 2021).
9. Dean, J.A.; Gallo, S.; Anderson, A.K. Factors associated with dietary acculturation among international students at the University of Georgia. *J. Am. Coll. Health* **2022**, 1–7. [CrossRef]
10. Van Hook, J.; Quiros, S.; Frisco, M.L.; Fikru, E. It is hard to swim upstream: Dietary acculturation among Mexican-origin children. *Popul. Res. Policy Rev.* **2016**, *35*, 177–196. [CrossRef]
11. Bowen, S.; Hardison-Moody, A.; Cordero Oceguera, E.; Elliott, S. Beyond Dietary Acculturation: How Latina Immigrants Navigate Exclusionary Systems to Feed Their Families. *Soc. Probl.* **2023**, spad013. [CrossRef]
12. Khan, S.A.; Jackson, R.T.; Momen, B. The relationship between diet quality and acculturation of immigrated South Asian American adults and their association with metabolic syndrome. *PLoS ONE* **2016**, *11*, e0156851. [CrossRef]
13. Vargas, P.; Leo-Felix, J. Dietary acculturation among Filipino Americans. *Int. J. Environ. Res. Public Health* **2016**, *13*, 16. [CrossRef]
14. Brown, A.G.; Houser, R.F.; Mattei, J.; Rehm, C.D.; Mozaffarian, D.; Lichtenstein, A.H.; Folta, S.C. Diet quality among US-born and foreign-born non-Hispanic blacks: NHANES 2003–2012 data. *Am. J. Clin. Nutr.* **2018**, *107*, 695–706. [CrossRef] [PubMed]
15. Centers for Disease Control and Prevention. National Health and Nutrition Examination Survey. Available online: https://www.cdc.gov/nchs/nhanes/index.htm (accessed on 13 February 2020).
16. U.S. Department of Agriculture. What We Eat in American (WWEIA) Database. Available online: https://data.nal.usda.gov/dataset/what-we-eat-america-wweia-database (accessed on 17 March 2020).
17. U.S. Department of Agriculture; U.S. Department of Health and Human Services. 2015–2020 Dietary Guidelines for Americans. 8th Edition. Available online: https://health.gov/our-work/nutrition-physical-activity/dietary-guidelines/previous-dietary-guidelines/2015 (accessed on 9 July 2020).
18. World Health Organization. Guideline: Sugars Intake for Adults and Children. Available online: https://www.who.int/publications/i/item/9789241549028 (accessed on 9 July 2020).
19. Reedy, J.; Lerman, J.L.; Krebs-Smith, S.M.; Kirkpatrick, S.I.; Pannucci, T.E.; Wilson, M.M.; Subar, A.F.; Kahle, L.L.; Tooze, J.A. Evaluation of the Healthy Eating Index-2015. *J. Acad. Nutr. Diet.* **2018**, *118*, 1622–1633. [CrossRef] [PubMed]
20. Krebs-Smith, S.M.; Pannucci, T.E.; Subar, A.F.; Kirkpatrick, S.I.; Lerman, J.L.; Tooze, J.A.; Wilson, M.M.; Reedy, J. Update of the Healthy Eating Index: HEI-2015. *J. Acad. Nutr. Diet.* **2018**, *118*, 1591–1602. [CrossRef]
21. National Cancer Institute. Healthy Eating Index: Overview of Methods & Calculations. Available online: https://epi.grants.cancer.gov/hei/hei-methods-and-calculations.html (accessed on 22 October 2020).
22. U.S. Census Bureau. How the Census Bureau Measures Poverty. Available online: https://www.census.gov/topics/income-poverty/poverty/guidance/poverty-measures.html (accessed on 12 November 2021).
23. Zhao, Y.; Araki, T. Diet quality and its associated factors among adults with overweight and obesity: Findings from the 2015–2018 National Health and Nutrition Examination Survey. *Br. J. Nutr.* **2023**, *in press*. [CrossRef]
24. SAS Institute Inc. *SAS/ACCESS®9.4 Interface to ADABAS: Reference*; SAS Institute, Inc.: Cary, NC, USA, 2013.
25. Thomson, J.L.; Landry, A.S.; Walls, T.I. Similarities and Dissimilarities in Diet Quality Differences by Acculturation Level Between Mexican Americans and Other Hispanic Americans: NHANES 2015-2018. *J. Nutr.* **2023**, *in press*.
26. Arandia, G.; Sotres-Alvarez, D.; Siega-Riz, A.M.; Arredondo, E.M.; Carnethon, M.R.; Delamater, A.M.; Gallo, L.C.; Isasi, C.R.; Marchante, A.N.; Pritchard, D.; et al. Associations between acculturation, ethnic identity, and diet quality among U.S. Hispanic/Latino Youth: Findings from the HCHS/SOL Youth Study. *Appetite* **2018**, *129*, 25–36. [CrossRef] [PubMed]

27. Yoshida, Y.; Scribner, R.; Chen, L.; Broyles, S.; Phillippi, S.; Tseng, T.S. Role of Age and Acculturation in Diet Quality among Mexican Americans-Findings From the National Health and Nutrition Examination Survey, 1999–2012. *Prev. Chronic Dis.* **2017**, *14*, E59. [CrossRef] [PubMed]
28. Paxton, A.; Pillai, A.; Phelan, K.P.Q.; Cevette, N.; Bah, F.; Akabas, S. Dietary Acculturation of Recent Immigrants from West Africa to New York City. Available online: https://journals.openedition.org/faceaface/1023 (accessed on 2 December 2020).
29. Jakub, K.E.; Turk, M.T.; Fapohunda, A.; Zoucha, R. Cultural beliefs, perceptions, and practices of young adult offspring of African immigrants regarding healthy eating and activity. *J. Transcult. Nurs.* **2018**, *29*, 548–554. [CrossRef]
30. Thompson, T.L.; Singleton, C.R.; Springfield, S.E.; Thorpe, R.J., Jr.; Odoms-Young, A. Differences in nutrient intake and diet quality between non-Hispanic black and non-Hispanic white men in the United States. *Public Health Rep.* **2020**, *135*, 334–342. [CrossRef] [PubMed]
31. U.S. Department of Agriculture. What We Eat in America: Usual Nutrient Intake from Food and Beverages among Non-Hispanic Black Individuals (NHANES 2015–2018). Available online: https://www.ars.usda.gov/ARSUserFiles/80400530/pdf/usual/Usual_Intake_Non_Hispanic_Black_WWEIA_2015_2018.pdf (accessed on 23 February 2022).
32. Bowen, K.J.; Sullivan, V.K.; Kris-Etherton, P.M.; Petersen, K.S. Nutrition and Cardiovascular Disease—An Update. *Curr. Atheroscler. Rep.* **2018**, *20*, 8. [CrossRef]
33. Obichi, C.C.; Dee, V. Acculturation, Cultural Beliefs, and Cardiovascular Disease Risk Levels among Nigerian, Ghanaian and Cameroonian Immigrants in the United States. *J. Immigr. Minor. Health* **2022**, *24*, 1154–1160. [CrossRef] [PubMed]
34. Lopez-Neyman, S.M.; Davis, K.; Zohoori, N.; Broughton, K.S.; Moore, C.E.; Miketinas, D. Racial disparities and prevalence of cardiovascular disease risk factors, cardiometabolic risk factors, and cardiovascular health metrics among US adults: NHANES 2011–2018. *Sci. Rep.* **2022**, *12*, 19475. [CrossRef] [PubMed]
35. Almoussa, M.; Mattei, J. Cardiovascular health and risk factors in African refugees and immigrants in the United States: A narrative review. *Ethn. Health* **2023**, *28*, 399–412. [CrossRef]
36. Horlyck-Romanovsky, M.F.; Huang, T.; Ahmed, R.; Echeverria, S.E.; Wyka, K.; Leung, M.M.; Sumner, A.E.; Fuster, M. Intergenerational differences in dietary acculturation among Ghanaian immigrants living in New York City: A qualitative study. *J. Nutr. Sci.* **2021**, *10*, e80. [CrossRef] [PubMed]

nutrients

MDPI

Article

Food Insecurity and Associated Factors among Households in Maputo City

Elias M. A. Militao [1,2,3,*], Olalekan A. Uthman [4,5], Elsa M. Salvador [3], Stig Vinberg [1] and Gloria Macassa [1,2,6,*]

1 Department of Health Sciences, Faculty of Humanities, Mid Sweden University, Holmgatan 10, 851 70 Sundsvall, Sweden; stig.vinberg@miun.se
2 Department of Public Health and Sports Science, Faculty of Occupational and Health Sciences, University of Gävle, Kungsbacksvägen 47, 801 76 Gävle, Sweden
3 Department of Biological Sciences, Faculty of Science, Eduardo Mondlane University, 3453 Julius Nyerere Avenue, Maputo 257, Mozambique; elsamariasalvador@gmail.com
4 Warwick Centre for Global Health, Division of Health Sciences, Warwick Medical School, University of Warwick, Coventry CV4 7AL, UK; olalekan.uthman@warwick.ac.uk
5 Department of Global Health, Division of Epidemiology and Biostatistics, Faculty of Health Sciences, Stellenbosch University, Francie van Zijl Drive, Cape Town 7505, South Africa
6 EPI Unit—Instituto de Saúde Pública, Universidade do Porto, Rua das Taipas 135, 4050-600 Porto, Portugal
* Correspondence: elias.militao@miun.se (E.M.A.M.); gloria.macassa@hig.se (G.M.)

Abstract: Food insecurity (FI) is a global concern and is one of the main causes of malnutrition in low- and middle-income countries. In Mozambique, the burden of FI and how various factors contribute to FI is not well known. This study aimed to investigate the prevalence of FI and its associated factors in southern Mozambique. Data from 1842 household heads in Maputo City were analyzed in a cross-sectional design. Food insecurity was measured using a modified version of the US Department of Agriculture Household Food Security scale, and its association with socio-demographic factors was assessed through multiple regressions. Altogether, 79% of the households were food insecure; of these, 16.6% had mild FI, 28.1% moderate and 34.4% severe FI. The study revealed that low-income households, those with less educated heads, and those engaged in informal work were significantly more prone to FI. Likewise, dietary diversity and the number of meals were also significant predictors of FI. These findings suggest the need for decent work and job creation, which calls for joint efforts from government, the private sector, and international institutions. Furthermore, these key drivers should be considered in the development of public health policies and programs designed to alleviate household FI and malnutrition in Mozambique.

Keywords: associated factors; food insecurity; prevalence; southern Mozambique

1. Introduction

Food insecurity (FI) is a global concern and a visible reality for most people in low- and middle-income countries (LMICs) [1], and has become an urgent public health issue that affects nourishment, health, and human well-being worldwide [2,3]. Food insecurity is defined as "a limited or uncertain availability of nutritionally adequate or safe foods or limited or uncertain ability to acquire food in socially acceptable ways" [4,5]. Others describe FI as a set of situations in which households compromise on the quality and variety or quantity of food as a consequence of deficient household resources and/or inability to afford food [3].

According to a report by FAO et al. [1] (pp. 14–15), about 768 million people worldwide (9.8% of the world's total population) are undernourished. Of these, 760 million are in developing countries, of whom 278 million live on the African continent and 261 million in Sub-Saharan Africa (SSA). Within SSA, Southern Africa emerges with a more favorable scenario while the Central appears with the worst picture, though the highest burden in numbers remains in the Eastern Africa region [1]. In addition, estimates indicate that about 2.3 billion people (29.3% of the global population) are moderately or severely food insecure. The number of undernourished people worldwide has increased, highlighting the challenge of achieving the United Nations' Sustainable Development Goal (SDG) of Zero Hunger, eradicating FI and all forms of malnutrition by 2030. In fact, projections indicate that nearly 670 million people will still face hunger in 2030, and currently, the number of people unable to afford a healthy diet has risen dramatically, especially because of conflicts, climate change and the COVID-19 pandemic [1]. The Russia–Ukraine war, the COVID-19 pandemic, along with climate change reinforce the need to rethink future actions towards global food security (FS) and nutrition, especially concerning staple foods [6,7]. Research evidence suggests that household FS and nutrition in many LMICs is much worse due to these factors combined with deficient socioeconomic and political conditions [1,6,8]. To this end, government policies along with agricultural investments (e.g., tax and tariff reductions, fertilizer subsidies, and rural infrastructure) are critical factors to protect domestic consumers and producers from rise in reference (border) price for imported food and agricultural inputs while ensuring that policy actions and investments needed for long-term agricultural development are not jeopardized, especially in African countries [9–11]. Likewise, rapid population growth is a serious challenge that needs to be considered when addressing global food security and nutrition [12,13].

In Mozambique, FI continues to be the primary challenge to economic growth and human well-being [14]. According to FAO [15], Mozambique is a low-income, high-inequality and food-deficit country with a largely rural population of 28 million. It ranked 181st out of 189 countries in the 2020 Human Development Index, 106th out of 116 in the 2021 Global Hunger Index and 127th out of 162 in the 2019 Gender Inequality Index [16]. The country achieved some progress under Millennium Development Goals target 1C of halving the number of undernourished people, but significant challenges remain that will hinder progress towards the targets of SDGs 2 [17]. About 80% of the Mozambican population cannot afford an adequate diet [18] and almost 60% live in extreme poverty [19]. Most households are at risk of FI and of adopting negative coping strategies [17,20]. Furthermore, Mozambique is prone to regular droughts, and floods occur virtually every year in large watersheds and poorly drained urban settlements. Roughly 70% of the rural population depends on subsistence agriculture, the markets are not integrated and post-harvest losses reach 30% due to limitations in storage, processing and handling [17,21]. However, the extent and severity of FI in general, as well as its associated factors, are not well known. Some reports suggest poverty, food unavailability, inadequate food intake and a non-diversified diet, high levels of infectious disease, poor knowledge of healthy foods, inadequate food preparation and eating habits as the underlying causes of undernourishment among the population [14,22]. A study by McCordic et al. [23] found female headship to be strongly linked to household FI, even though the degree of this relationship was somewhat dependent on employment and education. This study sought to investigate the prevalence of and factors associated with household FI in Maputo City, southern Mozambique.

2. Materials and Methods

2.1. Study Setting and Sampling

A cross-sectional study was conducted in Maputo, southern Mozambique. Maputo is the capital city of Mozambique and is divided into seven municipal districts that include KaNyaka Island and Katembe across the bay [24]. Maputo is the largest urban agglomeration in Mozambique. The city has a high level of underemployment, with most people being engaged in informal work [25]. Its urban landscape is usually divided into three areas. The first, the KaMpfumu district, is the wealthiest area of the city. The second consists of the poorer residential suburbs and covers Nlhamankulu and KaMaxaquene. The third covers the peri-urban districts of KaMavota and KaMubukwana [24]. According to the 2017 general census, Maputo has about 1,080,277 inhabitants (52% female and 48% male) and 235,750 households [26]. About 71% of the households are food insecure [23].

The selection of households included in this study relied on a two-stage design inspired by the National Institute of Statistics platform which was used by the Technical Secretariat for Food Security and Nutrition (SETSAN) in their 2013 Baseline Study [27]. Therefore, enumeration areas (located in a suburb or peri-urban district of Maputo) were randomly selected in the first stage. A total of 96 enumeration areas were selected, and each enumeration area provided a maximum of 20 households. Next, households within each enumeration area were selected using a systematic random sampling strategy (to sample every fifteenth household). Households whose heads (or other representative household members) did not meet the age criterion (18–60 years), or that did not agree to participate or decided to drop out were excluded from the study. In collaboration with the municipality, eligible households were approached and informed about the objectives and voluntary nature of the study. They were invited to participate and had up to 5 days to respond to the invitation letter. The total sample size was 1842 households based on approximate proportional allocation.

2.2. Data Collection and Procedure

Face-to-face structured interviews were performed at each participant's home between November 2021 and June 2022. Each interview lasted about 45–60 min. Data from households were collected using a questionnaire previously validated in Portuguese speaking populations [28–30] but adapted to the Mozambican context. The questionnaire consisted of eight items from the United States Department of Agriculture Household Food Security Survey Module (USDA HFSSM) designed to measure FI in the last 3 months. In addition, the questionnaire included background demographic and socioeconomic questions (education, work, income) as well as questions about: (a) physical health (diagnosed hypertension and type 2 diabetes); (b) mental health/psychiatric disease; (c) medication and health care utilization; (d) self-reported health; (e) food consumption patterns (dietary items, from oils, vegetables, meat, fish, starch to beverage); (f) barriers to food access; (g) food expenses and purchasing habits; (h) own food production or other ways to obtain food; (i) sleeping patterns; (j) life style/physical activity; and (k) health behavior (smoking and alcohol consumption). Before data collection, the questionnaire was piloted by the authors E.M. and E.S. in Manhiça district (a region outside the study setting) to ensure that it was accurate and effective.

The original, 14-item USDA HFSSM was modified to focus only on adult and household FI by excluding the six items related to children (Table 1). To make the scale easier to use, a "yes/no" response format was adopted. All "yes responses" were followed up by asking, "How often did it occur?", with three response options (often, sometimes, rarely). The responses "often" and "sometimes" were coded as 1, while "rarely" was coded as 0. Consequently, the scale had a maximum of 8 points. Households were considered food secure if they scored 0 or 1 and food insecure if they scored $\geq$2. Among food-insecure households, those that scored 2 or 3 were considered to have mild FI, while those scoring 4–6 were classed as having moderate FI, and scores of 7 or 8 were considered to represent severe FI. Similarly, regarding dietary patterns, three categories were considered (low, medium and high dietary diversity) based on food items consumed in the last 7 days [31]. Low dietary diversity included diets consisting largely of cereals, tubers and roots, vegetables and greens, oils, and fish and other seafood. The medium category added meat or poultry, spices, and eggs to the list. The last category, high dietary diversity, included diets composed of cereals, vegetables and greens, oils, spices and condiments, fish and other seafood, meat or poultry, eggs, fruits, beverages, and dairy products. With regard to occupation, the term "unpaid work" was used to categorize household heads engaged in informal work (insecure employment mostly self-employment), while "paid work" was used to categorize those engaged in formal work (secure employment mostly from the government and the private sector). Finally, both food transfers and money transfers from relatives (largely from South Africa) were considered to constitute remittance in this study.

Table 1. Adapted United States Department of Agriculture Household Food Security Survey Module (USDA HFSSM).

In the last three months:	
1.	Were you worried that your food would run out before you had money or other resources to buy more?
2.	Did you run out of food before you had enough money or other resources to buy more?
3.	Did you have to eat the same foods daily because you did not have money or other resources to buy other foods?
4.	Did you or any other adult in your household cut the size of your/their meals because you did not have enough money or other resources to buy food?
5.	Did you or any other adult in your household skip some of your/their daily meals because you did not have enough money or other resources for food?
6.	Did you ever eat less than you felt you should, because you did not have enough money or other resources to buy food?
7.	Were you ever hungry and did not eat because you did not have money or other resources to buy enough food?
8.	Did you or any other adult in your household ever not eat for a whole day because you did not have enough money or other resources to buy food?

2.3. Data Analysis

All data analyses were performed in IBM SPSS Statistics 27 [32]. Descriptive statistics was carried out and frequencies and percentages were used for categorical variables, and means for continuous variables. Before multiple regression was performed, preliminary analyses were conducted to ensure that the assumptions of normality, linearity, multicollinearity and homoscedasticity had not been violated. Multiple regression was performed to explore the predictive ability of a set of variables to explain the outcome variable (FI score), as well as to assess the relative contribution of each individual variable. Standard multiple regression was then performed to gain a quick insight into which predictors are relevant for explaining FI. Lastly, stepwise multiple regression was employed with all predictors as performed in standard multiple regression to check the consistency between the two techniques. In addition, as households were categorized as food secure versus food insecure, binary logistic regression was performed to explore the predictive power of the same set of variables (used on multiple regression) to explain the outcome variable (FI). A 95% confidence interval and p-value $\leq$0.05 were used to assess the statistical significance of the association between the explanatory variables and the outcome variable.

2.4. Ethical Approval

The study protocol was approved by the Institutional Committee of Bioethics in Health of the Faculty of Medicine, Eduardo Mondlane University, Maputo (registration No. CIBS FM&HCM/036/2019). Informed consent was obtained from each participant prior to the data collection, and all ethical requirements (e.g., voluntariness, confidentiality, anonymity) were followed.

3. Results

3.1. Characteristics of the Study Participants

This study included 1842 households located in Maputo City, representing a participation rate of about 97%. Table 2 illustrates the socio-demographic characteristics of the study population. Most households were male headed (71.6%), had five members, and 66.6% were married or living in marital union. In addition, 45.4% of the heads of households had primary or secondary education, and 48.5% did not have secure employment and were in the informal sector.

Table 2. Descriptive characteristics of the study participants, Maputo City, southern Mozambique.

Variables	Maputo Districts Covered by the Study				
	KaMaxaquene (n = 474)	KaMavota (n = 450)	KaMubukwana (n = 467)	Nlhamankulu (n = 451)	Total (n = 1842)
Head of household					
Male	331 (69.8%)	315 (70%)	316 (67.7%)	356 (78.9%)	1318 (71.6%)
Female	143 (30.2%)	135 (30%)	151 (32.3%)	95 (21.1)	524 (28.4)
Age of participant (mean ± SD)	34.57 ± 9.14	30.91 ± 8.53	32.58 ± 9.61	34.13 ± 8.79	33.05 ± 9.04
Household size (mean ± SD)	4.91 ± 0.9	4.66 ± 0.95	4.74 ± 0.96	4.85 ± 0.91	4.82 ± 0.75
Number of children (mean ± SD)	2.7 ± 0.77	2.41 ± 0.81	2.52 ± 0.86	2.43 ± 0.81	2.54 ± 0.74
Marital status					
Single/separated/divorced	188 (39.7%)	147 (32.7%)	165 (35.3%)	116 (25.7%)	616 (33.4%)
Married/marital union	286 (60.3%)	303 (67.3%)	302 (64.7%)	335 (74.3%)	1226 (66.6%)
Education					
Primary and secondary	200 (42.2%)	202 (44.9%)	221 (47.3%)	214 (47.5%)	837 (45.4%)
High school (Grade 11–12)	210 (44.3%)	182 (40.4%)	202 (43.3%)	168 (37.3%)	762 (41.4%)
University	64 (13.5%)	66 (14.7%)	44 (9.4%)	69 (15.3%)	243 (13.2%)
Type of work					
Unpaid work	233 (49.2%)	211 (46.9%)	229 (49%)	220 (48.8%)	893 (48.5%)
Paid work	241 (50.8%)	239 (53.1%)	238 (51%)	231 (51.2%)	949 (51.5%)
Monthly household income (in MZN)					
<9000	189 (39.9%)	189 (42%)	180 (38.5%)	175 (38.8%)	733 (39.8%)
9000–15,000	160 (33.8%)	139 (30.9%)	184 (39.4%)	151 (33.5%)	634 (34.4%)
>15,000	125 (26.4%)	122 (27.1%)	103 (22.1%)	125 (27.7%)	475 (25.8%)
Remittance from relatives					
No	357 (75.3%)	331 (73.6%)	333 (71.3%)	339 (75.2%)	1360 (73.8%)
Yes	117 (24.7%)	119 (26.4%)	134 (28.7%)	112 (24.8%)	482 (26.2%)
Dietary diversity					
Low	251 (53%)	225 (50%)	277 (59.3%)	222 (49.2%)	975 (52.9%)
Medium	128 (27%)	143 (31.8%)	143 (30.6%)	149 (33%)	563 (30.6%)
High	95 (20%)	82 (18.2%)	47 (10.1%)	80 (17.7%)	304 (16.5%)
Number of meals (mean ± SD)	2.2 ± 0.44	2.25 ± 0.43	2.24 ± 0.41	2.23 ± 0.42	2.23 ± 0.42

Mozambican metical (MZN); standard deviation (SD).

3.2. Prevalence of Household Food Insecurity

In this study, Cronbach's alpha was 0.871. Of the 1842 households that participated in the study, only 21% were food secure, while 79% were food insecure. Among food-insecure households, 16.6% were experiencing mild FI, while 28.1% and 34.4% were experiencing moderate and severe FI, respectively.

In the regression analyses, FI was associated with various factors. The final model was able to explain 75% of the variability (adjusted R Square = 0.752) in FI. Among ten variables included in the models, eight reached statistical significance with focus on household income, dietary diversity, education level, type of work and number of meals per day (Table 3). Likewise, the binary logistic regression revealed that household income, dietary diversity, education level, type of work and number of meals per day were the main predictors of FI (Table 4). The findings showed that households with a monthly income of <9000 Mozambican metical (equivalent to USD 140.86) were ten times more likely to be food insecure than their counterparts who had a monthly income of >15,000 metical (equivalent to USD 234.77). The households whose heads had primary or secondary education, for example, were twelve times more exposed to FI compared with those with university education. Likewise, households whose heads worked in the informal sector were three times more exposed to FI than their counterparts who had secure employment in the formal sector. On the other hand, households whose meals in the past 7 days were of medium diversity were eight times more likely to be food insecure than their counterparts whose meals were of high diversity. Similarly, households eating two meals a day were four times more likely to be food insecure compared with those eating three meals a day.

Table 3. Prevalence of household food insecurity by socio-demographic characteristics, Maputo City Household Survey, 2022.

Variables	Prevalence of Food Insecurity (%)		p-Value
	Food Insecure (%)	Food Secure (%)	
Head of household			
Female	85.5	14.5	0.001
Male	76.4	23.6	
Household size			
1–4 members	84.8	15.2	0.001
5 or more	75.2	24.8	
Number of children			
0–2 children	77.3	22.7	0.386
3 or more	79.7	20.3	
Marital status			
Single/separated/divorced	87.2	12.8	0.001
Married/marital union	74.9	25.1	
Education			
Primary and secondary	94.3	5.7	<0.001
High school (Grade 11–12)	77.8	22.2	
University	16	84	
Type of work			
Unpaid work	93.1	6.9	<0.001
Paid work	65.3	34.7	
Monthly household income (in MZN)			
<9000	95.95	4.05	<0.001
9000–15,000	86.1	13.9	
>15,000	37.1	62.9	
Remittance from relatives			
Yes	82.6	17.4	0.516
No	77.7	22.3	
Dietary diversity			
Low	97.85	2.15	<0.001
Medium	73.2	26.8	
High	23	77	
Number of meals			
1–2 meals	93.3	6.7	<0.001
3 or more	31.1	68.9	

Mozambican metical (MZN).

Table 4. Binary logistic regression analysis of food insecurity by socio-demographic characteristics, Maputo City Household Survey, 2022.

Variables	OR	95% CI	*p*-Value
Head of household			
Female	1.82	1.38–2.39	0.001
Male	1		
Household size			
1–4 members	1.63	1.14–2.31	0.007
5 or more	1		
Number of children			
0–2 children	0.79	0.53–1.14	0.196
3 or more	1		
Marital Status			
Single/separated/divorced	2.28	1.74–2.98	0.001
Married/marital union	1		
Education			
Primary and secondary	11.87	4.92–28.62	<0.001
High school (Grade 11–12)	4.17	2.19–7.91	
University	1		
Type of work			
Unpaid work	3.1	2.32–4.14	<0.001
Paid work	1		
Monthly household income (in MZN)			
<9000	10.54	7.84–14.01	<0.001
9000–15,000	2.04	1.32–3.15	
>15,000	1		
Remittance from relatives			
Yes	0.943	0.66–1.346	0.747
No	1		
Dietary diversity			
Low	–	–	<0.001
Medium	8.1	5.82–11.23	
High	1		
Number of meals			
1–2 meals	3.8	2.84–5.09	<0.001
3 or more	1		

Odds ratio (OR); confidence interval (CI); Mozambican metical (MZN).

4. Discussion

This study sought to investigate the prevalence of and factors associated with household FI in Maputo City, southern Mozambique. About 62.5% of the study population were experiencing moderate and severe FI, highlighting the challenges that Mozambique faces regarding food security and nutrition. This proportion may be conservative considering that about 60% of the Mozambican population live in extreme poverty [19], and the effects of the COVID-19 pandemic [20,33], as the data collection was carried out just after the pandemic. In any case, moderate and severe FI are a matter of concern for most households not only in Mozambique (and Maputo city in particular) as highlighted in this study, but also across SSA and other LMICs [1,34].

In fact, the SDGs, especially those aiming to end extreme poverty and eradicate hunger and all forms of malnutrition by 2030, are out of reach for many LMICs, including Mozambique [1,35]. This being a decade of informed actions, there is an urgent need to implement both emergency solutions, especially for the most vulnerable groups, and more sustainable solutions to combat household FI and malnutrition, and eventually achieve the

SDGs [34,36]. In addition, rapid population growth is a serious challenge that needs to be urgently considered when addressing global food security and nutrition, as overpopulation is expected to be the leading cause of FI worldwide by 2050 [13,37].

In this study, various variables were linked to FI, with a focus on socioeconomic and demographic factors (household income, dietary diversity, education level, type of work and number of meals). Food insecurity in Mozambique, and in Africa in general, is largely linked to poverty [38,39]. Therefore, there is a need to tackle those factors that contribute significantly to poverty and a rise in poverty. Research evidence in Africa indicates that flawed economic policies, corruption, poor governance and political conflicts [40,41] as well as poor land utilization are the main causes of poverty that need to be addressed [40]. Similarly, poor governance and political conflicts [42,43] have been highlighted as relevant determinants of FI in Africa. For instance, the quality of governance (e.g., government effectiveness, rule of law, accountability) and targeted policies are critical to promoting a stable environment that is suitable for economic investments, especially those related to improving food security and nutrition, social protection and the pace of economic growth [43]. To this end, effective interventions from major players such as governments, the private sector and international institutions are essential to stimulate decent work and build an inclusive economic growth for Africa as a whole [44].

Household income and food prices are critical determinants of FI in African cities, as most urban households buy most of their food rather than producing it themselves [38]. Urban FI tends to worsen with high food prices observed in cities. For instance, the cost of living and basic needs in Mozambique, especially in major urban settlements, has been worsening at a great pace [45]. Moreover, the COVID-19 pandemic has caused a rise in FI linked to food shortages and high food prices, job losses and a decrease in livelihoods [20]. A study by Rosenberg et al. [46] in 16 southern African countries found an association between the COVID-19 pandemic and increased risk of job loss. Therefore, the pandemic, in a unique way, has highlighted the weaknesses of food systems, and also of health systems in LMICs [47] as well as in high-income countries [48]. Altogether, the above-cited studies highlight the need to provide social and economic support to the most vulnerable groups [49,50] as well as to rethink future actions towards global food security and nutrition [48,49]. Furthermore, FI in urban settlements is largely a result of low income, often accompanied by a lack of secure employment as highlighted in this study, and by poor living conditions and limited access to clean water, sanitation and electricity [51]. In contrast to the African cities, seasonality and climate change can have a huge impact on household FI in rural areas. Most rural households depend on their own food production, which is heavily dependent on rainfall, which is becoming increasingly unreliable because of climate change [52]. Likewise, climate change may affect food systems and FI in various ways, from its direct effects on food production to changes in markets, food prices and food supply chain infrastructure [53].

On the other hand, various studies have shown a relationship between household FI and gender inequality in Africa and other LMICs, and the need for socioeconomic interventions to empower women and close the gender gap between female- and male-headed households [54,55]. Just as in the study by McCordic et al. [23], FI in the present study was associated with female headship depending mostly on their education level and employment. Similar results have been found across the world [54,56]. Indeed, gender inequality has been globally recognized as a significant determinant of household FI [56–58]. Due to inequalities in education and employment across female- and male-headed households, female-headed households are more likely to suffer from FI [23,57]. Likewise, there is inequality in social safety nets available to women [56,59]. Additionally, factors such as cultural norms and values, ownership of quality land and productive resources, including provision of extension services, compound the household FS situation in rural areas, as these factors tend to favor men over women [59]. Moreover, households with five or more members (including several adult members) were more likely to be food secure than their counterparts who had few members, which suggests that household size can have a protective effect against FI. Considering that most households were composed of members with considerable financial constraints, the dependency ratio could be more pronounced in smaller households than in larger ones. Indeed, a large household with more productive adults contributing to the affairs of that household exhibits improved household FS status [57,60]. In addition, there is substantial evidence showing the link between FI and dependency ratio [36,44]. Similarly, as highlighted in this study, research evidence across the world indicates that single parents, especially single mothers, are more likely to be food insecure than their counterparts who are married or in marital union [61–63].

At the same time, besides food quality and safety, food quantity and dietary diversity are a real concern for the vast majority of poor urban households [20,31]. In fact, households experiencing moderate and severe FI in this study were strongly associated with low dietary diversity and having very few meals a day. In any case, it is necessary to consider several factors together to get an overview of household FI, as one factor may not fully capture and explain the extent and severity of this complex phenomenon. In summation, the urgency of household FI and malnutrition in Mozambique should be recognized as a call for the country to develop multifaceted and multisectoral programs that include household FS and nutrition as an integral component to improve physical and mental health, especially among the most vulnerable groups. Likewise, these findings reinforce the need for social protection for the most vulnerable groups; in addition, they call for implementation of multifaceted programs to enhance food security and nutrition at a national, regional and global level [20,43,56].

Strengths and Limitations

This is one of the few quantitative studies that provide empirical and updated information on household FI and its associated factors in Maputo City in the context of the COVID-19 pandemic. In addition, a considerable number of household heads participated in the study, meaning that the findings can be generalized to the entire city of Maputo. Nonetheless, the study has some limitations to be considered. Besides using a cross-sectional design, the respondents' recall bias needs to be acknowledged, and the findings may not be fully applicable to other Mozambican cities whose characteristics (e.g., socio-cultural, demographic, and economic) are very different from the capital city.

5. Conclusions

This study aimed to investigate the prevalence of household FI and its associated factors in Maputo City. Almost four in every five households were food insecure, three of which were experiencing moderate or severe FI. Regarding associated factors, several variables were linked to household FI with a focus on poverty, low income, lack of secure employment, low education level, household size and dependency ratio, non-diversified diet and a very limited number of meals per day. This highlights the dynamic and complex nature of household FI, and the need for longitudinal studies (e.g., case–control studies, participatory action research and ethnographic studies) to gain a deeper understanding of the mechanisms linking demographic and socioeconomic factors to household FI and malnutrition, and to ascertain causality. On the other hand, these findings demand urgent informed actions from the government, the private sector and international institutions, not only to provide social and economic support to the most vulnerable groups, but also to implement multifaceted programs to combat household FI and malnutrition and create more job opportunities and promote decent work.

Author Contributions: Conceptualization, E.M.A.M. and G.M.; methodology, E.M.A.M., E.M.S. and G.M.; validation, E.M.A.M., E.M.S., G.M. and S.V.; formal analysis, E.M.A.M., O.A.U. and G.M.; investigation, E.M.A.M., E.M.S. and G.M.; data curation, E.M.A.M. and G.M.; writing—original draft preparation, E.M.A.M.; writing—review and editing, E.M.A.M., E.M.S., G.M., S.V. and O.A.U.; visualization, E.M.A.M. All authors have read and agreed to the published version of the manuscript.

Funding: This study was funded by SIDA, ISP 2018/28:6 Mozambique; SIDA Decision No.: 2017/11862 Subprogram 1.2.1. Food Technology and Food Safety; and PhD grant (Elias Militao) Project 8-71101-3283.

Institutional Review Board Statement: This research received ethical approval from the Institutional Committee of Bioethics in Health of the Faculty of Medicine, Eduardo Mondlane University, Maputo (registration No. CIBS FM&HCM/036/2019).

Informed Consent Statement: Informed consent was obtained from all participants involved in the study. The participants were reminded both verbally and in the invitation letter that they could withdraw from the study at any time with no consequences.

Data Availability Statement: The data presented in this paper are not publicly available owing to restrictions in the ethical approval for this study. Questions related to the data should be directed to the corresponding author.

Acknowledgments: The authors would like to thank Rocio Winersjö for statistical advice, Lúcia Muioche and Eleonora Nvumba for helping with data collection, all participants in the study and the Maputo City Council. Furthermore, the authors would like to thank Helena Canhão and Maria Gregório for providing us with the questionnaire.

Conflicts of Interest: The authors declare no conflict of interest.

References

1. FAO; IFAD; UNICEF; WFP; WHO. *The State of Food Security and Nutrition in the World 2022*; Repurposing Food and Agricultural Policies to Make Healthy Diets More Affordable; WHO: Rome, Italy, 2022; ISBN 978-92-5-136499-4.
2. Lee, J.S. Food Insecurity and Healthcare Costs: Research Strategies Using Local, State, and National Data Sources for Older Adults. *Adv. Nutr.* **2013**, *4*, 42–50. [CrossRef] [PubMed]
3. Gundersen, C.; Ziliak, J.P. Food Insecurity And Health Outcomes. *Health Aff.* **2015**, *34*, 1830–1839. [CrossRef]
4. Bickel, G.W.; Nord, M.; Price, C.; Hamilton, W.; Cook, J. *Guide to Measuring Household Food Security: Revised March*; USDA, Food and Nutrition Service: Alexandria, VA, USA, 2000; Volume 82.
5. FAO; IFAD; WFP. *The State of Food Insecurity in the World 2015*; Meeting the 2015 International Hunger Targets: Taking Stock of Uneven Progress; FAO: Rome, Italy, 2015; p. 62.
6. Yazbeck, N.; Mansour, R.; Salame, H.; Chahine, N.B.; Hoteit, M. The Ukraine–Russia War Is Deepening Food Insecurity, Unhealthy Dietary Patterns and the Lack of Dietary Diversity in Lebanon: Prevalence, Correlates and Findings from a National Cross-Sectional Study. *Nutrients* **2022**, *14*, 3504. [CrossRef] [PubMed]
7. Behnassi, M.; El Haiba, M. Implications of the Russia–Ukraine War for Global Food Security. *Nat. Hum. Behav.* **2022**, *6*, 754–755. [CrossRef] [PubMed]
8. Noland, M. North Korea as a Complex Humanitarian Emergency: Assessing Food Insecurity. *Asia Glob. Econ.* **2022**, *2*, 100049. [CrossRef]
9. Ackello-Ogutu, C. Managing Food Security Implications of Food Price Shocks in Africa. *J. Afr. Econ.* **2011**, *20*, i100–i141. [CrossRef]
10. Gustafson, D.J. Rising Food Costs & Global Food Security: Key Issues and Relevance for India. *IJMR* **2013**, *138*, 398–410.
11. Weinberger, K. Home and Community Gardens in Southeast Asia: Potential and Opportunities for Contributing to Nutrition-Sensitive Food Systems. *Food Sec.* **2013**, *5*, 847–856. [CrossRef]
12. Sadhguru, J.V. *Climate Action and Reducing Human Footprint*; UNCCD COP 14; UN Women, Global Mechanism of the UNCCD and IUCN: New Delhi, India, 2019.
13. FAO; IFAD; UNICEF; WFP; WHO. *The State of Food Security and Nutrition in the World 2021: Transforming Food Systems for Food Security, Improved Nutrition and Affordable Healthy Diets for All*; The State of Food Security and Nutrition in the World (SOFI); FAO: Rome, Italy, 2021; ISBN 978-92-5-134325-8.
14. MIC. Estratégia Nacional de Fortificação de Alimentos (2016–2021). Available online: https://pt.scribd.com/document/428418816/Estrategia-Nacional-de-Fortificacao-de-Alimentos (accessed on 1 November 2021).
15. FAO. Low-Income Food-Deficit Countries (LIFDCs). Available online: https://www.fao.org/countryprofiles/lifdc/en/ (accessed on 20 March 2023).
16. UNDP. *The Next Frontier: Human Development and the Anthropocene*; Human Development Report; United Nations Development Programme: New York, NY, USA, 2020; ISBN 978-92-1-005516-1.
17. WFP. *Mozambique Country Strategic Plan (2017–2021)*; WPF: Rome, Italy, 2017.
18. WFP. Mozambique. Available online: https://www.wfp.org/countries/mozambique (accessed on 11 March 2023).
19. Baez, J.E.; Olinto, P. *Accelerating Poverty Reduction in Mozambique: Challenges and Opportunities*; World Bank Group: Washington, DC, USA, 2016; p. 74.
20. Militao, E.M.A.; Salvador, E.M.; Silva, J.P.; Uthman, O.A.; Vinberg, S.; Macassa, G. Coping Strategies for Household Food Insecurity, and Perceived Health in an Urban Community in Southern Mozambique: A Qualitative Study. *Sustainability* **2022**, *14*, 8710. [CrossRef]

21. Paulo, A.; Mondlhane, A.; Buene, D. *Relatório da Avaliação de Segurança Alimentar e Nutricional*; Secretariado Técnico de Segurança Alimentar e Nutricional: Maputo, Moçambique, 2017; p. 19.
22. ROSC. *Reflectindo sobre a Desnutrição Crónica: Os Desafios da Construção de um Capital Humano Sustentável em Moçambique*; Forúm da Sociedade Civil para os Direitos da Criança: Maputo, Moçambique, 2014; p. 4.
23. McCordic, C.; Riley, L.; Raimundo, I. Household Food Security in Maputo: The Role of Gendered Access to Education and Employment. *Dev. S. Afr.* **2021**, *38*, 816–827. [CrossRef]
24. Raimundo, I.; Crush, J.S.; Pendleton, W. *The State of Food Insecurity in Maputo, Mozambique*; Urban Food Security Series; AFSUN: Cape Town, South Africa, 2014; ISBN 978-1-920597-11-5.
25. World Bank. *Greater Maputo: Urban Poverty and Inclusive Growth*; World Bank: Washington, DC, USA, 2017; p. 48.
26. INE. *IV Recenseamento Geral da População e Habitação, 2017: Resultados Definitivos—Moçambique*; INE: Maputo, Moçambique, 2019; p. 214.
27. de Koning, F.; Diogo, D.; Paulo, A. *Relatório do Estudo de Base de Segurança Alimentar e Nutricional de 2013*; Secretariado Técnico de Segurança Alimentar e Nutricional: Maputo, Moçambique, 2014; p. 185.
28. Gregório, M.J.; Graça, P.; Nogueira, P.J.; Gomes, S.; Santos, C.A.; Boavida, J. *Proposta Metodológica para a Avaliação da Insegurança Alimentar em Portugal*; Associação Portuguesa dos Nutricionistas: Porto, Portugal, 2014; pp. 4–11.
29. Gregório, M.J. *Desigualdades Sociais no Acesso a Uma Alimentação Saudável: Um Estudo na População Portuguesa*; Tese de Doutoramento, Universidade do Porto: Porto, Portugal, 2014.
30. Gregório, M.J.; Rodrigues, A.M.; Graça, P.; de Sousa, R.D.; Dias, S.S.; Branco, J.C.; Canhão, H. Food Insecurity Is Associated with Low Adherence to the Mediterranean Diet and Adverse Health Conditions in Portuguese Adults. *Front. Public Health* **2018**, *6*, 38. [CrossRef] [PubMed]
31. Verger, E.O.; Ballard, T.J.; Dop, M.C.; Martin-Prevel, Y. Systematic Review of Use and Interpretation of Dietary Diversity Indicators in Nutrition-Sensitive Agriculture Literature. *Glob. Food Secur.* **2019**, *20*, 156–169. [CrossRef]
32. IBM. IBM SPSS Statistics for Windows, Version 27.0. Available online: https://www.ibm.com (accessed on 10 December 2022).
33. Mugabe, V.A.; Gudo, E.S.; Inlamea, O.F.; Kitron, U.; Ribeiro, G.S. Natural Disasters, Population Displacement and Health Emergencies: Multiple Public Health Threats in Mozambique. *BMJ Glob. Health* **2021**, *6*, e006778. [CrossRef] [PubMed]
34. Picchioni, F.; Goulao, L.F.; Roberfroid, D. The Impact of COVID-19 on Diet Quality, Food Security and Nutrition in Low and Middle Income Countries: A Systematic Review of the Evidence. *Clin. Nutr.* **2021**, *10*, 2955–2964. [CrossRef] [PubMed]
35. United Nations. *The Sustainable Development Goals Report 2022*; United Nations: New York, NY, USA, 2022; p. 68.
36. Burchi, F.; Scarlato, M.; d'Agostino, G. Addressing Food Insecurity in Sub-Saharan Africa: The Role of Cash Transfers. *Poverty Public Policy* **2018**, *10*, 564–589. [CrossRef]
37. Hall, C.; Dawson, T.P.; Macdiarmid, J.I.; Matthews, R.B.; Smith, P. The Impact of Population Growth and Climate Change on Food Security in Africa: Looking Ahead to 2050. *Int. J. Agric. Sustain.* **2017**, *15*, 124–135. [CrossRef]
38. Crush, J.S.; Frayne, G.B. Urban Food Insecurity and the New International Food Security Agenda. *Dev. S. Afr.* **2011**, *28*, 527–544. [CrossRef]
39. Saha, S.; Behnke, A.; Oldewage-Theron, W.; Mubtasim, N.; Miller, M. Prevalence and Factors Associated with Food Insecurity among Older Adults in Sub-Saharan Africa: A Systematic Review. *J. Nutr. Gerontol. Geriatr.* **2021**, *40*, 171–196. [CrossRef]
40. Addae-Korankye, A. Causes of Poverty in Africa: A Review of Literature. *AIJSSc* **2014**, *3*, 147–153.
41. Kabuya, F.I. Fundamental Causes of Poverty in Sub-Saharan Africa. *IOSR-JHSS* **2015**, *20*, 78–81.
42. Ujunwa, A.; Okoyeuzu, C.; Kalu, E.U. Armed Conflict and Food Security in West Africa: Socioeconomic Perspective. *IJSE* **2019**, *46*, 182–198. [CrossRef]
43. Ogunniyi, A.I.; Mavrotas, G.; Olagunju, K.O.; Fadare, O.; Adedoyin, R. Governance Quality, Remittances and Their Implications for Food and Nutrition Security in Sub-Saharan Africa. *World Dev.* **2020**, *127*, 104752. [CrossRef]
44. Militao, E.M.A.; Salvador, E.M.; Uthman, O.A.; Vinberg, S.; Macassa, G. Food Insecurity and Health Outcomes Other than Malnutrition in Southern Africa: A Descriptive Systematic Review. *Int. J. Environ. Res. Public Health* **2022**, *19*, 5082. [CrossRef] [PubMed]
45. INE Índice de Preços no Consumidor. Available online: http://www.ine.gov.mz/estatisticas/estatisticas-economicas/indice-de-preco-no-consumidor/notas-de-imprensa/mocambique/ipcmocambique_8-cidades_nimprensa_fevereiro2023.pdf/view (accessed on 11 March 2023).
46. Rosenberg, J.; Strauss, I.; Isaacs, G. COVID-19 Impact on SADC Labour Markets: Evidence from High-frequency Data and Other Sources. *Afr. Dev. Rev.* **2021**, *33*, S177–S193. [CrossRef]
47. Erokhin, V.; Gao, T. Impacts of COVID-19 on Trade and Economic Aspects of Food Security: Evidence from 45 Developing Countries. *Int. J. Environ. Res. Public Health* **2020**, *17*, 5775. [CrossRef]
48. Toffolutti, V.; Stuckler, D.; McKee, M. Is the COVID-19 Pandemic Turning into a European Food Crisis? *Eur. J. Public Health* **2020**, *30*, 626–627. [CrossRef]
49. Laborde, D.; Martin, W.; Swinnen, J.; Vos, R. COVID-19 Risks to Global Food Security. *Science* **2020**, *369*, 500–502. [CrossRef]
50. Crush, J.; Si, Z. COVID-19 Containment and Food Security in the Global South. *J. Agric. Food Syst. Community Dev.* **2020**, *9*, 149–151. [CrossRef]
51. Anand, S.; Jagadeesh, K.; Adelina, C.; Koduganti, J. Urban Food Insecurity and Its Determinants: A Baseline Study of Bengaluru. *Environ. Urban.* **2019**, *31*, 421–442. [CrossRef]

52. Onyutha, C. African Food Insecurity in a Changing Climate: The Roles of Science and Policy. *Food Energy Secur.* **2019**, *8*, e00160. [CrossRef]
53. Sam, A.G.; Abidoye, B.O.; Mashaba, S. Climate Change and Household Welfare in Sub-Saharan Africa: Empirical Evidence from Swaziland. *Food Secur.* **2021**, *13*, 439–455. [CrossRef]
54. Jung, N.M.; De Bairros, F.S.; Pattussi, M.P.; Pauli, S.; Neutzling, M.B. Gender Differences in the Prevalence of Household Food Insecurity: A Systematic Review and Meta-Analysis. *Public Health Nutr.* **2017**, *20*, 902–916. [CrossRef] [PubMed]
55. Santos, M.P.; Brewer, J.D.; Lopez, M.A.; Paz-Soldan, V.A.; Chaparro, M.P. Determinants of Food Insecurity among Households with Children in Villa El Salvador, Lima, Peru: The Role of Gender and Employment, a Cross-Sectional Study. *BMC Public Health* **2022**, *22*, 717. [CrossRef] [PubMed]
56. Broussard, N.H. What Explains Gender Differences in Food Insecurity? *Food Policy* **2019**, *83*, 180–194. [CrossRef]
57. Drammeh, W.; Hamid, N.A.; Rohana, A.J. Determinants of Household Food Insecurity and Its Association with Child Malnutrition in Sub-Saharan Africa: A Review of the Literature. *Curr. Res. Nutr. Food. Sci.* **2019**, *7*, 610–623. [CrossRef]
58. Grimaccia, E.; Naccarato, A. Food Insecurity in Europe: A Gender Perspective. *Soc. Indic. Res.* **2022**, *161*, 649–667. [CrossRef]
59. Kassie, M.; Ndiritu, S.W.; Stage, J. What Determines Gender Inequality in Household Food Security in Kenya? Application of Exogenous Switching Treatment Regression. *World Dev.* **2014**, *56*, 153–171. [CrossRef]
60. Bogale, A.; Shimelis, A. Household Level Determinants of Food Insecurity in Rural Areas of Dire Dawa, Eastern Ethiopia. *AJFAND* **2009**, *9*, 1914–1926. [CrossRef]
61. Sulaiman, N.; Yeatman, H.; Russell, J.; Law, L.S. A Food Insecurity Systematic Review: Experience from Malaysia. *Nutrients* **2021**, *13*, 945. [CrossRef]
62. Maynard, M.; Andrade, L.; Packull-McCormick, S.; Perlman, C.; Leos-Toro, C.; Kirkpatrick, S. Food Insecurity and Mental Health among Females in High-Income Countries. *Int. J. Environ. Res. Public Health* **2018**, *15*, 1424. [CrossRef]
63. Smith, M.D.; Kassa, W.; Winters, P. Assessing Food Insecurity in Latin America and the Caribbean Using FAO's Food Insecurity Experience Scale. *Food Policy* **2017**, *71*, 48–61. [CrossRef]

nutrients

MDPI

Article

Beyond the Plate: Uncovering Inequalities in Fruit and Vegetable Intake across Indonesian Districts

Ede Surya Darmawan [1], Dian Kusuma [2,*], Vetty Yulianty Permanasari [1], Vilda Amir [3], Dwi Hapsari Tjandrarini [4] and Ika Dharmayanti [4]

1 Department of Health Administration and Policy, Faculty of Public Health, Universitas Indonesia, Depok 16424, Indonesia
2 Department of Health Services Research and Management, School of Health & Psychological Sciences, City University of London, London EC1V 0HB, UK
3 Center for Health Administration and Policy Studies, Faculty of Public Health, Universitas Indonesia, Depok 16424, Indonesia
4 Research Center for Public Health and Nutrition, National Research and Innovation Agency, Bogor 16915, Indonesia
* Correspondence: dian.kusuma@city.ac.uk

Abstract: Background: Non-communicable diseases (NCDs) are responsible for the deaths of 41 million individuals every year, with 77% of them occurring in low- and middle-income countries. Among the main NCD risk factors, inadequate intake of fruits and vegetables (FV) was one of the leading causes of death in 2019. Our study aims to identify disparities in inadequate FV intake among adults in 514 districts. We utilized the latest Indonesian Basic Health Survey 2018 to conduct geospatial and quantitative analyses. We used the World Health Organization's definition of inadequate FV intake, which refers to consuming less than five servings of fruit and vegetables daily. We analyzed inadequate FV intake among adults over the age of 18 years, as well as by gender and age group (including young adults 18–24 years, adults 25–59 years, and older adults 60+ years). Our study showed an alarmingly high prevalence of inadequate FV intake among adults, with 96.3% in 2018. The prevalence of inadequate FV intake drastically varied across 514 districts, ranging from 70.1% to 100%. Notable geographic and socioeconomic disparities were observed across the districts studied. Rural districts exhibited a higher prevalence of inadequate FV intake, translating to poorer diets, particularly among females and older adults, when compared to their urban counterparts. Interestingly, districts within more developed regions had poorer FV diets than those in less developed regions. Although districts with lower incomes generally had poorer FV diets, the association was not significant in multivariate analysis. However, districts with lower levels of education demonstrated poorer FV diets, especially among females, adults, and older adults. Despite its limitations, our study provides crucial insights for health policies in Indonesia and other LMICs.

Keywords: unhealthy diet; dietary risks; inequality; geographic; socioeconomic

1. Background

Non-communicable diseases (NCDs) claim the lives of 41 million people yearly, which constitutes 74% of total global deaths. Out of these fatalities, 77% are in low- and middle-income countries (LMICs) [1]. The two most critical NCDs are cardiovascular diseases (CVDs) and diabetes, causing 17.9 million and 2.0 million deaths, respectively [1]. The latest Global Burden of Disease Study identified CVDs, such as ischemic heart diseases and stroke, and diabetes, as among the top ten leading causes of global deaths and disabilities in 2019 [2]. Additionally, the study noted that dietary risks, including inadequate intake of fruits and vegetables (FV), were among the leading causes of death for both genders in 2019 [3].

Indonesia is currently facing an increasing burden of NCDs, while also dealing with maternal mortality and infectious diseases. According to the latest Basic Health Research (Riskesdas) by the Ministry of Health, the prevalence of NCDs and their risk factors has dramatically increased over the past five years [4]. For instance, the prevalence of diagnosed stroke among individuals aged 15 years and above surged by 56%, from 0.7% to 1.1%, while that of diabetes mellitus increased by 23%, from 6.9% to 8.5%, between 2013 and 2018. Additionally, an overwhelming 95.4% of the population aged 5 years and above had insufficient FV intake, consuming less than the WHO-recommended daily portions [4].

There can be several reasons for deficiencies in the FV consumption. First, fresh FV may not be readily available or accessible in some areas due to inadequate distribution systems or limited availability in local markets [5]. Second, fresh FV can be more expensive than other food options, making it challenging for some individuals to regularly afford them [6]. Third, many people may not be aware of the health benefits, or they may lack knowledge on how to incorporate them into their diets [7]. In addition, some cultural or social factors may discourage the consumption of certain FV or promote the consumption of other foods instead [8]. Fourth, many people may choose convenient, processed foods over fresh FV, which require more preparation and cooking time [9].

Several studies have demonstrated a link between inadequate FV intake and socioeconomic status and geographic location. In a 2019 systematic review that examined 40 studies on individuals aged 10–40 years in high-income countries, it was found that a higher FV intake was associated with better parental socioeconomic status, especially with regard to higher education levels [10]. Furthermore, studies utilizing geospatial analysis in the United States in 2008 revealed that neighborhood socioeconomic status was positively related to FV consumption [11]. An analysis conducted in Brazil in 2017 also discovered that areas with higher incomes and better-quality food stores had higher FV intake [12]. Similarly, a study in 2012, which used data from 232,056 adult participants in 48 LMICs from the 2002–2004 World Health Survey, found that inadequate FV intake was significantly higher among lower socioeconomic groups [13]. Similar findings were also observed in analyses conducted in the Netherlands and Brazil [14,15].

Reducing the inequality in inadequate FV intake is crucial in achieving Sustainable Development Goal Target 3.4.1, which aims to decrease premature mortality from NCDs. However, the current research on disparities in inadequate FV intake among adults has limitations. Firstly, most studies have used individual-level data [13–15], which are useful but may not capture locality-level factors in countries such as Indonesia. Secondly, previous research on geographic disparities has focused mainly on high-income countries, leaving limited studies in LMICs [10–16]. A 2014 study in Ghana compared FV intake across only three regions and found a higher consumption in the Forest zone due to better production [16]. Thus, our study aims to investigate disparities in FV intake among adults across 514 Indonesian districts, considering socioeconomic and geographic factors. Our study intends to fill the gap in the research by analyzing district-level data in Indonesia, a country with significant local decision-making power. Our research will provide valuable insights into addressing inadequate FV intake disparities, particularly in LMICs.

2. Methods

2.1. Study Design

This study aimed to investigate disparities in inadequate FV intake among adults aged 18 or older in Indonesia using geospatial and multivariate regression analyses. The study analyzed data from the 2018 Indonesian Basic Health Survey (Riskesdas), a nationwide health survey that collected information on FV intake from 514 districts across 34 provinces [4]. The survey aimed to include 300,000 households and utilized a 2-stage sampling method to select 30,000 census blocks in both urban and rural areas, followed by the selection of 10 households in each block based on the education level of the household head [4]. The study utilized both geospatial analysis and multivariate regression to analyze the collected data.

2.2. Independent Variables

The study examined four variables: region, urbanicity, income, and education, at the district level, and obtained the data from the World Bank database. The provinces and districts were classified into five regions, including Sumatera, Java and Bali, Kalimantan, Sulawesi, and Papua/Nusa Tenggara/Maluku. Java and Bali are more developed than the eastern regions [17–19]. The analysis was conducted for all districts, cities (urban districts), and regencies (rural districts).

In this study, poverty rates were used as a proxy for the income level of districts. The poverty rates for each district were divided into five groups, with the highest poverty rates assigned to the first quintile and the lowest poverty rates assigned to the fifth quintile. The basic needs approach, which is based on the Handbook on Poverty and Inequality published by the World Bank, was used by the Indonesia Statistics Bureau (BPS) to determine poverty levels. This approach defines poverty as the inability, from an economic perspective, to fulfill basic food and non-food needs, which are measured in terms of expenditure. Individuals are considered poor if their average monthly expenditure per capita falls below the poverty line [20]. Similarly, the net enrollment ratios for senior secondary education were grouped into five categories, with the first quintile representing the least educated and the fifth quintile representing the most educated [21,22]. Supplementary Figures S1 and S2 provide the country map and the district-level map by urban/rural, income level, and education level. Supplementary Table S1 shows the urban sample and the levels of education and poverty by urbanicity and region.

2.3. Dependent Variables

Our research focused on inadequate FV consumption as the outcome variable among all adults, males, females, young adults (18–24 years), adults (25–59 years), and older adults (60+ years). The FV questionnaire was adapted for use in Indonesia by the Ministry of Health and was based on the World Health Organization (WHO) STEPwise approach to NCD risk factor surveillance (STEPS) questionnaire, which is widely employed in global disease surveillance [23]. First, the respondents were asked about the number of days in a typical week on which they consume fruits (vegetables). Second, they were asked to specify the number of portions consumed in a typical day within the same week. For the analysis, we used the WHO's definition of inadequate FV intake, which refers to consuming less than five servings of fruit and vegetables daily [24]. We analyzed the prevalence of low intake among males and females separately to understand the differences. Furthermore, we also examined the prevalence of low intake among different age categories, which is crucial for controlling and preventing NCDs and developing effective health system responses [25].

2.4. Data Analysis

We utilized geospatial analysis and multivariable regressions to explore the link between inadequate FV intake and geographic/socioeconomic factors. The data were divided into quintiles using ArcMap 10.6 (Esri, Redlands, CA, USA), and we conducted Ordinary Least Square (OLS) regressions in STATA 15.1 (StataCorp LLC, College Station, TX, USA). Our analysis examined the connections between region, urbanicity, income, and education indicators, and each of the six outcome variables. We compared the variations between the most and least developed regions and the poorest and wealthiest/most educated quintiles. A statistical significance level of 5% or lower was deemed significant.

3. Results

3.1. Provincial-Level Results

Figure 1 displays the percentage of adults with inadequate FV intake across provinces. Figure 1a–f depict the data for all adults, male adults, female adults, young adults, adults, and older adults. The prevalence of inadequate FV intake varied among different provinces, with percentages ranging from 92.6% to 98.8% among all adults. The ranges were similar by sex (males and females) and age group (young adults, adults, and older adults). Moreover, the provinces with the highest prevalence (quintiles 4–5) of inadequate FV intake among all adults were mostly located in Sumatera, including Aceh, Jambi, Bangka Belitung, West Sumatera, South Sumatera, and Riau, as well as in some provinces in Kalimantan, Sulawesi, and Java. Such pattern was similar across sexes and age groups.

Table 1 displays the prevalence of inadequate FV intake among adults in each province. Sorted by poverty rates, the top box shows that wealthiest and the bottom box shows the poorest ten provinces. Grey-colored cells indicate a higher prevalence than the national average for each column (outcome indicator). Among the top ten wealthiest provinces, five had a higher-than-average prevalence for all six indicators, including South Kalimantan, Central Kalimantan, Banten, Bangka Belitung, and West Sumatera. However, only three of the ten poorest provinces had a higher-than-average prevalence.

3.2. District-Level Results

Table 2 presents the descriptive statistics of the districts included in our study, which includes the proportion of adults with inadequate FV intake. Out of the 514 districts, 97 (18.9%) were urban cities, and the remaining 417 (81.1%) were rural regencies. The cities were mainly situated in Java (36.1% of 97) and Sumatera (34.0%), while regencies were less concentrated, with 29.0% (of 417 regencies) in Java, 22.3% in Sumatera, 20.6% in Papua, 16.8% in Sulawesi, and 11.3% in Kalimantan. When analyzed based on income level, it was found that 79% of urban areas belonged to the wealthier group (quintiles 4–5), whereas almost half (47.2%) of the rural areas were part of the poorer group (quintiles 1–2). In terms of education level, 71.1% of cities belonged to the higher education group (quintiles 4–5), while almost half (46.8%) of the regencies were part of the lower education group (quintiles 1–2). Regarding the proportion of adults with inadequate FV intake, it was found that 96.3% of all adults had inadequate FV intake, with males and females having a prevalence of 97.6% and 96.0%, respectively. Moreover, young adults, adults, and older adults had an inadequate FV intake prevalence of 97.0%, 96.1%, and 97.6%, correspondingly. Compared to urban areas, rural areas had a higher prevalence of inadequate FV intake, and this difference was statistically significant in rural areas among females (p-value = 0.020) and older adults (p-value < 0.001). The prevalence of inadequate FV intake among females and older adults was 95.2% in urban areas, while in rural areas, it was 96.2% and 97.0%, respectively.

In Figure 2, there is a more detailed breakdown of the prevalence of inadequate FV intake by quintile at the district level. The prevalence of inadequate FV intake varied among different districts, with percentages ranging from 70.1% to 100% among all adults. Figure 2 provides a more detailed view than at the provincial level. For example, despite showing a relatively lower prevalence of inadequate FV intake at the provincial level, many districts in various provinces, such as North Sumatera and Lampung, Central Java and East Java, West and North Kalimantan, and Papua and West Papua, had a high prevalence of inadequate FV intake (quintiles 4–5) among all adults. Similarly, despite showing a relatively higher prevalence at the provincial level, many districts in Riau and Jambi, Central and South Kalimantan, and Banten and West Java had a lower prevalence of inadequate FV intake (quintiles 1–2). This pattern was consistent for the prevalence among males, females, young adults, adults, and older adults.

Supplementary Tables S2 and S3 show the ten districts with the lowest and highest prevalence of inadequate FV intake among adults, respectively, revealing significant socioeconomic disparities. Among all adults, inadequate FV intake ranged from 70.1% in Kolaka Timur (Sulawesi region) to 100% in several rural regencies in the Sumatera, Sulawesi, and Papua regions. Moreover, many districts with the lowest prevalence of inadequate FV intake were rural, while all districts with the highest prevalence were also rural. The average poverty rates among the districts with the lowest prevalence of inadequate FV intake were up to 20%, while the rates among the districts with the highest prevalence were up to 35%.

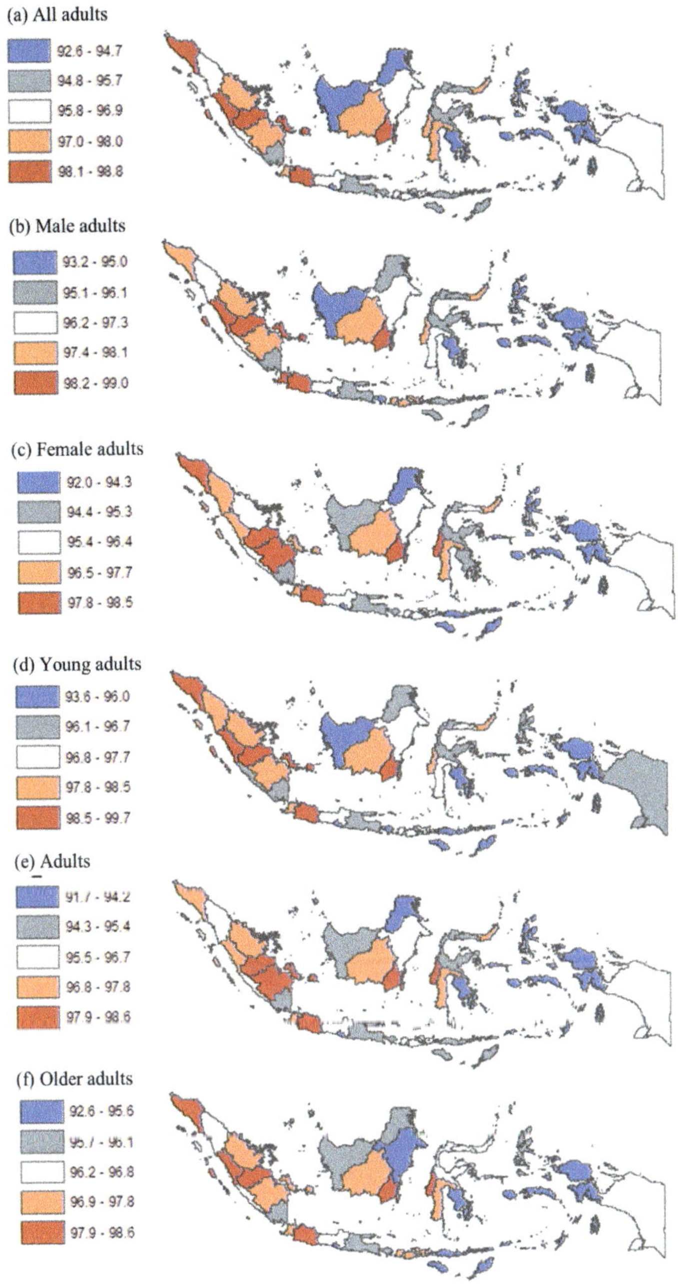

Figure 1. Disparity in inadequate FV intake among adults by province in Indonesia, 2018. FV = fruit and vegetable. Numbers show the prevalence of inadequate FV intake among all adults, males, females, young adults, adults, and older adults. The prevalence was grouped by quintile.

Table 1. Prevalence of inadequate FV intake among adults by province in Indonesia, 2018.

	Poverty Rates (%)	Low FV Intake Prevalence (%)					
		All	Males	Females	Young Adults	Adults	Older Adults
	(1)	(2)	(3)	(4)	(5)	(6)	(7)
Bali	4.5	94.8	95.0	94.5	95.6	94.4	95.6
South Kalimantan	4.8	98.8	99.1	98.5	99.7	98.6	98.6
Central Kalimantan	5.0	97.5	97.9	97.1	98.2	97.4	97.0
Jakarta	5.0	95.9	96.6	95.3	97.7	96.1	92.6
Banten	5.3	97.7	98.3	97.1	98.3	97.5	97.8
Bangka Belitung	5.4	98.1	98.4	97.7	98.9	97.9	97.7
West Sumatera	6.6	98.0	98.3	97.7	98.5	97.8	98.1
North Kalimantan	7.0	94.6	95.4	93.7	96.4	94.0	95.7
East Kalimantan	7.1	96.2	96.3	96.0	97.2	96.0	95.6
Riau Islands	7.6	94.7	95.3	94.1	96.9	94.2	95.9
Jambi	7.8	98.1	98.2	98.0	98.6	97.9	98.6
North Maluku	7.9	94.5	94.7	94.3	96.2	93.9	96.1
West Java	7.9	98.6	98.8	98.3	99.1	98.4	98.6
West Kalimantan	8.1	94.7	95.0	94.4	95.4	94.4	95.6
North Sulawesi	8.5	97.3	97.7	96.9	98.0	97.3	96.8
Riau	8.8	97.0	97.5	96.4	97.7	96.8	97.0
South Sulawesi	9.8	97.9	97.9	97.9	97.9	97.9	98.0
West Sulawesi	10.3	95.0	95.4	94.6	96.0	94.6	95.7
East Java	10.9	96.0	96.4	95.7	96.8	95.8	96.2
Central Java	10.9	96.9	97.2	96.5	98.1	96.6	96.6
North Sumatera	11.3	95.5	95.9	95.0	96.4	95.2	95.6
Lampung	12.6	92.6	93.2	92.0	95.5	91.7	93.4
Yogyakarta	12.7	94.4	94.4	94.5	96.0	93.9	95.1
Southeast Sulawesi	13.0	96.9	97.3	96.6	97.1	96.8	97.6
South Sumatera	13.1	98.0	98.0	97.9	98.5	97.9	97.8
Central Sulawesi	14.6	95.7	96.1	95.3	96.3	95.4	96.4
West Nusa Tenggara	14.8	96.7	97.7	95.9	96.8	96.7	96.8
Bengkulu	15.0	96.1	96.2	95.9	96.7	95.9	96.5
Aceh	16.4	98.1	98.1	98.0	98.7	97.8	98.6
Gorontalo	16.8	95.7	95.9	95.6	97.0	95.3	96.1
Maluku	21.8	94.2	94.2	94.1	94.8	93.8	95.4
East Nusa Tenggara	22.0	94.9	95.4	94.3	95.9	94.6	94.9
West Papua	26.5	93.1	93.2	92.9	93.6	92.8	94.4
Papua	29.4	96.3	96.5	96.0	96.2	96.3	96.3
Average		96.2	96.5	95.8	97.1	95.9	96.4

Note: FV = fruit and vegetable. Ordered by the average poverty rates (column 1), the provinces in the top box are the richest and those in the bottom box are the poorest. Shaded values show higher than the national average for each group.

Tables 3 and 4 display the associations between geographic (e.g., region) and socioeconomic indicators (e.g., income and education) with inadequate FV intake. Table 3 shows the prevalence of inadequate FV intake by region, income, and education, while Table 4 illustrates the results of multivariable regressions. The prevalence of inadequate FV intake was higher in Sumatera, Java, Sulawesi, and Kalimantan, by 1.69%, 1.86%, 1.18%, and 2.59%, respectively, in contrast to Papua. This trend was consistent across sex and age group. Inadequate FV intake was somewhat greater among districts with higher incomes, although the differences were not statistically significant in the multivariable regression. In comparison to districts with the least education, districts with the most education, especially among females, adults, and older adults, had a significantly lower prevalence of inadequate FV intake, by 1.28%, 1.28%, and 1.25%, respectively.

Table 2. Characteristics of districts and inadequate FV intake among adults in Indonesia, 2018.

	All		Urban		Rural		Difference	
	n	%	n	%	n	%	%	*p*-Value
	(1)	(2)	(3)	(4)	(5)	(6)	(7) = (4–6)	
(a) Characteristics (#)								
Sample size district	514	100%	97	100%	417	100%	0%	
Region								
Papua	95	18.5%	9	9.3%	86	20.6%	11.3%	0.008
Java	128	24.9%	35	36.1%	93	22.3%	−13.8%	
Sumatera	154	30.0%	33	34.0%	121	29.0%	−5.0%	
Kalimantan	56	10.9%	9	9.3%	47	11.3%	2.0%	
Sulawesi	81	15.8%	11	11.3%	70	16.8%	5.4%	
	514		97		417			
Income								
Q1 poor	102	19.8%	3	3.1%	99	23.7%	20.6%	<0.001
Q2	103	20.0%	5	5.2%	98	23.5%	18.3%	
Q3	103	20.0%	13	13.4%	90	21.6%	8.2%	
Q4	103	20.0%	22	22.7%	81	19.4%	−3.3%	
Q5 rich	103	20.0%	54	55.7%	49	11.8%	−43.9%	
	514		97		417			
Education								
Q1 least	103	20.0%	0	0.0%	103	24.7%	24.7%	<0.001
Q2	103	20.0%	11	11.3%	92	22.1%	10.7%	
Q3	103	20.0%	17	17.5%	86	20.6%	3.1%	
Q4	103	20.0%	29	29.9%	74	17.7%	−12.2%	
Q5 most	102	19.8%	40	41.2%	62	14.9%	−26.4%	
	514		97		417			
(b) Inadequate FV intake (%)								
All adults	n/a	96.3%	n/a	95.8%	n/a	96.5%	−0.7%	0.093
Male adults	n/a	96.7%	n/a	96.4%	n/a	96.7%	−0.3%	0.375
Female adults	n/a	96.0%	n/a	95.2%	n/a	96.2%	−1.0%	0.020
Young adults	n/a	97.0%	n/a	97.4%	n/a	97.0%	0.4%	0.309
Adults	n/a	96.1%	n/a	95.4%	n/a	96.3%	−0.9%	0.050
Older adults	n/a	96.7%	n/a	95.2%	n/a	97.0%	−1.8%	<0.001

Note: Q = quintile, n = number, FV = fruit and vegetable, % = proportion of column total, urban = city, rural = regency. Data on district characteristics are from the World Bank and fruit/vegetable intake data are from the Basic Health Survey 2018. For *p*-values, chi-square tests were used in panel (a) and OLS regressions were used in panel (b). See Supplementary Table S4 for the regression outputs.

Table 3. Prevalence of inadequate FV intake by region, income, and education among adults in Indonesia, 2018.

	Inadequate FV Intake (N = 514 Districts)					
	All Adults	Males	Females	Young Adults	Adults	Older Adults
Region						
Papua	94.9%	95.1%	94.6%	95.2%	94.6%	95.9%
Sulawesi	96.5%	96.8%	96.3%	97.0%	96.3%	96.9%
Kalimantan	96.8%	97.2%	96.4%	97.6%	96.6%	97.1%
Sumatera	97.2%	97.5%	97.0%	98.0%	97.1%	97.2%
Java	96.1%	96.5%	95.6%	97.0%	95.8%	96.2%
Absolute	1.2%	1.4%	1.0%	1.8%	1.2%	0.3%
Relative	1.01	1.01	1.01	1.02	1.01	1.00
Income						
Q1 poor	95.7%	95.8%	95.6%	95.9%	95.6%	96.5%

Table 3. *Cont.*

	Inadequate FV Intake (N = 514 Districts)					
	All Adults	Males	Females	Young Adults	Adults	Older Adults
Q2	95.9%	96.3%	95.5%	96.6%	95.6%	96.6%
Q3	96.7%	97.1%	96.4%	97.5%	96.5%	96.8%
Q4	96.9%	97.2%	96.5%	97.6%	96.7%	97.0%
Q5 rich	96.5%	96.9%	96.2%	97.6%	96.3%	96.4%
Absolute	0.8%	1.1%	0.6%	1.7%	0.7%	−0.1%
Relative	1.01	1.01	1.01	1.02	1.01	1.00
Education						
Q1 least	96.6%	96.8%	96.5%	96.8%	96.5%	97.2%
Q2	96.5%	96.8%	96.1%	97.1%	96.2%	97.0%
Q3	96.0%	96.3%	95.7%	96.7%	95.8%	96.2%
Q4	96.2%	96.5%	95.9%	97.0%	96.0%	96.5%
Q5 most	96.4%	96.8%	96.0%	97.6%	96.1%	96.4%
Absolute	−0.2%	0.0%	−0.5%	0.8%	−0.4%	−0.8%
Relative	1.00	1.00	0.99	1.01	1.00	0.99

Note: FV = fruit and vegetable, Q = quintile. Java region includes Bali, Papua region includes Maluku and Nusa Tenggara. Income quintile used district-level poverty rate (e.g., Q1 = 20% of districts with highest poverty rate). Absolute (relative) = difference (ratio) between Papua and Java, as well as Q1 and Q5. For education, absolute (relative) was between Q1 and Q5, except among urban (Q2 and Q5). Outcome variables are inadequate FV intake among all adults, males, females, young adults (18–24 years), adults (25–59 years), and older adults (60+ years).

Table 4. Multivariate regression results for geographic and socioeconomic disparity in inadequate FV intake among adults in Indonesia, 2018.

	Inadequate FV intake (N = 514 districts)					
	All Adults	Males	Females	Young Adults	Adults	Older Adults
	Coef (*p*-Value)	Coef (*p*-Value)	Coef (*p*-Value)	Coef (*p*-Value)	Coef (*p*-Value)	Coef (*p*-Value)
Region						
Papua	Reference					
Java	1.176 *	1.130 *	1.228 *	1.274 *	1.194 *	0.583
	(0.042)	(0.047)	(0.047)	(0.037)	(0.047)	(0.343)
Sumatera	2.587 **	2.332 **	2.828 **	2.524 **	2.715 **	1.776 **
	(0.000)	(0.000)	(0.000)	(0.000)	(0.000)	(0.003)
Kalimantan	1.691 *	1.617 *	1.714 *	1.633 *	1.740 *	1.365
	(0.020)	(0.023)	(0.027)	(0.032)	(0.021)	(0.077)
Sulawesi	1.859 **	1.647 **	2.075 **	1.618 *	1.956 **	1.262
	(0.002)	(0.006)	(0.001)	(0.011)	(0.002)	(0.051)
Income						
Quintile 1 poor	Reference					
Quintile 2	−0.359	−0.040	−0.683	0.013	−0.491	−0.135
	(0.521)	(0.942)	(0.254)	(0.983)	(0.401)	(0.822)
Quintile 3	0.374	0.653	0.089	0.791	0.297	0.055
	(0.523)	(0.258)	(0.887)	(0.200)	(0.626)	(0.930)
Quintile 4	0.389	0.710	0.058	0.808	0.321	0.094
	(0.507)	(0.218)	(0.926)	(0.191)	(0.598)	(0.881)
Quintile 5 rich	0.341	0.601	0.076	1.014	0.242	−0.301
	(0.585)	(0.328)	(0.909)	(0.123)	(0.710)	(0.651)
Education						
Quintile 1 least	Reference					
Quintile 2	−0.628	−0.482	−0.790	−0.323	−0.750	−0.451
	(0.235)	(0.356)	(0.162)	(0.562)	(0.174)	(0.424)
Quintile 3	−1.171 *	−1.030 *	−1.319 *	−0.763	−1.285 *	−1.336 *
	(0.027)	(0.048)	(0.019)	(0.170)	(0.020)	(0.018)
Quintile 4	−1.059 *	−0.925	−1.195 *	−0.581	−1.197 *	−1.007
	(0.045)	(0.076)	(0.035)	(0.297)	(0.030)	(0.074)
Quintile 5 most	−1.066	−0.855	−1.284 *	−0.262	−1.280 *	−1.246 *
	(0.057)	(0.122)	(0.032)	(0.657)	(0.029)	(0.038)

Note: FV = fruit and vegetable, Coef = coefficient, Q = quintile. Java region includes Bali, Papua region includes Maluku and Nusa Tenggara. Income quintile used district-level poverty rate (e.g., Q1 = 20% of districts with highest poverty rate). Outcome variables are inadequate FV intake among all adults, males, females, young adults (18–24 years), adults (25–59 years), and older adults (60+ years). * = Significant at the 5% level, and ** = significant at the 1% level.

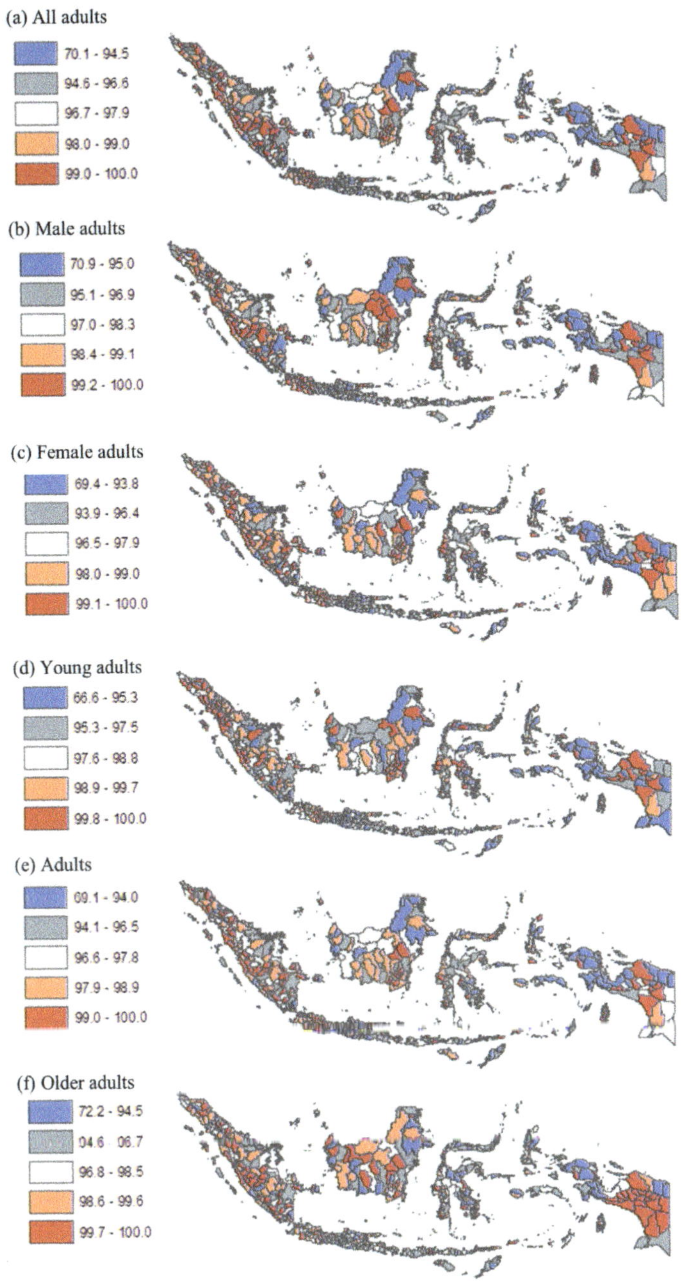

Figure 2. Disparity in inadequate FV intake among adults by district in Indonesia, 2018. FV = fruit and vegetable. Numbers show the prevalence of low FV intake among all adults, males, females, young adults, adults, and older adults. The prevalence was grouped by quintile.

4. Discussion

In 2018, we found an alarmingly high prevalence of inadequate FV intake among Indonesian adults aged 18 and above. At the district level, the prevalence of inadequate FV intake was 96.3%, 97.6%, and 96.0% for all adults, males, and females, respectively. Across age groups, the prevalence was 97.0%, 96.1%, and 97.6% for young adults (18–24 years), adults (25–59 years), and older adults (60 years and above), respectively. These findings are comparable to other LMICs, such as India (95.8%), Pakistan (96.5%), Nepal (99%), Ethiopia (98.5%), and Kenya (94%) [26–30].

Our research revealed that there was a significant disparity in inadequate FV intake among adults in Indonesia based on both geography and socioeconomic status across 514 districts. Rural districts had, on average, a higher prevalence of inadequate FV intake (i.e., poorer FV diet), especially among females and older adults, compared to urban districts. However, note that many districts with the lowest prevalence of inadequate FV intake (i.e., better FV diet) were rural regencies. In high-income countries, FV intake can vary between urban and rural areas due to factors such as access to fresh produce, income, education, and cultural practices. However, there are some general trends that urban areas tend to have greater access to a variety of fruits and vegetables due to the presence of supermarkets, grocery stores, and specialty shops. This can lead to a higher overall consumption of fruits and vegetables in urban areas compared to rural areas [11,31]. In LMICs, FV intake in urban and rural areas can be quite different due to various factors, such as access to markets, availability, affordability, cultural practices, and overall dietary patterns [32]. In many LMICs, urban residents may have better access to markets and a wider variety of fruits and vegetables due to the concentration of shops, supermarkets, and local vendors. However, urban populations can also experience disparities in access to healthy food options, particularly in low-income neighborhoods or informal settlements [27,29]. In rural areas of LMICs, residents might have more opportunities to grow their own fruits and vegetables, leading to increased consumption of fresh produce. However, the diversity of fruits and vegetables available may be limited due to seasonality, geographic constraints, or a lack of market access to a wider variety of fresh produce [16,27,29].

Our study also found that districts in more developed regions (Java, Sumatera, Kalimantan, and Sulawesi) had poorer FV diets than those in less developed regions (Papua, Maluku, and Nusa Tenggara). In LMICs, FV intake can significantly vary between regions and within communities due to various factors. Some less developed regions might have a lower FV intake due to factors such as limited access to markets, lower income levels, and fewer diverse food options. Analysis among 18 countries from the Prospective Urban Rural Epidemiology (PURE) study found the cost of two servings of fruits and three servings of vegetables per day per individual accounted for 52.0% of the household income in low-income countries, 18.1% in lower-middle income countries, 15.9% in upper-middle income countries, and 1.9% in high-income countries [33]. However, local agricultural practices and traditional diets in some LMICs might lead to higher levels of FV consumption. A 2014 study in Ghana found that the FV intake was notably higher in the Forest zone, where the production of fruits and vegetables was more advanced compared to the Savannah and Coastal zones [16].

Our findings showed that districts with lower incomes tended to have poorer FV diets, but the associations were not significant in the multivariate regression. Moreover, we found that districts with less education had poorer FV diets, particularly among females, adults, and older adults. These results align with previous studies. A geospatial analysis from the United States found that poorer socioeconomic status at the neighborhood level was associated with lower FV intake [11]. Another study in Brazil showed that average FV intake was higher in neighborhoods with higher incomes and concentration of food stores, and a better index of access to healthy foods [12]. Similarly, a multilevel study in the Netherlands found significant disparities in FV intake, with odds ratios of not consuming FV at 5.47 among the lowest-educated groups [14].

For policy, inadequate FV intake among adults in Indonesia is a significant public health concern and is associated with high rates of CVDs and diabetes, and their main risk factors, such as obesity and hypertension [18,22,34]. There are several policy implications that can be drawn. First, policymakers should consider incorporating the study's evidence-based insights into the development of targeted interventions, in order to bridge the gap in FV intake between rural and urban areas, as well as between different socioeconomic groups in Indonesia. This may include enhancing access to diverse and affordable FV options in rural and low-income areas through improved transportation and market infrastructure, as well as supporting local agricultural practices [35,36]. Additionally, public health campaigns should emphasize the importance of FV consumption and aim to increase awareness, particularly among females, older adults, and those with lower levels of education. These campaigns can be tailored to the cultural practices and dietary patterns of specific regions, taking into account the unique challenges faced by communities in both developed and less developed areas [32,33]. Lastly, further research is needed to identify and address barriers to FV intake in specific districts and to evaluate the effectiveness of interventions in improving dietary habits among the Indonesian population.

Our study is the first to investigate disparities in inadequate FV intake among adults across more than 500 districts. However, it has at least three limitations, which may be due to at least two reasons. Firstly, we were unable to examine a sub-group analysis by ethnicity as we lacked relevant data in our dataset [37]. Secondly, the study was conducted using cross-sectional data, and trends over time could not be assessed. Thirdly, there was only a small urban area (i.e., 95 cities of 514 districts), which may limit the comparison. Our definition of urban/rural (cities = urban and regencies = rural) may not capture the most accurate variations in terms of more/less developed regions as well as education/income levels. For instance, some regencies that are adjacent or closer to cities may have a similar development/education/income level to the cities. Nevertheless, our findings are essential for informing health policies in Indonesia and other LMICs.

5. Conclusions

Our study in Indonesia showed an alarmingly high prevalence of inadequate FV intake among adults, with 96.3% in 2018. The prevalence of inadequate FV intake drastically varied across the 514 districts, ranging from 70.1% to 100%. Notable geographic and socioeconomic disparities were observed across the districts studied. Rural districts exhibited a higher prevalence of inadequate FV intake, translating to poorer diets, particularly among females and older adults, when compared to their urban counterparts. Interestingly, districts within more developed regions had poorer FV diets than those in less developed regions. Although districts with lower incomes generally had poorer FV diets, the association was not significant in multivariate analysis. However, districts with lower levels of education demonstrated poorer FV diets, especially among females, adults, and older adults. Although our study has limitations, it provides crucial insights for health policies in Indonesia and other LMICs.

Supplementary Materials: The following supporting information can be downloaded at: https://www.mdpi.com/article/10.3390/nu15092160/s1, Figure S1: Map of provinces in Indonesia; Figure S2: Map of Districts by urbanicity, income level, and educational level, Table S1. Urban sample and educational/poverty level by urbanicity and region; Table S2: Ten districts with LOWEST prevalence of inadequate FV intake in Indonesia, 2018; Table S3: Ten districts with HIGHEST prevalence of inadequate FV intake in Indonesia, 2018; Table S4: Regression outputs for urban/rural differences.

Author Contributions: Conceptualization, D.K., V.A. and E.S.D.; formal analysis, D.K., V.A., D.H.T. and I.D.; data curation, D.H.T., I.D. and V.Y.P.; writing—original draft preparation, D.K.; writing—review and editing, D.K., E.S.D., V.Y.P., V.A., D.H.T. and I.D.; project administration, E.S.D. and V.Y.P.; funding acquisition, D.K., V.A., E.S.D. and V.Y.P. All authors have read and agreed to the published version of the manuscript.

Funding: Our research was funded by the Directorate of Research and Community Service, Universitas Indonesia (NKB-1402/UN2.RST/HKP.05.00/2022). The funder had no role in the study design, data collection and analysis/interpretation, or preparation of the manuscript.

Institutional Review Board Statement: Not applicable.

Informed Consent Statement: Not applicable.

Data Availability Statement: Available from the authors upon reasonable request.

Conflicts of Interest: The authors have no conflict of interest to declare.

References

1. World Health Organization (WHO). Noncommunicable Diseases: Childhood Overweight and Obesity. 2020. Available online: https://www.who.int/news-room/questions-and-answers/item/noncommunicable-diseases-childhood-overweight-and-obesity (accessed on 22 February 2023).
2. GBD 2019 Diseases and Injuries Collaborators. Global burden of 369 diseases and injuries in 204 countries and territories, 1990–2019: A systematic analysis for the Global Burden of Disease Study 2019. *Lancet* **2020**, *396*, 1204–1222. [CrossRef] [PubMed]
3. GBD 2019 Risk Factors Collaborators. Global burden of 87 risk factors in 204 countries and territories, 1990–2019: A systematic analysis for the Global Burden of Disease Study 2019. *Lancet* **2020**, *396*, 1223–1249. [CrossRef] [PubMed]
4. National Institute of Health Research and Development (NIHRD). Report of Riskesdas. 2018. Available online: http://repository.bkpk.kemkes.go.id/3514/1/Laporan%20Riskesdas%202018%20Nasional.pdf (accessed on 15 April 2023).
5. Jones, A.D.; Shrinivas, A.; Bezner-Kerr, R. Farm production diversity is associated with greater household dietary diversity in Malawi: Findings from nationally representative data. *Food Policy* **2014**, *46*, 1–12. [CrossRef]
6. Drewnowski, A.; Darmon, N. The economics of obesity: Dietary energy density and energy cost. *Am. J. Clin. Nutr.* **2005**, *82*, 265S–273S. [CrossRef]
7. Gibson, E.L.; Wardle, J.; Watts, C.J. Fruit and Vegetable Consumption, Nutritional Knowledge and Beliefs in Mothers and Children. *Appetite* **1998**, *31*, 205–228. [CrossRef]
8. Bodor, J.N.; Rose, D.; AFarley, T.; Swalm, C.; Scott, S.K. Neighbourhood fruit and vegetable availability and consumption: The role of small food stores in an urban environment. *Public Health Nutr.* **2008**, *11*, 413–420. [CrossRef]
9. Reicks, M.; Trofholz, A.C.; Stang, J.S.; Laska, M.N. Impact of Cooking and Home Food Preparation Interventions Among Adults: Outcomes and Implications forFuture Programs. *J. Nutr. Educ. Behav.* **2014**, *46*, 259–276. [CrossRef]
10. Desbouys, L.; Méjean, C.; De Henauw, S.; Castetbon, K. Socio-economic and cultural disparities in diet among adolescents and young adults: A systematic review. *Public Health Nutr.* **2020**, *23*, 843–860. [CrossRef]
11. Dubowitz, T.; Heron, M.; E Bird, C.; Lurie, N.; Finch, B.K.; Basurto-Dávila, R.; Hale, L.; Escarce, J.J. Neighborhood socioeconomic status and fruit and vegetable intake among whites, blacks, and Mexican Americans in the United States. *Am. J. Clin. Nutr.* **2008**, *87*, 1883–1891. [CrossRef]
12. Menezes, M.C.; Costa, B.V.L.; Oliveira, C.D.L.; Lopes, A.C.S. Local food environment and fruit and vegetable consumption: An ecological study. *Prev. Med. Rep.* **2017**, *5*, 13–20. [CrossRef]
13. Hosseinpoor, A.R.; Bergen, N.; Kunst, A.; Harper, S.; Guthold, R.; Rekve, D.; D'Espaignet, E.T.; Naidoo, N.; Chatterji, S. Socioeconomic inequalities in risk factors for non communicable diseases in low-income and middle-income countries: Results from the World Health Survey. *BMC Public Health* **2012**, *12*, 912. [CrossRef] [PubMed]
14. Giskes, K.; Van Lenthe, F.J.; Kamphuis, C.B.M.; Huisman, M.; Brug, J.; MacKenbach, J.P. Household and food shopping environments: Do they play a role in socioeconomic inequalities in fruit and vegetable consumption? A multilevel study among Dutch adults. *J. Epidemiol. Community Health* **2009**, *63*, 113–120. [CrossRef]
15. de Azevedo Barros, M.B.; Lima, M.G.; Medina LD, P.B.; Szwarcwald, C.L.; Malta, D.C. Social inequalities in health behaviors among Brazilian adults: National Health Survey, 2013. *Int. J. Equity Health* **2016**, *15*, 148. [CrossRef]
16. Amo-Adjei, J.; Kumi-Kyereme, A. Fruit and Vegetable Consumption by Ecological Zone and Socioeconomic Status in Ghana. *J. Biosoc. Sci.* **2015**, *47*, 613–631. [CrossRef] [PubMed]
17. Ayuningtyas, D.; Hapsari, D.; Rachmalina, R.; Amir, V.; Rachmawati, R.; Kusuma, D. Geographic and Socioeconomic Disparity in Child Undernutrition across 514 Districts in Indonesia. *Nutrients* **2022**, *14*, 843. [CrossRef] [PubMed]
18. Ayuningtyas, D.; Kusuma, D.; Amir, V.; Tjandrarini, D.H.; Andarwati, P. Disparities in Obesity Rates among Adults: Analysis of 514 Districts in Indonesia. *Nutrients* **2022**, *14*, 3332. [CrossRef]
19. Bella, A.; Akbar, M.T.; Kusnadi, G.; Herlinda, O.; Regita, P.A.; Kusuma, D. Socioeconomic and Behavioral Correlates of COVID-19 Infections among Hospital Workers in the Greater Jakarta Area, Indonesia: A Cross-Sectional Study. *Int. J. Environ. Res. Public Health* **2021**, *18*, 5048. [CrossRef]
20. Indonesian Statistics Bureau (BPS). [Poverty and Inequality Concept]. 2020. Available online: https://www.bps.go.id/subject/23/kemiskinan-dan-ketimpangan.html (accessed on 1 April 2023).
21. Megatsari, H.; Kusuma, D.; Ernawaty, E.; Putri, N.K. Geographic and Socioeconomic Inequalities in Delays in COVID-19 Vaccinations: A Cross-Sectional Study in Indonesia. *Vaccines* **2022**, *10*, 1857. [CrossRef]
22. Oktamianti, P.; Kusuma, D.; Amir, V.; Tjandrarini, D.H.; Paramita, A. District-Level Inequalities in Hypertension among Adults in Indonesia: A Cross-Sectional Analysis by Sex and Age Group. *Int. J. Environ. Res. Public Health* **2022**, *19*, 13268. [CrossRef]
23. Song, P.; Gupta, A.; Goon, I.Y.; Hasan, M.; Mahmood, S.; Page, P.; Pradeepa, R.; Siddiqui, S.; Silva, W.; Aarthi, G.R.; et al. Data Resource Profile: Understanding the patterns and determinants of health in South Asians-South Asia Biobank. *Int. J. Epidemiol.* **2021**, *50*, 717–718e. [CrossRef]

24. Kusuma, D.; Pradeepa, R.; Khawaja, K.I.; Hasan, M.; Siddiqui, S.; Mahmood, S.; Shah, S.M.A.; De Silva, C.K.; de Silva, L.; Gamage, M.; et al. Low uptake of COVID-19 prevention behaviours and high socioeconomic impact of lockdown measures in South Asia: Evidence from a large-scale multi-country surveillance programme. *SSM—Popul. Health* **2021**, *13*, 100751. [CrossRef] [PubMed]
25. Di Cesare, M.; Khang, Y.-H.; Asaria, P.; Blakely, T.; Cowan, M.J.; Farzadfar, F.; Guerrero, R.; Ikeda, N.; Kyobutungi, C.; Msyamboza, K.P.; et al. Inequalities in non-communicable diseases and effective responses. *Lancet* **2013**, *381*, 585–597. [CrossRef] [PubMed]
26. Mwenda, V.; Mwangi, M.; Nyanjau, L.; Gichu, M.; Kyobutungi, C.; Kibachio, J. Dietary risk factors for non-communicable diseases in Kenya: Findings of the STEPS survey, 2015. *BMC Public Health* **2018**, *18*, 1218. [CrossRef]
27. Gelibo, T.; Amenu, K.; Taddele, T.; Taye, G.; Getnet, M.; Getachew, T.; Defar, A.; Teklie, H.; Bekele, A.; Shiferaw, F.; et al. Low fruit and vegetable intake and its associated factors in Ethiopia: A community based cross sectional NCD steps survey. *Ethiop. J. Health Dev.* **2018**, *31*, 355–361.
28. Rafique, I.; Saqib, M.A.; Munir, M.A.; Qureshi, H.; Rizwanullah, K.S.; Khan, S.A.; Fouad, H. Prevalence of risk factors for noncommunicable diseases in adults: Key findings from the Pakistan steps survey. *East. Mediterr. Health J.* **2018**, *24*, 33–41. [CrossRef]
29. Tripathy, J.P.; Thakur, J.S.; Jeet, G.; Chawla, S.; Jain, S.; Prasad, R. Urban rural differences in diet, physical activity and obesity in India: Are we witnessing the great Indian equalisation? Results from a cross-sectional STEPS survey. *BMC Public Health* **2016**, *16*, 816. [CrossRef] [PubMed]
30. Aryal, K.K.; Mehata, S.; Neupane, S.; Vaidya, A.; Dhimal, M.; Dhakal, P.; Rana, S.; Bhusal, C.L.; Lohani, G.R.; Paulin, F.H.; et al. The Burden and Determinants of Non Communicable Diseases Risk Factors in Nepal: Findings from a Nationwide STEPS Survey. *PLoS ONE* **2015**, *10*, e0134834. [CrossRef]
31. Widener, M.J.; Metcalf, S.S.; Bar-Yam, Y. Dynamic Urban food environments: A temporal analysis of access to healthy foods. *Am. J. Prev. Med.* **2011**, *41*, 439–441. [CrossRef]
32. Hawkes, C.; Smith, T.G.; Jewell, J.; Wardle, J.; Hammond, R.A.; Friel, S.; Thow, A.M.; Kain, J. Smart food policies for obesity prevention. *Lancet* **2015**, *385*, 2410–2421. [CrossRef]
33. Miller, V.; Yusuf, S.; Chow, C.K.; Dehghan, M.; Corsi, D.J.; Lock, K.; Popkin, B.; Rangarajan, S.; Khatib, R.; A Lear, S.; et al. Availability, affordability, and consumption of fruits and vegetables in 18 countries across income levels: Findings from the Prospective Urban Rural Epidemiology (PURE) study. *Lancet Glob. Health* **2016**, *4*, e695–e703. [CrossRef]
34. Adisasmito, W.; Amir, V.; Atin, A.; Megraini, A.; Kusuma, D. Geographic and socioeconomic disparity in cardiovascular risk factors in Indonesia: Analysis of the Basic Health Research 2018. *BMC Public Health* **2020**, *20*, 1004. [CrossRef] [PubMed]
35. FAO. Nutrition and Food Systems. A Report by the High Level Panel of Experts on Food Security and Nutrition of the Committee on World Food Security. September 2017. Available online: https://www.fao.org/documents/card/en/c/I7846E (accessed on 8 April 2023).
36. Story, M.; Kaphingst, K.M.; Robinson-O'Brien, R.; Glanz, K. Creating Healthy Food and Eating Environments: Policy and Environmental Approaches. *Annu. Rev. Public Health* **2008**, *29*, 253–272. [CrossRef] [PubMed]
37. Drobniewski, F.; Kusuma, D.; Broda, A.; Castro-Sánchez, E.; Ahmad, R. COVID-19 Vaccine Hesitancy in Diverse Groups in the UK—Is the Driver Economic or Cultural in Student Populations. *Vaccines* **2022**, *10*, 501. [CrossRef] [PubMed]

nutrients

MDPI

Article

Association between Disability and Unmet Food Needs in the Venezuelan Migrant and Refugee Population: Analysis of a Population-Based Survey, 2022

Akram Hernández-Vásquez [1,*], Alicia Bartra Reátegui [2], Keller Sánchez-Dávila [2] and Rodrigo Vargas-Fernández [3]

[1] Centro de Excelencia en Investigaciones Económicas y Sociales en Salud, Vicerrectorado de Investigación, Universidad San Ignacio de Loyola, Lima 15046, Peru
[2] Vicerrectorado de Investigación, Universidad Nacional de San Martín, Tarapoto 22201, Peru; abartra@unsm.edu.pe (A.B.R.); ksanchezd@unsm.edu.pe (K.S.-D.)
[3] Faculty of Health Sciences, Universidad Científica del Sur, Lima 15067, Peru; jvargasf@cientifica.edu.pe
* Correspondence: ahernandez@usil.edu.pe

Abstract: In Peru, Venezuelan migrants and refugees have been exposed to food shortages before their emigration. This problem could have worse outcomes in vulnerable populations (such as people with disabilities); however, the literature on the basic needs of this population is still scarce. The objective was to determine the association between the presence of disability and the unmet need for access to food in the household of the Venezuelan migrant and refugee population residing in Peru. A cross-sectional study was conducted using data from the Second Survey of the Venezuelan Population Residing in Peru (ENPOVE 2022). The outcome variable was unmet need for food, while the independent variable was the presence of disability. Poisson log generalized linear regression models (crude and adjusted for potential confounding variables) were fitted to evaluate the association between the variables of interest, reporting prevalence ratios (PR) and 95% confidence intervals (CIs). A total of 7739 migrants and refugees from Venezuela were included. The proportion of unmet need for access to food in the household was 45.2%, while the proportion of disability was 2.1%. People with disabilities were found to be more likely to have an unmet need for access to food at home (adjusted PR [aPR]: 1.25; 95% CI: 1.08–1.46; $p = 0.003$). According to our findings, almost half of Venezuelan households were found to have an unmet need for access to food. In addition, Venezuelan migrants and refugees with disabilities were more likely to have an unmet need for this basic need.

Keywords: immigrants; refugees; food; people with disability; Peru

1. Introduction

People with disabilities are a vulnerable and underserved group who experience difficulties in accessing health, education, employment, and social support services [1]. It is estimated that more than one billion people around the world live with disabilities (representing 15% of the world's population) [1,2], and about 80% of this population resides in low- and middle-income countries (LMIC) [3]. In Latin America and the Caribbean (LAC), the highest proportion of migrants and refugees with disabilities and their families reside in Peru (31.5%), followed by Colombia (15.1%) and the Dominican Republic (11.8%). Forty percent are male, aged 36 to 59 years (43.2%), and they are illegal immigrants in the city where they reside (53.8%) [4]. Despite the fact that government institutions seek to ensure that people with disabilities have access to health services, education, employment, and other basic needs, this population experiences worse health outcomes and inequalities in access to food compared to the general population, which could be further accentuated by their migratory status [1,5]. However, data on the proportion of migrants and refugee population are scarce and vary considerably from one region to another [6,7], which could be attributed to the lack of recognition of forms of disability; lack of uniform definitions of disability; and cultural, social and economic barriers that hinder the migration of people with disabilities.

In LAC, the Venezuelan migrant and refugee population have maintained an unsatisfied need for food since before their emigration, because in their cities of origin, they experienced food shortages and high costs, demonstrated by a hypocaloric diet low in nutrients [8]. In addition, in LMIC (as in the countries that make up the LAC region), people with disabilities live in conditions of poverty and extreme poverty, with a lack of access to health services, inadequate sources of drinking water and sanitation, and a lack of food [9]. Specifically, the lack of access to food in people with disabilities is associated with poverty, which results in higher rates of malnutrition and it is has even been observed that people with disabilities have a higher risk of this condition due to their nutritional requirements [9–11]. This problem could further increase the lack of access to adequate quantity and quality of food in the migrant and refugee population with disabilities, leading to an increase in the prevalence of nutritional diseases and worse health outcomes due to their disability status. Although inequalities in access to food is a priority in the Sustainable Development Goals in vulnerable populations (such as people with disabilities) [7], epidemiological studies conducted in LMIC have only focused on the relationship between disability and access to food [12], without considering the migratory status of people in their evaluations.

In Peru, about 10% of the national population has some type of disability [13]. On the other hand, Peru is the second Latin American country that hosts the largest number of Venezuelan migrants since 2016, reaching a figure of more than one million migrants in the last year [13]. In this regard, a previous study conducted in the Venezuelan migrant and refugee population residing in Peru reported that food insecurity in this population exceeded 60% (11% with a severe food insecurity and 52% with moderate food insecurity) [14]. Although studies show high rates of lack of access to food in the migrant and refugee population in Peru, there is little scientific evidence on this outcome in people with disabilities according to their migratory status. In fact, the scarce biomedical literature only focuses on studies that evaluate the disadvantages of people with disabilities in terms of public policies on food and access to health services [15,16]. Therefore, the aim of this study was to determine the association between the presence of disability and the unmet need for access to food in the household of the Venezuelan migrant and refugee population residing in Peru.

2. Materials and Methods

2.1. Design and Data Source

This study involved a secondary data analysis based on data from the Second Survey of the Venezuelan Population Residing in Peru (ENPOVE 2022—acronym in Spanish) that used a cross-sectional study design to collect the data [17]. The objective of the ENPOVE is to obtain demographic and socioeconomic information on the Venezuelan refugee and migrant population in Peru. The survey was carried out by the National Institute of Statistics and Informatics (INEI—acronym in Spanish) of Peru during the months of February and March 2022. ENPOVE 2022 was sponsored and financed by the World Bank, the United Nations Refugee Agency (UNHCR), the International Organization for Migration (IOM), the United Nations Population Fund (UNFPA), the United Nations Children's Fund (UNICEF), and the World Food Program (WFP) [17].

The sampling frame was based on information from the Registry of Dwellings and Establishments of the National Labor Market Survey (ENAMEL) and the National Superintendence of Migration of Peru [18]. A sample frame of 236,074 households of the Venezuelan population in Peru was constructed and a total of 195,710 households were obtained, representing 82.9% of the total number of households of the Venezuelan population at the national level. The target population were people of Venezuelan nationality (refugees, refugee applicants, migrants, and people with protection needs), who usually reside in private and collective households in urban areas of the main cities of Peru (Tumbes, Piura,

Chiclayo, Trujillo, Chimbote, Ica, Arequipa, Metropolitan Lima) [18]. The ENPOVE 2022 defines a household as a group of people, whether or not they are relatives, who share the main meals and attend to their vital needs together. The information was collected by direct interview and the information was recorded on a tablet by interviewers who were previously trained [18].

The sample selection was probabilistic, stratified, and independent in each study city [18]. The total sample size was 3680 households of the Venezuelan population. A total of 12,487 participants were included in the ENPOVE 2022 database of individuals. Further specifications on the sample design, procedures, and data collection can be found in the ENPOVE 2022 data sheet and report [17,18]. The sample selected for this study consisted of 7739 Venezuelan migrants and refugees aged 18 years or older with complete data on the variables studied.

2.2. *Variables*

2.2.1. Outcome

Based on the response to the question "What would be the three main needs, which are not being met in your household today?", we defined the dependent variable of the study as "Unmet need for access to food in the household" being a "Yes" when the participants answered that "Food" would be one of the main needs not being met in the household, and as "No" otherwise.

2.2.2. Exposition

The disability variable was constructed from the Washington Group's disability questions [19]. The questions were: Do you have permanent limitations in moving or walking, in using arms and legs? Do you have permanent limitations in seeing, even when wearing glasses? Do you have permanent limitations in speaking or communicating, even when using sign language or other? Do you have permanent limitations in hearing, even when using hearing aids? Do you have permanent limitations in understanding or learning (concentrating and remembering)? Do you have permanent limitations in relating to others, because of your thoughts, feelings, emotions, or behaviors? The possible response categories were yes or no. We considered a person to have a disability if they answered yes to at least one of the questions.

2.2.3. Covariates

The following variables were selected as potential confounders: age in age groups (18–59 years, 60 or older), gender (male, female), educational level (up to primary education, secondary education, higher education), chronic disease (no, yes), migration permit (no, yes), work in the last week (no, yes), wealth index (low, middle, high), period of arrival to Peru (pre-pandemic, during the COVID-19 pandemic), and city of residence (Tumbes, Piura, Chiclayo, Trujillo, Chimbote, Ica, Arequipa, Metropolitan Lima).

The creation of the wealth index took into consideration housing characteristics (walls, roofs, floors, water, drainage and lighting) and household goods or services (internet, television, stove, blender, iron, computer, cell phone, landline, radio, refrigerator and washing machine). Each characteristic was recategorized as a dichotomous variable (yes, no), assigning it a score generated through principal component analysis and each household was assigned a score for each characteristic, and the scores for each household were summed [20]. From the results that included the sample weights, households were classified according to the total score of the household, and three equal categories (terciles) were created: "low", "middle", and "high".

2.3. *Statistical Analysis*

Stata 17.0 (StataCorp, College Station, TX, USA) was used to clean, recode, and analyze the data. All analyses included the complex sampling characteristics and sampling weights of the ENPOVE 2022, in addition to the *subpop* command (respondents aged 18 years or older).

Summary statistics and cross tabulations were used to describe the study sample. Chi-square tests with Rao–Scott correction were performed to determine the differences between the proportions of the variables included in the study. Poisson log generalized linear regression models (crude and adjusted for potential confounding variables) were fitted to evaluate the association between disability and food need, reporting prevalence ratios (PR) and 95% confidence intervals (CIs) as measures of association. Finally, a p value less than 0.05 was considered statistically significant.

2.4. Ethical Considerations

The ENPOVE 2022 surveyors obtained informed consent from the participants at the beginning of the survey. The ENPOVE 2022 databases do not contain information that would allow respondents to be identified. The ENPOVE 2022 databases and other relevant documents are freely available in the INEI's microdata repository (https://iinei.inei.gob.pe/microdatos/ (accessed on 26 January 2023)) and no formal ethical clearance was obtained since we conducted a secondary analysis of publicly available data.

3. Results

A total of 7739 migrants and refugees from Venezuela were included in the analysis. The mean age was 33.1 years (standard deviation [SD]: 10.5), and more female than male respondents were included (3999 vs. 3740, respectively). The sociodemographic and economic characteristics of both groups (men and women) are shown in Table 1.

Table 1. Characteristics of the Venezuelan migrants and refugees included in this study, ENPOVE 2022.

Characteristic	Males *n* (%) *	Females *n* (%) *
Overall	3740 (100)	3999 (100)
Age, mean (+/− SD)	33.1 (10.5)	35.0 (12.2)
Age group (years)		
18–59	3633 (97.5)	3807 (95.1)
60 or more	107 (2.5)	192 (4.9)
Educational level		
Higher education	1422 (41.2)	1843 (50.7)
Secondary education	1782 (48.5)	1669 (40.4)
Up to primary education	536 (10.3)	487 (8.9)
Chronic disease		
No	3327 (90.1)	3075 (77.2)
Yes	413 (9.9)	924 (22.8)
Migration permit		
No	1307 (27.2)	1560 (32.1)
Yes	2433 (72.8)	2439 (67.9)
Work in the last week		
Yes	3341 (89.8)	2498 (63.9)
No	399 (10.2)	1501 (36.1)
Wealth index		
Low	1235 (30.2)	1182 (27.2)
Middle	1260 (34.2)	1366 (33.2)
High	1242 (35.6)	1442 (39.7)
Period of arrival to Peru		
During the COVID-19 pandemic	892 (22.1)	1113 (26.0)
Pre-pandemic	2848 (77.9)	2886 (74.0)

Table 1. *Cont.*

Characteristic	Males *n* (%) *	Females *n* (%) *
City of residence		
Arequipa	215 (3.5)	213 (3.3)
Chiclayo	198 (1.4)	242 (1.6)
Chimbote	258 (1.6)	262 (1.5)
Ica	217 (2.7)	188 (2.2)
Metropolitan Lima	2004 (83.0)	2162 (83.3)
Piura	215 (2.2)	234 (2.2)
Trujillo	410 (4.8)	449 (5.0)
Tumbes	223 (0.9)	249 (1.0)

* The weighting factor and sample specifications of ENPOVE were included. ENPOVE: Encuesta dirigida a la población venezolana que reside en el Perú. SD: standard deviation, CI: confidence interval. Values are the number of participants and percentages, unless stated otherwise.

Table 2 shows that the proportion of unmet need for access to food at home was 45.2% (95% CI: 43.0–47.4). Among migrants and refugees without disability, 44.8% reported unmet food need; in those with disability, 61.4% reported unmet food need. The highest proportions of this outcome were found in people aged 60 years or older (52.5%); females (48.0%); in those with a high school education (52.2%); chronic illness (49.4%); without a legal stay permit (52. 2%); who did not work in the week prior to the survey (54.2%); had a low wealth index (54.0%); had migrated during the pandemic (48.5%); and resided in the city of Tumbes (58.2%), Piura (50.6%), or Chimbote (49.4%).

Table 2. Frequency of unmet need for access to food in the household among Venezuelan migrants and refugees by background characteristics, ENPOVE 2022.

Characteristics	Unmet Need for Access to Food in the Household		
	No (*n* = 4242) % * (95% CI)	Yes (*n* = 3497) % * (95% CI)	*p*-Value **
Overall	54.8 (52.6–57.0)	45.2 (43.0–47.4)	
Disability			
No	55.2 (52.9–57.4)	44.8 (42.6–47.1)	0.001
Yes	38.6 (29.6–48.4)	61.4 (51.6–70.4)	
Age group (years)			
18–59	55.1 (52.9–57.3)	44.9 (42.7–47.1)	0.046
60 or more	47.5 (40.2–55.0)	52.5 (45.0–59.8)	
Gender			
Male	57.8 (55.3–60.3)	42.2 (39.7–44.7)	<0.001
Female	52.0 (49.4–54.6)	48.0 (45.4–50.6)	
Educational level			
Higher education	61.8 (58.9–64.5)	38.2 (35.5–41.1)	<0.001
Secondary education	47.8 (44.7–50.8)	52.2 (49.2–55.3)	
Up to primary education	54.0 (48.9–59.1)	46.0 (40.9–51.1)	
Chronic disease			
No	55.7 (53.3–58.0)	44.3 (42.0–46.7)	0.013
Yes	50.6 (46.8–54.4)	49.4 (45.6–53.2)	
Migration permit			
No	47.8 (44.6–51.0)	52.2 (49.0–55.4)	<0.001
Yes	57.8 (55.3–60.2)	42.2 (39.8–44.7)	
Work in the last week			
Yes	57.6 (55.3–59.9)	42.4 (40.1–44.7)	<0.001
No	45.8 (42.5–49.1)	54.2 (50.9–57.5)	

Table 2. *Cont.*

Characteristics	Unmet Need for Access to Food in the Household		p-Value **
	No (n = 4242) % * (95% CI)	Yes (n = 3497) % * (95% CI)	
Wealth index			
Low	46.0 (42.4–49.7)	54.0 (50.3–57.6)	<0.001
Middle	51.1 (47.7–54.5)	48.9 (45.5–52.3)	
High	64.9 (61.5–68.1)	35.1 (31.9–38.5)	
Period of arrival to Peru			
During the COVID-19 pandemic	51.5 (48.0–55.0)	48.5 (45.0–52.0)	0.019
Pre-pandemic	55.9 (53.5–58.3)	44.1 (41.7–46.5)	
City of residence			
Arequipa	64.2 (57.1–70.7)	35.8 (29.3–42.9)	<0.001
Chiclayo	55.0 (46.8–62.9)	45.0 (37.1–53.2)	
Chimbote	50.6 (43.8–57.3)	49.4 (42.7–56.2)	
Ica	62.7 (54.5–70.2)	37.3 (29.8–45.5)	
Metropolitan Lima	54.1 (51.5–56.7)	45.9 (43.3–48.5)	
Piura	49.4 (41.6–57.2)	50.6 (42.8–58.4)	
Trujillo	63.1 (57.5–68.3)	36.9 (31.7–42.5)	
Tumbes	41.8 (35.4–48.6)	58.2 (51.4–64.6)	

Data are displayed as weighted % of the row unless indicated otherwise. * The weighting factor and sample specifications of ENPOVE were included. ** Estimated p-value using the chi-square test with Rao–Scott adjustment. ENPOVE: Encuesta dirigida a la población venezolana que reside en el Perú. CI: confidence interval.

The proportion of disability among Venezuelan migrants and refugees was 2.1%. The highest proportions of disability were found in those 60 years of age or older (8.5%), had up to primary education (4.2%), had a chronic illness (5.0%), had not worked in the week prior to the survey (4.2%), had migrated during the pandemic period (3.0%), and resided in Chiclayo (5.0%) (Table 3).

Table 3. Frequency of disability among Venezuelan migrants and refugees by background characteristics, ENPOVE 2022.

Characteristics	Disability		p-Value **
	No (n = 7583) % * (95% CI)	Yes (n = 156) % * (95% CI)	
Overall	97.9 (97.5–98.3)	2.1 (1.7–2.5)	
Age group (years)			
18–59	98.2 (97.7–98.6)	1.8 (1.4–2.3)	<0.001
60 or more	91.5 (87.2–94.4)	8.5 (5.6–12.8)	
Gender			
Male	98.1 (97.5–98.6)	1.9 (1.4–2.5)	0.346
Female	97.8 (97.0–98.3)	2.2 (1.7–3.0)	
Educational level			
Higher education	98.7 (98.1–99.1)	1.3 (0.9–1.9)	<0.001
Secondary education	97.6 (96.8–98.2)	2.4 (1.8–3.2)	
Up to primary education	95.8 (93.5–97.4)	4.2 (2.6–6.5)	
Chronic disease			
No	98.5 (98.0–98.9)	1.5 (1.1–2.0)	<0.001
Yes	95.0 (93.4–96.3)	5.0 (3.7–6.6)	

Table 3. *Cont.*

Characteristics	Disability		
	No (n = 7583) % * (95% CI)	Yes (n = 156) % * (95% CI)	p-Value **
Migration permit			
No	97.5 (96.6–98.2)	2.5 (1.8–3.4)	0.200
Yes	98.1 (97.6–98.6)	1.9 (1.4–2.4)	
Work in the last week			
Yes	98.6 (98.1–99.0)	1.4 (1.0–1.9)	<0.001
No	95.8 (94.4–96.9)	4.2 (3.1–5.6)	
Wealth index			
Low	98.1 (97.1–98.8)	1.9 (1.2-2.9)	0.542
Middle	98.1 (97.4–98.7)	1.9 (1.3–2.6)	
High	97.7 (96.7–98.3)	2.3 (1.7–3.3)	
Period of arrival to Peru			
During the COVID-19 pandemic	97.0 (95.8–97.9)	3.0 (2.1–4.2)	0.011
Pre-pandemic	98.2 (97.7–98.7)	1.8 (1.3–2.3)	
City of residence			
Arequipa	97.7 (95.6–98.8)	2.3 (1.2-4.4)	0.005
Chiclayo	95.0 (91.6–97.0)	5.0 (3.0–8.4)	
Chimbote	99.1 (97.7–99.6)	0.9 (0.4–2.3)	
Ica	99.7 (98.7–99.9)	0.3 (0.1–1.3)	
Metropolitan Lima	97.9 (97.3–98.3)	2.1 (1.7-2.7)	
Piura	98.7 (96.8–99.5)	1.3 (0.5-3.2)	
Trujillo	98.4 (96.9–99.2)	1.6 (0.8–3.1)	
Tumbes	99.1 (97.0–99.7)	0.9 (0.3–3.0)	

Data are displayed as weighted % of the row unless indicated otherwise. * The weighting factor and sample specifications of ENPOVE were included. ** Estimated p-value using the chi-square test with Rao–Scott adjustment. ENPOVE: Encuesta dirigida a la población venezolana que reside en el Perú. CI: confidence interval.

Regarding the association of interest, the crude analysis showed that there was an association between having a disability and an unmet need for access to food at home (PR: 1.37; 95% CI: 1.17–1.61; $p < 0.001$). This same association was observed in the analysis adjusted for the covariates gender, age, educational level, chronic diseases, work in the last week, wealth index, period to arrival to Peru, and city of residence, with people with disabilities being more likely to have an unmet need for access to food in the household (adjusted PR [aPR]: 1.25; 95% CI: 1.08–1.46; $p = 0.003$) (Table 4).

Table 4. Association between disability and unmet need for access to food in the household among Venezuelan migrants and refugees, ENPOVE 2022.

Variable	Crude		Adjusted *	
	PR (95% CI)	p-Value	aPR (95% CI)	p-Value
Disability				
No	Reference		Reference	
Yes	1.37 (1.17–1.61)	<0.001	1.25 (1.08–1.46)	0.003

Weighting factors and sample specifications of ENPOVE were included for all analysis. ENPOVE: Encuesta dirigida a la población venezolana que reside en el Perú. PR: prevalence ratio. aPR: adjusted prevalence ratio. CI: confidence interval. * Model adjusted for gender, age, educational level, chronic disease, work in the last week, wealth index, period of arrival to Peru, and city of residence.

4. Discussion

The objective of this study was to determine the association between the presence of disability and the unsatisfied need for access to food in the households of the Venezuelan migrant and refugee population residing in Peru. It was found that 2 out of 100 Venezuelan migrants and refugees have a disability. On the other hand, almost half of the households in which migrants and refugees from Venezuela reside have an unmet need for access to food. In addition, it was found that migrants and refugees from Venezuela with disabilities were more likely to have an unmet need for access to food at household level.

In relation to the outcome of the present study, approximately 5 out of 10 Venezuelan migrants and refugees in Peru had an unsatisfied need for access to food in their households. This finding is lower than that reported in the official reports conducted in Ecuador and Colombia, in which 82.8% and 85% of households with migrants and refugees from Venezuela had an unmet need for food in 2022 and 2021, respectively [21,22]. These differences could be attributed to the lack of a sampling frame (since they used the databases of non-governmental organizations), the form of telephone interview, and particularly, the Colombian survey was conducted in the context of the COVID-19 pandemic, during which there was a higher proportion of unmet basic needs. These characteristics could increase the proportion of this outcome. Our finding could be attributed to various factors experienced by the Venezuelan migrant and refugee population when they migrate to another country, such as their illegal migratory status, lack of employment, low income, food insecurity, and informality in employment [23,24]. On the other hand, our result reflects a cyclical problem that the population from Venezuela had been experiencing since before their emigration due to the constant lack of adequate food, which could translate into worse nutritional indicators and an increase in diseases or deficiencies.

Regarding the presence of disability, 2% of Venezuelan migrants and refugees reported having a disability at the time of the survey. This finding is in contrast to that reported by the UNHCR and the Latin American Network of Persons with Disabilities and their Families (RIADIS), which estimated that 39.0% of the Venezuelan population with disabilities and their families reside in Peru [4]. This difference could be attributed to the fact that healthier people with greater economic resources are more likely to migrate to other countries [25,26], which could explain the advantage in terms of disability of these migrants compared to other populations. On the other hand, this figure could expose a social and public health problem because people with disabilities who have migrated to other countries experience situations of discrimination, violation of human rights, and unmet basic needs of access to health services and food [4,27,28], which could be reflected in worse living standards for a population that, due to its characteristics, has greater needs. In this sense, the main non-governmental institutions, such as UNHCR, seek to guarantee access to vital services for migrants with disabilities and encourage the application of their skills for their own benefit. Nonetheless, there are still problems of social inclusion of this population due to the lack of access to disability certificates or incorporation of this population in humanitarian programs [4,29,30]. Therefore, strategies for the support and social inclusion of this vulnerable population should be reinforced with the objective of reducing the social and economic inequality they experience due to their migrant and disability status.

As a main finding, our study found that Venezuelan migrants and refugees with disabilities were more likely to have an unmet need for access to food. While the Venezuelan migrant and refugee population already had a lack of food access and availability prior to emigration [8], our finding could be attributed to the impact of emigration coupled with the health and economic crisis caused by the COVID-19 pandemic [4]. Both precedents have generated inadequate living conditions in the migrant and refugee population with disabilities due to the loss of income sources and eviction from their homes, resulting in poor access to basic needs such as food [4,31]. In addition, there is a possibility that given the lack of resources, these households consume hypercaloric and nutrient-poor foods, which according to the biomedical literature, are associated with obesogenic dietary behavior, worse nutritional indicators, and an increase in the incidence of chronic noncommunicable diseases [32].

The public health implications of this study are based on three main considerations. First, intersectoral work should be carried out on migrants and refugees with disabilities to promote their social inclusion, access to basic needs, and legal permanence in the city where they reside. Second, Peruvian governmental institutions should focus on the fulfillment of Sustainable Development Goal 2.1, which seeks to ensure access to all populations, especially people who experience greater vulnerability (such as people with disabilities) [7] to reduce the prevalence and burden of disease due to nutritional diseases. Finally, governmental and non-governmental institutions should redouble their efforts to continue humanitarian support to migrants and refugees with disabilities, which is one of the main recommendations issued by UNHCR and RIADIS, in order to cover basic needs such as employment, access to health services, and food [4].

One of the main strengths of this study is the use of a survey, including a large number of Venezuelan migrants and refugees residing in Peru, that was designed by INEI in conjunction with the main international organizations that seek the protection of migrants and refugees, and thereby provides a current overview of the disability status of this migrant and refugee population. Nevertheless, this study has limitations. First, the lack of temporality in the measurement of the variables due to its cross-sectional design prevents establishing causality. Second, there could be an information bias when considering specific events that occurred in the past. Third, it is possible that there was an over-report or under-report of disabilities by the participants, as previously described [33]. Finally, some variables may not have been included as potential confounders, such as the migrants having food insecurity before moving to Peru.

5. Conclusions

In conclusion, it was found that approximately 50% of migrants and refugees from Venezuela have an unmet need for access to food, while 2% have a disability. In addition, having a disability increased the probability of having an unmet need for food access in this Venezuelan population. Considering these findings, non-governmental institutions together with the Peruvian state should focus their strategies on social inclusion and economic and humanitarian support for migrants and refugees with disabilities to improve their access to basic needs such as food, in order to reduce negative nutritional indicators and the occurrence of chronic non-communicable diseases. In addition, our research provides evidence on the main dietary requirements of a minority population that has been understudied and neglected in recent decades.

Author Contributions: A.H.-V. Conceptualization, Methodology, Validation, Formal analysis, Investigation, Data Curation, Writing—Original Draft, Writing—Review and Editing, Visualization, Supervision; A.B.R. Validation, Investigation, Writing—Review and Editing; K.S.-D. Validation, Investigation, Writing—Review and Editing; R.V.-F. Methodology, Validation, Investigation, Writing—Original Draft, Writing—Review and Editing; A.H.-V., A.B.R., K.S.-D. and R.V.-F. All authors have read and agreed to the published version of the manuscript.

Funding: This research received no external funding.

Institutional Review Board Statement: Not applicable.

Informed Consent Statement: Not applicable.

Data Availability Statement: Not applicable.

Acknowledgments: The authors are grateful to Donna Pringle for reviewing the language and style.

Conflicts of Interest: The authors declare no conflict of interest.

References

1. World Health Organization. *World Bank World Report on Disability 2011*; World Health Organization: Geneva, Switzerland, 2011.
2. *United Nations Policy Brief: A Disability-Inclusive Response to COVID-19 2020*; United Nations: New York, NY, USA, 2020.
3. Mitra, S.; Posarac, A.; Vick, B.C. *Disability and Poverty in Developing Countries: A Snapshot from the World Health Survey*; World Bank: Washington, DC, USA, 2011.
4. Agencia de las Naciones Unidas para los Refugiados (ACNUR). *Estudio Regional Sobre La Situación de Las Personas Con Discapacidad Refugiadas, Desplazadas y Migrantes En América Latina 2021*; ACNUR: Geneva, Switzerland, 2021.

5. Assi, L.; Deal, J.A.; Samuel, L.; Reed, N.S.; Ehrlich, J.R.; Swenor, B.K. Access to Food and Health Care during the COVID-19 Pandemic by Disability Status in the United States. *Disabil. Health J.* **2022**, *15*, 101271. [CrossRef]
6. Stilwell, B.; Diallo, K.; Zurn, P.; Dal Poz, M.R.; Adams, O.; Buchan, J. Developing Evidence-Based Ethical Policies on the Migration of Health Workers: Conceptual and Practical Challenges. *Hum. Resour. Health* **2003**, *1*, 8. [CrossRef]
7. United Nations Disability and Development Report. *Realizing the Sustainable Development Goals by, for and with Persons with Disabilities 2018*; United Nations: New York, NY, USA, 2018.
8. Landaeta-Jiménez, M.; Herrera Cuenca, M.; Vásquez, M.; Ramírez, G. La alimentación y nutrición de los venezolanos: Encuesta Nacional de Condiciones de Vida 2014. *An. Venez. Nutr.* **2017**, *30*, 99–111.
9. Banks, L.M.; Kuper, H.; Polack, S. Poverty and Disability in Low- and Middle-Income Countries: A Systematic Review. *PLoS ONE* **2017**, *12*, e0189996. [CrossRef]
10. Mitra, S.; Posarac, A.; Vick, B. Disability and Poverty in Developing Countries: A Multidimensional Study. *World Dev.* **2013**, *41*, 1–18. [CrossRef]
11. Groce, N.; Challenger, E.; Berman-Bieler, R.; Farkas, A.; Yilmaz, N.; Schultink, W.; Clark, D.; Kaplan, C.; Kerac, M. Malnutrition and Disability: Unexplored Opportunities for Collaboration. *Paediatr. Int. Child Health* **2014**, *34*, 308–314. [CrossRef]
12. Bright, T.; Kuper, H. A Systematic Review of Access to General Healthcare Services for People with Disabilities in Low and Middle Income Countries. *Int. J. Environ. Res. Public. Health* **2018**, *15*, 1879. [CrossRef] [PubMed]
13. United Nations Children's Fund (UNICEF). UNICEF Peru Humanitarian Situation Report (Venezuela Migration): 30 March 2022. Available online: https://reliefweb.int/report/peru/unicef-peru-humanitarian-situation-report-venezuela-migration-30-march-2022 (accessed on 19 February 2023).
14. Vargas-Vásquez, A.; Aparco, J.P.; Hernández-Vásquez, A.; Pisfil-Benites, N.; Fuentes-Rivera, H. Food Insecurity among the Migrant Venezuelan Population in Peru during the COVID-19 Pandemic. *Rev. Chil. Nutr.* **2022**, *49*, 524–525. [CrossRef]
15. Reher, S. Mind This Gap, Too: Political Orientations of People with Disabilities in Europe. *Polit. Behav.* **2020**, *42*, 791–818. [CrossRef]
16. Schwartz, N.; Buliung, R.; Wilson, K. Disability and Food Access and Insecurity: A Scoping Review of the Literature. *Health Place* **2019**, *57*, 107–121. [CrossRef]
17. Instituto Nacional de Estadística e Informática. *Condiciones de Vida de la Población VENEZOLANA que Reside en el Perú. Resultados de la "Encuesta Dirigida a la Polación Venezolana que Reside en el País" II ENPOVE 2022*; Instituto Nacional de Estadística e Informática: Lima, Peru, 2023.
18. Instituto Nacional de Estadística e Informática. *Segunda Encuesta Dirigida a la Población Venezolana que Reside en el País. II ENPOVE 2021–2022. Ficha Técnica*; Instituto Nacional de Estadística e Informática: Lima, Peru, 2022.
19. Madans, J.H.; Loeb, M.E.; Altman, B.M. Measuring Disability and Monitoring the UN Convention on the Rights of Persons with Disabilities: The Work of the Washington Group on Disability Statistics. *BMC Public Health* **2011**, *11*, S4. [CrossRef]
20. Vyas, S.; Kumaranayake, L. Constructing Socio-Economic Status Indices: How to Use Principal Components Analysis. *Health Policy Plan.* **2006**, *21*, 459–468. [CrossRef]
21. Grupo de Trabajo para Refugiados y Migrantes (GTRM). *GTRM Ecuador: Evaluación Conjunta Necesidades 2022*; GTRM: Ecuador, 2022.
22. Grupo Interagencial sobre Flujos Migratorios Mixtos (GIFMM). *GIFMM Colombia: Evaluación Conjunta de Necesidades*; GIFMM: Ecuador, 2021.
23. Ortemberg, P. *Inclusión Laboral de Personas Migrantes Con Discapacidad: El Caso de La Migración Venezolana En La República Argentina*; Organización Internacional para las Migraciones: Ciudad Autónoma de Buenos Aires, Argentina, 2022.
24. Saint Ville, A.; Francis-Granderson, I.; Bhagwandeen, B.; Mohammed, M. Food Insecurity in Venezuelan Migrants in Trinidad and Tobago Using the Food Insecurity Experience Scale. *Front. Public Health* **2022**, *10*, 925813. [CrossRef] [PubMed]
25. Klein, J.; Von dem Knesebeck, O. Inequalities in Health Care Utilization among Migrants and Non-Migrants in Germany: A Systematic Review. *Int. J. Equity Health* **2018**, *17*, 160. [CrossRef]
26. Bernabe-Ortiz, A.; Carrillo-Larco, R.M. Multimorbidity and Disability Among Venezuelan Migrants: A Population-Based Survey in Peru. *J. Immigr. Minor. Health* **2022**, *24*, 1206–1213. [CrossRef] [PubMed]
27. Mendoza, W.; Miranda, J.J. La Inmigración Venezolana En El Perú: Desafíos y Oportunidades Desde La Perspectiva de La Salud. *Rev. Peru. Med. Exp. Salud Pública* **2019**, *36*, 497. [CrossRef] [PubMed]
28. Hernández-Vásquez, A.; Vargas-Fernández, R.; Rojas-Roque, C.; Bendezu-Quispe, G. Factores Asociados a La No Utilización de Servicios de Salud En Inmigrantes Venezolanos En Perú. *Rev. Peru. Med. Exp. Salud Pública* **2019**, *36*, 583–591. [CrossRef]
29. Bregaglio Lazarte, R.; Camino Morgado, P. Problemas En La Frontera: Retos Migratorios En El Perú Desde Un Enfoque Interseccional de Discapacidad. *Anu. Mex. Derecho Int.* **2021**, *1*, 895. [CrossRef]
30. Blouin, C. Complejidades y contradicciones de la política migratoria hacia la migración venezolana en el Perú. *Colomb. Int.* **2021**, 141–164. [CrossRef]
31. Sanabria-Rojas, H.; Tarqui-Mamani, C.; Portugal-Benavides, W.; Pereyra-Zaldívar, H.; Mamani-Castillo, L. The physical activity level of people working at a regional health office in Lima, Peru. *Rev. Salud Publica Bogota Colomb.* **2014**, *16*, 53–62.

32. Giskes, K.; Van Lenthe, F.; Avendano-Pabon, M.; Brug, J. A Systematic Review of Environmental Factors and Obesogenic Dietary Intakes among Adults: Are We Getting Closer to Understanding Obesogenic Environments?: Environmental Factors and Obesogenic Dietary Behaviours. *Obes. Rev.* **2011**, *12*, e95–e106. [CrossRef] [PubMed]
33. Elkasabi, M. Differences in Proxy-Reported and Self-Reported Disability in the Demographic and Health Surveys. *J. Surv. Stat. Methodol.* **2021**, *9*, 335–351. [CrossRef]

nutrients

MDPI

Article

Foods and Nutrients at Risk for Insufficient Intake by Community-Dwelling Healthy Older Women Eating Alone and Together in Japan—A Preliminary Finding

Tomoya Takiguchi [1], Muneko Nishijo [1,*], Noriko Kaneko [2], Katsushi Yoshita [3], Yusuke Arai [4], Noboru Demura [5] and Yoshikazu Nishino [1]

1 Department of Public Health, Kanazawa Medical University, Uchinada 920-0293, Japan; ttakiguc@kanazawa-med.ac.jp (T.T.); ynishino@kanazawa-med.ac.jp (Y.N.)
2 Faculty of Nursing, Ishikawa Prefectural Nursing University, Kahoku 929-1210, Japan; kaneko@ishikawa-nu.ac.jp
3 Department of Public Health, Nutrition, School of Human Life and Ecology, Osaka Metropolitan University, Osaka 558-8585, Japan; yoshita@omu.ac.jp
4 Department of Nutrition, Chiba Prefectural University of Health Sciences, Chiba 260-0801, Japan; yusuke.arai@cpuhs.ac.jp
5 Department of Oral and Maxillofacial Surgery, Kanazawa Medical University, Uchinada 920-0293, Japan; n-demura@kanazawa-med.ac.jp
* Correspondence: ni-koei@kanazawa-med.ac.jp; Tel.: +81-76-218-8093

Abstract: Eating alone and poor dental status have been reported to influence dietary intake in older adults. First, we compared nutrient and food intake and dental markers between women eating alone and together, who participated in a home health management program conducted by Kanazawa Medical University. The results showed the significantly higher intake of fresh fruit and some micronutrients and a lower decayed, missing, and filled teeth (DMFT) index (better dental status) in women eating alone after adjusting for age, suggesting that dental status may mediate the association between commensality and dietary intake. Then, we investigated nutrients and foods at risk for insufficient intake and associated with increasing dental markers. The risks for the insufficient intake of protein and *n*-3 and *n*-6 polyunsaturated fatty acids (PUFAs) were significantly increased with an increasing DMFT index. The risk for *n*-3 PUFA intake also increased with increasing numbers of missing teeth in women. Foods at risk for insufficient consumption included beans for women with an increasing DMFT index and green and yellow vegetables, fresh fruits, and meat and fish for women with increasing numbers of missing teeth. These findings suggest that good health management, including the treatment of decayed teeth, is important for the prevention of malnutrition in community-dwelling healthy older women.

Keywords: eating alone; dental status; nutrient intake; food consumption; older adults

1. Introduction

Older adults are at risk for malnutrition because of physiological and metabolic changes that progress during aging, particularly those that occur in the digestive organs, such as decreased gastric acid secretion and salivary production, which lead to the insufficient digestion and absorption of nutrients, and appetite loss due to a diminished sense of smell and taste [1]. In a population-based study in Germany of more than 1000 community-dwelling older adults aged ≥65 years, frequent subclinical micronutrient deficiencies, such as the lower intake of iron, folate, vitamin D, and vitamin B12, were reported, although malnutrition indicated by a low body mass index (BMI) due to insufficient protein and energy intake (macronutrient deficiency) was not common [2]. In the same study, physical inactivity and frailty were indicated as relevant factors associated with subclinical microdeficiencies in this older German population [2].

In 2021, Bjorwall et al. reviewed the literature and found that eating alone and eating together (commensality) were key factors related to eating behavior that could lead to malnutrition in community-dwelling older adults [3]. In older Japanese adults aged ≥65 years, Tani et al. reported in 2015 that men eating alone were more likely to be underweight (BMI < 18.5) than men eating together, although no clear association was found between eating alone and the prevalence of underweight in women [4]. These findings suggest macronutrient deficiency only in men. However, the authors of this Japanese study suggested that micronutrient deficiency might be possible in women who eat alone as a result of more frequent unhealthy dietary habits, such as skipping meals, in comparison with women eating together [4].

The alteration of oral health status with aging, such as the increased prevalence of caries, periodontal disease, and edentulism, and consequent decreased chewing ability due to the increased loss of teeth directly affects nutrition in older adults [5,6]. In this regard, many studies that investigate associations between dental status and dietary intake have been conducted in the United Kingdom (UK), the United States, and Asian countries including Japan. Dental parameters including edentate/dentate, the numbers of present teeth or missing teeth [7–10], self-reported chewing ability [11,12], and observational chewing ability [13,14] have been reported to be associated with lower dietary intakes in community-dwelling older adults. Particularly in Japanese studies, chewing ability evaluated by color-changeable chewing gum [13] or small numbers of posterior occluding pairs of teeth [14] have been investigated in relation to lower intakes of various kinds of foods and nutrients, including minerals and vitamins, in older adults in comparison with their counterparts with normal oral health status.

Among older adults aged ≥75 years who participated in the Adult Dental Health Survey 2009 in the UK, older adults who lived alone more frequently wore dentures, self-reported a poor oral status, and had poor dental care attendance in comparison with their co-habiting counterparts [15]. In Sweden, a Swedish National Quality Register Study to investigate relationships between quality of life and oral health among older adults aged ≥65 years reported that living alone was one of the relevant factors in having a higher risk of oral health problems [16]. These results suggest that older adults living alone and, ipso facto, eating alone may have an insufficient intake of foods and nutrients, and that this may be related to oral health problems.

Against this background, we first compared food and nutrient intake and dental markers among Japanese older women living and eating alone and together and found different dietary and dental statuses between them, suggesting an association between commensality (eating alone and together) and dental status. Because the subjects enrolled were participants in a home health management program organized by our department at Kanazawa Medical University, the number of men who ate alone was too small for statistical analysis, with only one man. We then investigated the risks associated with dental parameters for insufficient food and nutrient intake in women under the hypothesis that dental status may mediate the association between commensality and dietary intake. At this time, the reference levels of nutrients recommended from the standpoint of good health in healthy older adults by the Japanese government [17] were used for defining cut-off values of insufficient intake.

2. Materials and Methods

2.1. Study Subjects

A total of 84 independent older adults (29 men and 55 women) aged 65 years and older who resided in Uchinada town, Japan, and participated in home health management conducted by the Department of Public Health and Epidemiology, Kanazawa Medical University, were invited to participate the health impact survey consisting of a health check-up, dietary survey, and dental examination in May 2019. All of them underwent a health check-up including body size measurement, blood and urinary tests, blood pressure measurement, electrocardiogram, and chest X-ray examination (Figure 1). The number of participants of the dietary survey after the health check-up were 76 older adults (25 men and 51 women) who had completed dietary records at home (Figure 1).

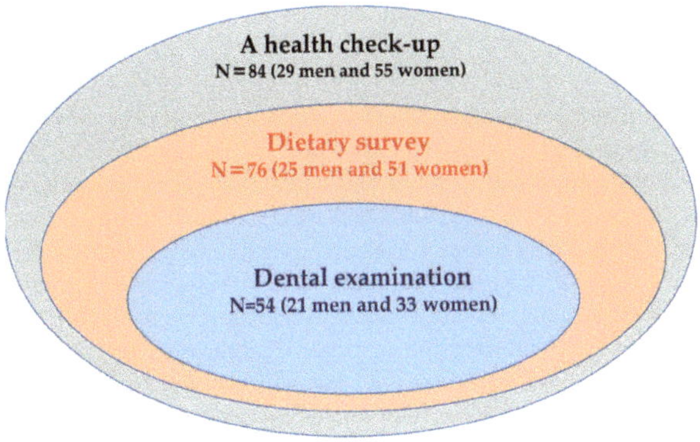

Figure 1. Participants of the health impact survey consisting of a health check-up, dietary survey, and dental examination.

A total of 54 older adults (21 men and 33 women) from participants to the dietary survey underwent an oral examination (Figure 1). The participant rate of the dental survey was lower, particularly in women (60%), compared to that of the dietary survey because women who visited dentists for regular dental check-up did not want to be examined again in the current survey.

The information on living alone or together with family, smoking habits, and educational history were obtained from records of home health management. In the dietary survey, the information on eating alone or together was collected by dietitians.

The study design and all procedures were approved by the Medical Research Ethics Review Committee of Kanazawa Medical University (No. I522, 24 June 2020). Written informed consent was obtained from all subjects.

2.2. Measurements

2.2.1. Dental Examination

An intra-oral examination was conducted by a single dentist using a dental mirror and a dental probe. Participants' teeth were recorded as sound, decayed, missing, and filled according to the diagnostic criteria of the Japanese national survey titles "Survey of Dental Diseases" [18]. Third molars, extractions for orthodontic treatment, and areas considered innate defects were excluded from missing teeth. The DMFT index numerically expresses the prevalence of dental caries and is calculated from the sum of numbers of decayed teeth, missing teeth, and filled teeth. A higher value of DMFT index indicates poorer dental status [19,20].

2.2.2. Dietary Survey

Subjects were required to record all foods and beverages including ingredients and portion sizes for 2 days. At the site of the survey, dietitians interviewed the subjects to confirm their records and the amount of each ingredient, using standard food models (Iwai Sample, Osaka, Japan) to improve accuracy and estimate their dietary intake. Total energy intake, macronutrient intake and energy ratios (balances), and micronutrients including minerals and fatty acids were estimated by the nutritional calculation software "Shokuji-Shirabe 2011", developed by the National Institute of Health and Nutrition. At this time, intakes were calculated after accounting for changes in weight and nutrient content arising from cooking. To define the lower limit of recommended intakes, we used the Dietary Reference Intakes for Japanese (2015) [17] for each nutrient. The cutoff values for beans, fruit, and vegetables were set according to intake levels recommended in the national health promotion named Healthy Japan 21 [21]. For other foods, such as meat and fish, intakes were set by referring to the recommended intakes (for 1600 calories per day) in the handbook based on the 4-food-groups scoring method [22].

2.3. Statistical Analysis

STATA/MP 16.1 (Stata, College Station, TX, USA) was used for statistical analysis. Adjusted comparisons of demographic factors, dental parameters, and nutrient and food intakes were compared between older adults eating alone and together after adjusting for age using general linear model (analysis of covariance with age as a covariate) in women alone because of the small number of men eating alone. A logistic regression model was used to analyze the risks (odds ratios) for insufficient nutrient and food intakes associated with increasing dental parameters after adjusting for age in women alone because recommended values for nutrients were different between men and women [17]. In the current analysis, smoking status and educational history, which are well-known confounding factors in dental and nutrition status, were not adjusted at this time because there were very few smokers (two men and no women) and no significant correlations between dental markers or nutrients and educational history in our subjects. The significance level was set at 5% ($p < 0.05$).

3. Results

One man (4.2%) and nineteen women (37.3%) were living alone. All older adults living alone prepared food by themselves and ate alone on almost all days except for a few days per month when meeting family members or friends living in different areas. Almost all older adults who lived with others (95.8% men and 90.6% women) were eating with their spouse, except for one man and two women who lived and ate with their children and one woman who lived and ate with her sister. Taken together, in the current study, all subjects living alone ate alone, and all subjects living together ate together. In the results that follow, "eating alone or together" means "living and eating alone or together".

3.1. Comparisons of Body Size and Food and Nutrient Intake between Older Adults Eating Alone and Together in Each Sex

According to sex and commensality (eating alone or together), the means with standard deviations (SD) of age and BMI and the frequencies (%) of underweight (BMI < 18.5) and overweight (BMI $\geq$ 25.0), as defined by the Japan Society for the Study of Obesity, are shown in Table 1.

Only one man ate alone; therefore, no comparison could be made between men eating alone and those eating together. In women, no significant differences in age, body size, or the frequency of cases with low and high bodyweight were found between older adults eating alone and together. Daily food intake (g) in each food group was also compared between women living and eating alone and together (Table 1). However, only fresh fruit intake was significantly higher in women eating alone, even after adjusting for age ($p < 0.05$), in comparison with women eating together.

No significant difference in macronutrient intake was found between women eating alone and together (Table 1). With regard to micronutrients, however, the intakes of potassium, magnesium, Vitamin K, folate, and total dietary fiber were significantly lower in women eating together after adjusting for age in comparison with women eating alone (Table 1).

Table 1. Comparisons of body size and food and nutrient intake between older adults eating alone and together.

Category	Health and Nutrition Markers	Men				Women				p
		Alone (N = 1)		Together (N = 24)		Alone (N = 18)		Together (N = 33)		
		Mean, %	SD	Mean, %	SD	Mean, %	SD	Mean, %	SD	
Age and habits	Age (years)	82.0		77.1	4.6	77.7	4.9	75.3	5.8	
	Present smokers (%)	100.0		20.8		0.0		0.0		
Body size	Height (cm)	167.0		164.2	5.8	149.7	4.6	151.4	5.4	
	Weight (kg)	72.5		63.7	9.6	50.4	7.7	49.7	8.4	
	BMI	26.0		23.6	3.3	22.4	3.0	21.7	3.3	
	BMI < 18.5 (%)	0.0		8.3		5.6		9.1		
	BMI ≥ 25 (%)	100.0		41.7		16.7		12.1		
Food intake	Rice (g)	560.0		282.3	107.7	233.9	124.2	199.9	105.4	
	Beans (g)	10.0		51.3	38.9	75.6	69.4	58.1	52.7	
	Green vegetables (g)	217.5		129.5	90.0	157.1	75.4	133.9	83.6	
	Other vegetables (g)	24.0		122.6	71.9	151.2	90.6	137.4	73.0	
	Fresh fruits (g)	15.0		90.4	47.9	151.2	81.6	97.7	62.9	*
	Seaweed (g)	9.0		16.6	19.7	27.5	28.0	17.1	18.5	
	Seafood (g)	120.5		82.0	51.0	78.3	41.5	76.9	58.5	
	Meat (g)	166.5		60.9	35.5	57.9	38.5	55.5	36.3	
	Meat and seafood (g)	287.0		142.9	56.5	132.6	56.7	134.5	62.8	
	Eggs (g)	69.5		39.8	36.4	39.3	27.1	39.6	34.1	
Macronutrient intake	Energy (kcal)	2691		1980	383	1796.9	429.8	1635	367	
	Protein (g)	98.9		68.9	15.1	72.7	18.8	63.9	17.7	
	Protein density (%kcal)	14.8		14.0	2.3	16.3	2.0	15.7	2.3	
	Total fat (g)	80.6		50.8	13.7	57.0	23.7	49.8	16.9	
	Fat density (%kcal)	26.9		23.2	5.8	27.7	6.9	27.1	6.3	
	Carbohydrate (g)	380.6		269.5	66.8	244.2	57.5	223.9	51.6	
	Carbohydrate density (%kcal)	58.4		62.7	6.2	56.0	7.4	57.3	7.3	
Micronutrient intake	Potassium (mg)	2701		2622	925	3100	1133	2436	697	*
	Calcium (mg)	899		524	193	663.2	313.0	538.5	260.6	
	Magnesium (mg)	300		270	100	320.9	116.3	242.8	73.2	**
	Phosphorus (mg)	1543		1024	245	1112.3	331.2	964.9	282.1	
	Iron (mg)	9.3		7.6	1.9	9.2	3.3	7.3	2.4	*
	Zinc (mg)	12.4		7.7	1.6	8.3	2.7	7.0	1.9	*
	Copper (mg)	1.5		1.2	0.5	1.2	0.4	1.0	0.3	
	Vitamin A (μgRAE)	623.0		752.6	1414	656.6	314.4	465.9	281.6	
	Vitamin D (μg)	13.4		7.1	5.3	8.5	6.0	8.9	7.3	
	Vitamin E (mg)	7.9		6.9	2.5	7.7	2.3	6.5	2.1	
	Vitamin K (μg)	339.5		221.3	150.0	304.0	189.0	194.6	112.6	*
	Folate (μg)	292.0		353.8	170.9	393.8	123.8	303.2	106.1	**
	Vitamin C (mg)	343.5		107.3	57.3	135.4	55.2	104.7	50.2	
	n-3 PUFA (g)	3.1		2.1	1.0	2.3	1.2	2.0	1.1	
	n-6 PUFA (g)	10.5		8.6	3.7	9.4	4.4	7.7	3.9	
	Total dietary fiber (g)	13.3		14.5	4.3	17.5	6.3	13.9	4.4	*

*: $p < 0.05$; **: $p < 0.01$: age-adjusted p-value; N: number of subjects; SD: standard deviation; SFA: saturated fatty acid; PUFA: polyunsaturated fatty acid.

3.2. Comparisons of Body Size and Food and Nutrient Intake between Men and Women Eating Together

To estimate the gender differences of nutritional status, body size and food and nutrient intake were compared between men and women eating together (Table 1; statistical test results not shown in the table).

The prevalence of overweight (BMI ≥ 25) and mean rice intake were significantly higher ($p = 0.025$ and $p = 0.006$, respectively) in men eating together compared with women after adjusting for age. Additionally, men eating together showed significantly higher energy ($p = 0.001$), carbonate ($p = 0.001$), and carbonate balance ($p = 0.005$) and significantly lower protein balance ($p = 0.008$) and fat balance ($p = 0.028$) compared with women eating together. These results indicate that higher energy intake due to higher rice intake might be related to a high prevalence of overweight in men eating together in this cohort.

3.3. Comparisons of BMI, Dental Parameters, and Food and Nutrient Intake between Female Dental Examination Participants Eating Alone and Together

Because of the smaller number of participants in the dental examination, including only one male participant who ate alone, the comparisons of health and nutritional markers including dental parameters between groups eating alone and together were, once again, only performed in women (Table 2).

Table 2. Comparisons of BMI, dental parameters, and food and nutrient intake between female dental examination participants eating alone and together.

Category	Health Marker and Foods	Alone (N = 10)		Together (N = 23)		p
		Mean, %	SD	Mean, %	SD	
Age and body size	Age (years)	76.5	4.6	73.9	5.9	
	Height (cm)	150.6	5.6	151.5	5.5	
	Weight (kg)	50.9	9.4	49.9	7.9	
	BMI	22.3	3.3	21.7	2.9	
	BMI < 18.5 (%)	10.0		4.3		
	BMI ≥ 25 (%)	20.0		13.0		
Dental status	Present teeth	21.0	7.6	19.9	7.3	
	DMFT Index	16.7	9.4	23.2	5.8	*
	Decayed (untreated)	0.1	0.3	1.0	1.3	*
	Missing teeth	6.8	7.5	8.2	7.3	
	Treated teeth	9.8	6.2	14.0	6.5	
Food intake	Rice (g)	233.9	124.2	199.9	105.4	
	Beans (g)	75.6	69.4	58.1	52.7	
	Green vegetables (g)	157.1	75.4	133.9	83.6	
	Other vegetables (g)	151.2	90.6	137.4	73.0	
	Fresh fruits (g)	151.2	81.6	97.7	62.9	*
	Seaweed (g)	27.5	28.0	17.1	18.5	*
	Seafood (g)	78.3	41.5	76.9	58.5	
	Meat (g)	57.9	38.5	55.5	36.3	
	Meat and seafood (g)	132.6	56.7	134.5	62.8	
	Eggs (g)	39.3	27.1	39.6	34.1	
Macronutrient intake	Energy (kcal)	2011.2	419.0	1623.1	388.0	**
	Protein (g)	82.8	18.6	63.0	17.7	**
	Protein density (%kcal)	16.5	1.6	15.5	2.1	
	Total fat (g)	72.2	20.4	46.5	13.4	***
	Fat density (%kcal)	31.8	5.3	25.6	5.2	**
	Carbohydrate (g)	255.2	57.8	229.4	56.9	
	Carbohydrate density (%kcal)	51.7	5.4	58.9	6.2	**
	Potassium (mg)	3369.6	1075.1	2369.5	629.7	**
	Calcium (mg)	831.8	310.6	507.1	202.4	**
	Magnesium (mg)	351.8	109.1	234.7	64.2	***
	Phosphorus (mg)	1284.4	343.8	946.3	279.9	**
	Iron (mg)	10.9	3.5	6.9	2.1	***
	Zinc (mg)	9.9	2.4	6.8	1.9	***
	Copper (mg)	1.4	0.5	1.0	0.3	*
	Vitamin A (μgRAE)	811.2	322.4	415.0	213.1	**
	Vitamin D (μg)	9.6	5.5	8.4	6.7	
	Vitamin E (mg)	8.4	2.3	6.0	2.4	**
	Vitamin K (μg)	390.5	218.0	183.9	114.0	**
	Folate (μg)	451.5	127.6	294.2	104.1	**
	Vitamin C (mg)	146.6	43.0	104.7	52.7	*
	n-3 PUFA (g)	2.8	1.3	1.9	1.0	
	n-6 PUFA (g)	11.2	5.1	6.9	2.6	**
	Total dietary fiber (g)	20.0	7.2	13.1	4.1	**

*: $p < 0.05$; **: $p < 0.01$; ***: $p < 0.001$: age-adjusted p-value; N: number of subjects; SD: standard deviation; DMFT index: the sum of decayed, missing, and filled teeth; SFA: saturated fatty acid; PUFA: polyunsaturated fatty acid.

Although there was no difference in BMI-related markers between the two groups, dental status, such as that defined by the DMFT index, and, particularly, the number of untreated, decayed teeth, was significantly lower in women eating alone after adjusting for age. Regarding food intake, women eating alone ingested significantly more fresh fruits and seaweed than women eating together. These results suggest that dental and nutritional status are better in women eating alone.

Regarding nutrient intake, women eating alone ingested significantly more sources of energy, protein, and fat compared with women eating together. Fat balance was significantly higher and carbonate balance significantly lower in women eating alone than in women eating together. Similarly, the intakes of vitamin A, E, K, and C; folate; *n*-3, *n*-6 polyunsaturated fatty acids (PUFAs); and total dietary fiber were significantly higher in women eating alone compared with women eating together after adjusting for age (Table 2).

3.4. Increased Risks for Insufficient Nutrient and Food Intake Associated with Dental Status in Women

Significant inverse associations between macronutrient parameters, such as protein and/or fat intakes and balance, and dental parameters were found in female participants of the dental examination, whereas there were no significant associations between them in all women. With regard to micronutrients, the intake levels of phosphorus, iron, zinc, *n*-3 and *n*-6 PUFAs, vitamin A, vitamin E, folic acid, and total dietary fiber were also significantly and inversely associated with both the DMFT index and/or the number of missing teeth.

Then, we analyzed the risks (odds ratios) for insufficient nutrient intake associated with increasing dental parameters using binary logistic analysis, and the results for women are shown in Table 3. In addition, a risk analysis for insufficient intake was performed only for protein because of the lack of reference values for good health from other macronutrients [17].

In women, after adjusting for age, the risk (odds ratio) of the insufficient intake of protein (<55 g/day) was 1.2 and significantly associated with an increasing DMFT index. The odds ratios for the insufficient intakes of *n*-3 PUFA (<1.9 g/day) and *n*-6 PUFA (<7 g/day) were 1.18 and 1.16, respectively, and significantly increased with an increasing DMFT index in women (Table 3). The number of missing teeth was also significantly associated with an increased odds ratio for the insufficient intake of *n*-3 PUFA, suggesting a 1.19 times higher risk with the increasing number of missing teeth in women (Table 3).

The numbers of decayed_teeth were significantly associated with a lower intake of Vitamin B12 with an increased odds ratio of 3.45 in women.

Regarding the risk analysis for insufficient food intake, a lower intake of beans (<100 g/day) was significantly associated with an increasing DMFT index, with an odds ratio of 1.14 for an increase in the DMFT index. The numbers of missing teeth were significantly associated with the lower intake of green and yellow vegetables (<120 g/day), fresh fruits (<150 g/day), and meat and seafood (<100 g/day), with increased odds ratios of 1.17, 1.25, and 1.35, respectively (Table 3).

Table 3. Adjusted increased risks for insufficient dietary intake < lower limit of reference values associated with increasing dental parameters (poorer dental status) in women (N = 33).

Category	Nutrients	Lower Limit	Insufficient (%)	DMFT Index			N of Decayed Teeth			N of Missing Teeth		
				OR	95%CI	p	OR	95%CI	p	OR	95%CI	p
Macronutrient intake	Protein	55 (g)	27.3	1.21	1.00, 1.46	*	2.58	0.96, 6.95		1.08	0.96, 1.22	
	Protein density	14.5 (%kcal)	27.3	1.17	0.98, 1.40		1.54	0.79, 2.97		1.15	1.00, 1.32	
Micronutrient intake	Calcium	500 (mg)	36.4	1.05	0.94, 1.16		1.35	0.72, 2.54		1.07	0.96, 1.20	
	Phosphorus	800 (mg)	24.2	1.04	0.92, 1.17		1.78	0.88, 3.61		1.05	0.93, 1.18	
	Iron	5.5 (mg)	30.3	1.14	0.98, 1.31		1.21	0.65, 2.25		1.02	0.91, 1.14	
	Zinc	6 (mg)	30.3	1.19	1.00, 1.42		1.92	0.88, 4.18		1.09	0.97, 1.22	
	Vitamin A	450 (μgRAE)	51.5	1.07	0.96, 1.18		1.48	0.72, 3.06		1.09	0.96, 1.23	
	Vitamin D	5.5 (μg)	36.4	1.02	0.93, 1.13		1.33	0.71, 2.51		1.06	0.95, 1.19	
	Vitamin E	6.0 (mg)	42.4	1.13	1.00, 1.27		1.60	0.77, 3.30		1.14	0.99, 1.30	
	Vitamin K	150 (μg)	39.4	1.14	1.00, 1.29		1.72	0.81, 3.64		1.09	0.97, 1.23	
	Vitamin B2	1.1 (mg)	27.3	1.12	0.97, 1.30		1.65	0.83, 3.27		1.08	0.96, 1.21	
	Vitamin B12	2.4 (μg)	9.1	1.24	0.80, 1.92		3.45	1.17, 10.1	*	1.13	0.95, 1.35	
	Folate	240 (μg)	24.2	1.07	0.94, 1.21		1.07	0.55, 2.10		1.02	0.90, 1.14	
	Pantothenic acid	5 (mg)	33.3	1.07	0.96, 1.20		1.50	0.77, 2.91		1.09	0.97, 1.22	
	Vitamin C	100 (mg)	36.4	1.04	0.94, 1.16		1.03	0.55, 1.91		1.05	0.94, 1.18	
	n-3 PUFA	1.9 (g)	45.5	1.18	1.02, 1.37	*	1.73	0.79, 3.80		1.19	1.01, 1.41	*
	n-6 PUFA	7 (g)	48.5	1.16	1.02, 1.32	*	1.64	0.76, 3.54		1.07	0.96, 1.20	
	Total dietary fiber	17 (g)	75.8	1.04	0.94, 1.15		1.04	0.51, 2.14		1.12	0.95, 1.31	
Food intake	Beans	100 (g)	72.7	1.14	1.02, 1.28	*	2.13	0.62, 7.28		1.12	0.96, 1.31	
	Green vegetables	120 (g)	42.4	1.10	0.99, 1.24		1.22	0.65, 2.26		1.17	1.01, 1.36	*
	Other vegetables	230 (g)	87.9	1.05	0.92, 1.19		1.92	0.48, 7.72		1.08	0.89, 1.30	
	Fresh fruits	150 (g)	69.7	1.11	1.00, 1.24		1.59	0.62, 4.07		1.24	1.01, 1.51	*
	Seafood	60 (g)	33.3	1.13	0.98, 1.31		1.77	0.84, 3.71		1.10	0.97, 1.25	
	Meat	50 (g)	42.4	1.05	0.95, 1.16		1.19	0.64, 2.21		1.11	0.98, 1.26	
	Meat and seafood	100 (g)	27.3	1.24	0.99, 1.56		1.66	0.84, 3.31		1.35	1.04, 1.76	*
	Eggs	50 (g)	39.4	0.97	0.88, 1.08		1.32	0.62, 2.82		0.97	0.86, 1.09	

*: $p < 0.05$; age-adjusted p-value; N: number of subjects; SD: standard deviation; OR: odds ratio; 95%CI: 95% confidence interval; DMFT index: the sum of decayed, missing, and filled teeth; SFA: saturated fatty acid; PUFA: polyunsaturated fatty acid.

4. Discussion

4.1. Commensality (Eating Alone or Together) and Food and Nutrient Intake

No significant difference in macronutrient intake or the frequency of underweight and overweight was found between women eating alone and together. However, fresh fruit consumption and the intakes of folate, total dietary fiber, and several micronutrients, including potassium, magnesium, and Vitamin K, were significantly higher in women eating alone compared to women eating together. In addition, the risks (odds ratios) for insufficient fresh fruit intake (<150 g/day) and folate intake (<240 g/day) in women eating alone were significantly lower than in women eating together. These results suggest better nutrient intake in older women eating alone than in those eating together, which is inconsistent with the study results of increased malnutrition risks associated with eating alone in previous reports involving older adults [3,4].

One probable reason for these unexpected results is that women in the current study have participated in our home health management program, including the nutrition survey, and practice good dietary behavior. In particular, women living and eating alone are taking care of themselves regarding their diet because they have come to recognize that they should remain healthy enough to stay at home independently. In contrast, women eating together prepare food primarily for their families and consider others' tastes and health statuses. Almost all of them were living with their husbands, whose micronutrient intakes were similar to theirs, although husbands consumed more carbohydrates due to higher rice intake.

More specifically, the mean macronutrient intake in women eating alone who participated in the dental examination was higher than that in all women eating alone (Table 2), suggesting that women who saw an opportunity to improve their health status and eat nutritional foods may have agreed to participate in the dental examination.

Dental status as a health indicator was also better in women eating alone than in those eating together because of the significantly lower number of untreated, decayed teeth. These results also support the notion that the women living alone in the current study were more inclined toward self-care, including dental care attendance, than women living together.

In the UK, it was previously reported that men living and eating together who were responsible for preparing food but had poorer cooking skills had lower energy intake and specific nutrients [23]. However, in the current study, we were unable to analyze the association between commensality and nutritional status in men because only one male participant was living and eating alone. Future recruitment should be extended to more men living and eating alone among the older adult population, and their food consumption and nutrient intake should be investigated using methods that are easier than the "dietary diary" approach, such as taking photos of meals.

4.2. Associations between Dietary Intake and Dental Parameters

4.2.1. Nutrient Intake and Dental Parameters

In women, the intake of various kinds of macro- and micronutrients, including protein, trace elements, n-3 and n-6 PUFAs, and vitamins, significantly decreased with an increasing DMFT index and increasing numbers of missing teeth. The risk for insufficient intake of protein and n-3 and n-6 PUFAs increased significantly with an increasing DMFT index. Particularly for n-3 PUFA intake in women, this risk increased with increasing numbers of missing teeth. Regarding foods, the increased risk for insufficient meat and fish consumption was associated with increasing numbers of missing teeth, and the risk for the insufficient consumption of beans increased significantly with an increasing DMFT index, albeit only in women.

Consistently with these results, Yoshihara et al. performed a survey of nutritional intake using a precise weighing method for ≥74-year-old residents in another coastal area in Japan and reported that numbers of present teeth were significantly associated with various nutrients, including protein, minerals, and vitamins, among subjects of both sexes after adjusting for sex, smoking habit, and education [10]. They also reported that the ingestion of seafood and vegetables was significantly lower in subjects with <20 present teeth compared with their counterparts with ≥20 teeth. These results suggest that increasing numbers of missing teeth may influence intakes of vegetables and seafood, which contribute to sufficient protein intake in Japanese older adults.

Although no previous studies investigated the association between nutritional intake and the DMFT index in older adults, in the current study, women with a higher DMFT index had an increased risk for the insufficient intake of protein, *n*-6, and beans, suggesting that not only numbers of missing teeth but also numbers of decayed and filled teeth caused by dental caries may influence chewing ability and thus decrease nutritional intake in healthy older women.

4.2.2. *n*-3 and *n*-6 PUFA Intake and Dental Parameters

Iwasaki et al. followed up adults aged 74 years and older who participated in the survey performed by Yoshihara et al. [10] and reported that subjects with a lower intake of docosahexaenoic acid, one of the *n*-3 PUFAs, developed progressive periodontal disease because of the aggravated inflammation of the oral environment during a follow-up period of 5 years [24]. Iwasaki et al. also showed that *n*-3 PUFA intake from fish was significantly lower among ≥80-year-olds with ill-fitting dentures or compromised dentition compared to similarly aged people with good dentition [14]. However, among the present subjects, seafood intake was not insufficient, and *n*-3 PUFA intake was highly correlated with seafood intake. In general, oily fish, which contains *n*-3 PUFA, was not often eaten by older adults because they prefer to consume white-flesh fish with a lower fat content. Taken together, older women with poor dental status, even when living in a coastal area, should be advised to increase their intake of *n*-3 PUFA via fish for the prevention of not only cardiovascular diseases [25] but also oral inflammatory diseases such as periodontitis [24].

The insufficient intake of *n*-6 PUFA associated with dental parameters was also suggested to occur in women. Because of the high correlation of *n*-6 PUFA intake with the consumption of beans, which is a food at risk of insufficient consumption, *n*-6 PUFA intake may be insufficient in women with an increased DMTF index. In addition, insufficient protein intake was also significantly associated with a higher DMFT index. Therefore, the consumption of tofu and bean products should be recommended for older women with a high DMFT index to increase both protein and *n*-6 PUFA intake.

4.2.3. Fruit and Vegetable Intake and Dental Parameters

The increased risk of lower fresh fruit intake associated with both dental markers was observed, although our subjects had no increased risk of lower vitamin C intake because there was no significant increased risk of lower total vegetable intake, which is another source of vitamin C. The lower intakes of fruits, vegetables, vitamin C, and potassium have been reported in Korea, where older adults self-reported chewing difficulties [12]. These authors also compared their percentages of nutrient intakes, relative to the recommended levels of dietary reference intakes, for Koreans between groups with and without chewing difficulty, and they reported lower intakes of total energy and nutrients other than vitamin C and potassium, including calcium, which was inconsistent with our results that showed an increased risk for the lower intake of only limited nutrients. The difference between our results and those of Kwon et al. may be related to differences in dental status, which was worse in their subjects who reported chewing difficulty [12].

In the United States, people wearing dentures were reported to eat less fruit compared with dentate individuals, although psychosocial factors such as attitude and self-identity contributed more than chewing ability to this increased fruit intake [26]. In Japan, self-efficacy for designing meals and the awareness of recommendations for fruit and vegetable intake were reported to be important for the entire aged population [27]. In the present study, however, dental status including dental caries may be an important factor in fruit intake among women who have had the opportunity to improve their lifestyle using the home health management program.

The risk of low intakes of green and yellow vegetables was significantly associated only with women with a high DMFT index and a significantly lower intake of vitamin A and vitamin E, which are ubiquitous in green and yellow vegetables. In the total cohort, there were significantly increased odds ratios for the insufficient intake of green and yellow vegetables alongside an increase in both renal markers (DNFT index > number of missing teeth) and an inverse correlation between dental markers and vitamin E intake, suggesting that poor dental status in both sexes may decrease vitamin E because of the lower consumption of green and yellow vegetables.

4.3. Strengths and Limitations

The main strength of this study is the dietary survey method; diet records, which are not easy for older adults, were successfully achieved. Additionally, dietitians who interviewed the current cohort have supported our home health management program for more than 10 years and know their eating habits and common diet well enough to improve the accuracy of their records and estimate their dietary intake. With these records, we could perform a risk analysis of the insufficient intake of these micronutrients for which reference levels are established for each sex. Another strength is our cohort of targeted subjects comprising older healthy adults with an interest in health management, including oral health. In the present study, we showed that key micronutrients and foods were at risk of insufficient intake even in older adults living a healthy lifestyle.

Despite these strengths, the small sample size, particularly for men, is a limitation of the study because it decreases statistical power, especially in an analysis with multiple covariates. Indeed, the number of men eating alone amounted to only a single individual. Even for women, the sample size was too small for statistical analysis using the model with two main factors, the commensality factor and dental factor. In future surveys, we will enroll larger numbers of older adults to include more men living and eating alone.

5. Conclusions

In older women living a healthy lifestyle with good health management, poor commensality (i.e., living and eating alone) was not a risk factor for insufficient food consumption and nutrient intake. However, poor dental status, indicated by the DMFT index and the numbers of missing teeth, decreased the ingestion of beans, green and yellow vegetables, and fresh fruits and increased the risk for the insufficient intake of protein and n-3 and n-6 PUFAs. These findings suggest that good health management, including the treatment of decayed teeth, is important for the prevention of malnutrition in community-dwelling older adults.

Author Contributions: Conceptualization, Y.N. and M.N.; methodology, N.D. and K.Y.; validation, K.Y., Y.A. and T.T.; formal analysis, T.T. and M.N.; investigation, Y.A., T.T. and N.K.; resources, N.D. and Y.A.; data curation, Y.A. and M.N.; writing—original draft preparation, T.T., M.N. and K.Y.; writing—review and editing, Y.N.; visualization, M.N.; supervision, Y.N.; project administration, M.N. and N.K.; funding acquisition, Y.N. All authors have read and agreed to the published version of the manuscript.

Funding: This research received no external funding.

Institutional Review Board Statement: The study was conducted in accordance with the Declaration of Helsinki and approved by the Institutional Review Board (or Ethics Committee) of Kanazawa Medical University (No. I522, 24 June 2020).

Informed Consent Statement: Written informed consent was obtained from all subjects involved in the study.

Data Availability Statement: The datasets used and/or analyzed during the current study are available from the corresponding author on reasonable request.

Acknowledgments: We thank Mikiko Muroi, a secretary of our laboratory, for their support and assistance rendered in the study.

Conflicts of Interest: The authors declare no conflict of interest.

References

1. Amarya, S.; Singh, K.; Sabharwal, M. Changes during aging and their association with malnutrition. *J. Clin. Gerontol. Geriatr.* **2015**, *6*, 78–84. [CrossRef]
2. Conzade, R.; Koenig, W.; Heier, M.; Schneider, A.; Grill, E.; Peters, A.; Thorand, B. Prevalence and Predictors of Subclinical Micronutrient Deficiency in German Older Adults: Results from the Population-Based KORA-Age Study. *Nutrients* **2017**, *9*, 1276. [CrossRef] [PubMed]
3. Björnwall, A.; Mattsson Sydner, Y.; Koochek, A.; Neuman, N. Eating Alone or Together among Community-Living Older People—A Scoping Review. *Int. J. Environ. Res. Public Health* **2021**, *18*, 3495. [CrossRef]
4. Tani, Y.; Kondo, N.; Takagi, D.; Saito, M.; Hikichi, H.; Ojima, T.; Kondo, K. Combined effects of eating alone and living alone on unhealthy dietary behaviors, obesity and underweight in older Japanese adults: Results of the JAGES. *Appetite* **2015**, *95*, 1–8. [CrossRef]
5. Kazemi, S.; Savabi, G.; Khazaei, S.; Savabi, O.; Esmaillzadeh, A.; Keshteli, A.H.; Adibi, P. Association between food intake and oral health in elderly: SEPAHAN systematic review no. 8. *Dent. Res. J.* **2011**, *8*, S15–S20.
6. Gil-Montoya, J.A.; de Mello, A.L.; Barrios, R.; Gonzalez-Moles, M.A.; Bravo, M. Oral health in the elderly patient and its impact on general well-being: A nonsystematic review. *Clin. Interv. Aging* **2015**, *10*, 461–467. [CrossRef]
7. Sheiham, A.; Steele, J. Does the condition of the mouth and teeth affect the ability to eat certain foods, nutrient and dietary intake and nutritional status amongst older people? *Public Health Nutr.* **2001**, *4*, 797–803. [CrossRef]
8. Nowjack-Raymer, R.E.; Sheiham, A. Numbers of natural teeth, diet, and nutritional status in US adults. *J. Dent. Res.* **2007**, *86*, 1171–1175. [CrossRef]
9. Hung, H.C.; Colditz, G.; Joshipura, K.J. The association between tooth loss and the self-reported intake of selected CVD-related nutrients and foods among US women. *Community Dent. Oral Epidemiol.* **2005**, *33*, 167–173. [CrossRef]
10. Yoshihara, A.; Watanabe, R.; Nishimuta, M.; Hanada, N.; Miyazaki, H. The relationship between dietary intake and the number of teeth in elderly Japanese subjects. *Gerodontology* **2005**, *22*, 211–218. [CrossRef]
11. Mann, T.; Heuberger, R.; Wong, H. The association between chewing and swallowing difficulties and nutritional status in older adults. *Aust. Dent. J.* **2013**, *58*, 200–206. [CrossRef] [PubMed]
12. Kwon, S.H.; Park, H.R.; Lee, Y.M.; Kwon, S.Y.; Kim, O.S.; Kim, H.Y.; Lim, Y.S. Difference in food and nutrient intakes in Korean elderly people according to chewing difficulty: Using data from the Korea National Health and Nutrition Examination Survey 2013 (6th). *Nutr. Res. Pract.* **2017**, *11*, 139–146. [CrossRef]
13. Kimura, Y.; Ogawa, H.; Yoshihara, A.; Yamaga, T.; Takiguchi, T.; Wada, T.; Sakamoto, R.; Ishimoto, Y.; Fukutomi, E.; Chen, W.; et al. Evaluation of chewing ability and its relationship with activities of daily living, depression, cognitive status and food intake in the community-dwelling elderly. *Geriatr. Gerontol. Int.* **2013**, *13*, 718–725. [CrossRef] [PubMed]
14. Iwasaki, M.; Taylor, G.W.; Manz, M.C.; Yoshihara, A.; Sato, M.; Muramatsu, K.; Watanabe, R.; Miyazaki, H. Oral health status: Relationship to nutrient and food intake among 80-year-old Japanese adults. *Community Dent. Oral Epidemiol.* **2014**, *42*, 441–450. [CrossRef] [PubMed]
15. Aminu, A.Q. Adult Dental Health Survey 2009: Association between oral health outcomes and living arrangements of older adults in the UK. *Br. Dent. J.* **2019**, *227*, 115–120. [CrossRef]
16. Lindmark, U.; Ernsth Bravell, M.; Johansson, L.; Finkel, D. Oral health is essential for quality of life in older adults: A Swedish National Quality Register Study. *Gerodontology* **2021**, *38*, 191–198. [CrossRef]
17. Ministry of Health, Labour and Welfare of Japan. Dietary Reference Intakes for Japanese (2015). 2018. Available online: https://www.mhlw.go.jp/stf/seisakunitsuite/bunya/0000208970.html (accessed on 10 March 2023).
18. Ministry of Health, Labour and Welfare. Survey of Dental Diseases. 2016. Available online: https://www.mhlw.go.jp/toukei/list/dl/62-28-02.pdf (accessed on 10 March 2023). (In Japanese)
19. Petersen, P.E.; Baez, R.J.; World Health Organization. *Oral Health Surveys: Basic Methods*; World Health Organization: Geneva, Switzerland, 2013.
20. Klein, H.; Palmer, C.E.; Knutson, J.W. Studies on Dental Caries: I. Dental Status and Dental Needs of Elementary School Children. *Public Health Rep. (1896–1970)* **1938**, *53*, 751–765. [CrossRef]
21. Sakurai, H. Healthy Japan 21. *JMA Policies* **2003**, *46*, 47–49.
22. Kagawa Nutrition University Publishing Division. *Encyclopedia of Nutrition and Calories of Foods*; Kagawa Nutrition University Publishing Division: Tokyo, Japan, 1988; p. 143. (In Japanese)
23. Holmes, B.A.; Roberts, C.L.; Nelson, M. How access, isolation and other factors may influence food consumption and nutrient intake in materially deprived older men in the UK. *Nutr. Bull.* **2008**, *33*, 212–220. [CrossRef]
24. Iwasaki, M.; Yoshihara, A.; Moynihan, P.; Watanabe, R.; Taylor, G.W.; Miyazaki, H. Longitudinal relationship between dietary omega-3 fatty acids and periodontal disease. *Nutrition* **2010**, *26*, 1105–1109. [CrossRef]

25. Visioli, F.; Hagen, T.M. Nutritional strategies for healthy cardiovascular aging: Focus on micronutrients. *Pharmacol. Res.* **2007**, *55*, 199–206. [CrossRef] [PubMed]
26. Bradbury, J.; Thomason, J.M.; Jepson, N.J.; Walls, A.W.; Mulvaney, C.E.; Allen, P.F.; Moynihan, P.J. Perceived chewing ability and intake of fruit and vegetables. *J. Dent. Res.* **2008**, *87*, 720–725. [CrossRef] [PubMed]
27. Wang, D.H.; Kogashiwa, M.; Mori, N.; Yamashita, S.; Fujii, W.; Ueda, N.; Homma, H.; Suzuki, H.; Masuoka, N. Psychosocial Determinants of Fruit and Vegetable Consumption in a Japanese Population. *Int. J. Environ. Res. Public Health* **2016**, *13*, 786. [CrossRef] [PubMed]

nutrients MDPI

Article

Eating Patterns among Emergency Medical Service Providers in the United States: A Qualitative Interview Study

Tegan Mansouri [1,*], George Ghanatios [1], Lori Hatzinger [1,2], Rachel Barich [1,3], Ebriama Dampha [1], Jennifer L. Temple [1], Brian M. Clemency [1,4] and David Hostler [1,4]

1 Department of Exercise and Nutrition Sciences, University at Buffalo, Buffalo, NY 14214, USA
2 Department of Population and Public Health Sciences, University of Southern California, Los Angeles, CA 90007, USA
3 Department of Foods and Nutrition, University of Prince Edward Island, Charlottetown, PE C1A 4P3, Canada
4 Department of Emergency Medicine, University at Buffalo, Buffalo, NY 14203, USA
* Correspondence: teganman@buffalo.edu; Tel.: +1-716-829-2941; Fax: +1-716-829-2428

Abstract: Emergency medical service (EMS) providers experience demanding work conditions in addition to shift work, which increases risk for nutrition related chronic disease such as metabolic syndrome, diabetes, obesity, and cardiovascular disease. The high stress, emergent, and unpredictable nature of EMS may interfere with healthy eating patterns on and off shift, however little is known about how these conditions impact dietary patterns among EMS providers. This study aimed to understand factors impacting dietary patterns through semi-structured interviews with 40 EMS providers throughout the United States. Interviews were conducted virtually via Zoom video conference. Inductive coding was used to identify themes throughout the interviews. Salient factors mentioned in the interviews included hunger, fatigue, stress, coworker influence, ambulance posting, geographical location, agency policy, and culture. Factors were grouped into 4 domains: physiological factors, psychosocial factors, physical environment, and organizational environment, represented by an adapted version of the social ecological model of health behaviors to include factors influencing eating patterns specific to EMS, which may contribute to overall health. Various barriers to healthy eating exist within EMS, and future studies should explore interventions at each level of our proposed model to improve conditions and reduce nutrition related disease risk in this essential population.

Keywords: emergency medical services; EMS; eating patterns; nutrition; paramedics; nutrition related disease

1. Introduction

Emergency medical service (EMS) providers, including paramedics and emergency medical technicians (EMT) provide essential services 24 h a day. They work in shifts ranging in duration from 8.5 to 24+ hours, and up to 80% of EMS providers report working multiple jobs and/or overtime hours with variable shift rotations [1,2]. Shiftwork is associated with circadian misalignment [3–6] poor sleep quality [7] and increased risk of metabolic syndrome, type 2 diabetes, obesity and cardiovascular disease [8–13]. EMS providers also experience elevated rates of these diseases relative to the general population [14–16].

In addition to the stress of shift work, EMS providers' work environment is unpredictable and inconsistent, contributing to erratic sleep and eating patterns [16]. They face high levels of stress and occupational fatigue [1] and are at greater risk of work-related injury compared to the general population and other public safety professionals [15–17]. EMS professionals provide an essential service and are responsible for carrying out fast paced procedures including ventilating patients, administering cardiopulmonary resuscitation, administration of potentially dangerous drugs, and assisting with childbirth [18]. Maintaining an experienced, specialized workforce will contribute to the quality and efficiency of our healthcare system. It is crucial to protect the health of this work force.

Diet is a modifiable factor that can reduce metabolic disease risk [19]. Previous research reports that shift workers tend to eat more meals and snacks at later hours of the day, and their diets are higher in snacks, sweets, alcohol, sugar sweetened beverages, and lower in dietary fiber [20]. Some studies report no difference in energy intake between day and night shift workers [21,22], however, we previously reported that among EMS providers, those working the night shift consume more overall energy (kilocalories) and grams of total fat compared to providers working the day shift [23]. Work environment may be an important consideration when assessing impact of diet on health outcomes in the shift working population. Little is known about what specific barriers to healthy eating currently exist among EMS providers.

The unpredictable nature of EMS causes significant variation in daily job demands and conditions [24]. Depending on the agency, providers may remain posted in their ambulance during a shift with minimal room for food storage and no access to refrigeration [25]. Alternatively, those who reside at the station between calls may have abundant access to meals and snacks during their down time. Call volume also varies depending on the agency and the day, posing unique challenges to healthy eating and sleep patterns [16].

The social ecological model of health explains that health is impacted by the interaction between the individual, the group/community, and the physical, social, and political environments [26–28]. Health behaviors in the context of EMS have been described previously by researchers in Australia, where the paramedicine system differs from the United States (US) [3]. Increasingly, agencies in the US are governed by a private system and are implementing new, more efficient response systems, incurring arduous conditions for providers. This study aimed to describe the lived experience of EMS providers in the United States to understand the impact of a rapidly changing system providers' health and overall wellbeing.

2. Methods

2.1. Participants

A combination of purposive and snowball sampling was used to recruit participants. EMS coordinators throughout the United States were identified from their respective State's Department of Health website. We contacted all EMS coordinators where updated contact information was available on their website. A brief overview of the study, a study flyer, and a link to the screening survey were emailed to EMS coordinators to forward to EMS providers in their county. Participants were also asked to forward the email to anyone they thought would be interested. Interested providers were asked to complete a screening survey, which inquired about inclusion and exclusion criteria, and we contacted eligible participants to schedule a 1 h interview via Zoom (Zoom, San Jose, CA, USA, Version 5.4.6). We used data from the screening survey to describe the characteristics of the final sample (Table 1). Eligible participants were 18 years or older, worked in EMS, and provided patient care as their primary duty. Of those who completed the screening survey, 3 were ineligible, 30 did not respond to the invitation to participate, 40 participated in the interview, and no one dropped out. A portion of participants were involved in a previous study in our lab, but otherwise had no relationship with the study team prior to the interviews.

2.2. Data Collection

This study used a phenomenological approach to understand and describe individuals' experience working in EMS, specifically related to eating patterns. The study was approved by the University at Buffalo's Institutional Review Board. At the beginning of the appointment, participants were told the reason for the research and informed consent was obtained and documented electronically via RedCap [29] Using an interview guide (Supplementary Table S1), a registered dietitian conducted semi-structured interviews to inquire about participants' lived experience working in EMS. Questions were informed by previous findings from our lab [23] and designed based on the theoretical domain framework, which was developed to examine influences on behavior of health professionals [30].

The questions were specifically related to work conditions, sleep, and eating patterns. The interview lasted 45–80 min and took place over Zoom from a private location of the participants' choice, and the interviewer was in a private room in the Nutrition and Health Research lab at the University at Buffalo. Following the interview, the interviewer took notes to document key topics discussed in the interview. The interviews were audio and video recorded and transcripts were generated by Zoom.

2.3. Analysis

All transcripts were reviewed and compared to interview recordings to verify accuracy and allow for familiarization with the data prior to coding. Transcripts were coded using Atlas.ti 9 (Atlas.ti Scientific Software Development, Berlin, Germany). Inductive thematic analysis coding was employed to identify major themes in the data following the steps suggested by Braun and Clarke [31]. Forty transcripts were divided among five independent coders. Coders were trained by the study leader, including random selection of one transcript to be coded by each, followed by reconciliation of disagreements to ensure consistency across coders. The initial round of coding involved in vivo coding and informed the initial codebook, which was then applied in a second round of coding by a separate coder. Throughout the coding process, reliability was met through weekly meetings with all coders to review each transcript, allowing for full agreement among coders (inter-coder agreement = 1). Finally, similar codes were categorized into groups and through an iterative process, major themes were identified based on those groups. Using the codes and major themes, we developed a conceptual model based on the social ecological model of health to inform future interventions in this population [32].

3. Results

Participants were 50% female, predominantly white, with a mean age of 33 $\pm$ 10 years and mean body mass index (BMI) in the overweight range (28.2 $\pm$ 5.7 kg/m^2). We identified common factors discussed throughout the interviews that influenced eating patterns. The factors could all be grouped into the following overarching themes: physiological factors, psychosocial factors, physical environment, and organizational environment. These themes informed a conceptual model based on the social ecological model of health to reflect the interrelated factors influencing eating patterns among EMS providers (Figure 1). Within each theme, factors uniquely experienced by EMS providers included hunger, fatigue, stress, coworker influence, ambulance posting, geographical location, agency policy, and culture. We discuss these factors below.

3.1. Physiological Factors

Physiological factors included fatigue and hunger. Participants reported being too tired to cook after work and were more likely to rely on convenience food during a shift and on days off. Participants mentioned that their food choice differed when they were tired compared to when they were well rested, and some mentioned eating as a tool to help them stay awake during a shift.

> *Participant #1: I definitely noticed when i'm like super tired, then I would eat like much more poorly so I definitely go for more like sugary things and coffee, and so it kind of depends on how intense of a workload I have how tired, I am.*

> *Participant #2: And i'll eat to stay awake while I am doing [patient notes], and I would love to tell you that eat carrots right, but instead I am eating ranch doritos.*

Hunger level was mentioned by participants as influencing their food choice. Participants mentioned having to go long periods of time without eating during work and that their hunger level affected their mood.

> *Participant #3: Like you're so busy that you forget to eat and that's like something that happens, like so often like it just it becomes like your secondary priority.*

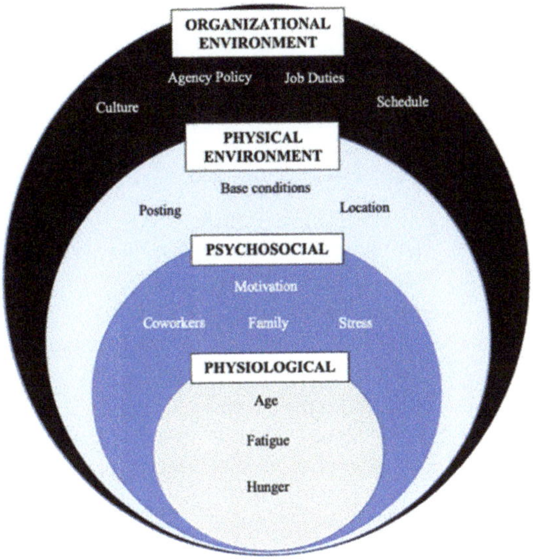

Figure 1. Conceptual model—From the major themes, we developed the following conceptual model informed by the social ecological model. The model displays the four overarching, interrelated themes, each containing commonly discussed factors describing the context in which food choice and eating occur for EMS providers.

Table 1. Participant Characteristics.

	N/Mean ± SD	%
Job title		
Paramedic	23	57.5
EMT *	9	22.5
Flight paramedic	2	5
AEMT-CC **	2	5
Firefighter	3	92.5
Volunteer	1	2.5
Age	33 ± 10.8	
Sex	20 female	50
BMI (kg/m^2)	28.2 ± 5.7	
Race		
American Indian or Alaskan Native	0	0
Asian	1	2.5
White	40	100
Black or African American	1	2.5
Native Hawaiian or other Pacific Islander	0	0
More than 1 race	2	5
Ethnicity		
Hispanic or Latino	1	2.5
Not Hispanic or Latino	39	97.5

* EMT = Emergency Medical Technician. ** AEMT-CC = Advanced Emergency Medical Technician-Critical Care.

3.2. Psychosocial Factors

Psychosocial factors included stress and coworker influence. Participants discussed stress related to call volume, call severity, COVID-19 precautions, sleep deprivation, and their work schedule. Stress often led to eating more and was discussed as a factor impairing ability to plan and prepare meals ahead of time. Planning was a factor that facilitated eating during work, and those who did not plan relied on acquiring food during their shift, which was unpredictable. The effort involved with planning was discussed as a barrier to consistent meal preparation.

Participant #4: If it's like an overly stressful week or something ... Sometimes you eat more just to like stress eat pretty much.

Participant #5: So right now I don't really have the time to actually sit down and think about and plan out a meal for the week this just grab and go for right now until my life gets a little bit less stressful.

In some, stress leads to decreased appetite and reduced energy intake resulting in unintentional weight loss.

Participant #6: It just got to the point, I was getting so stressed, I just couldn't eat you know it's like now it's like I have to force myself to eat.

Providers typically work in crews of at least two on an ambulance, and report that their partner influences their food choice. Others report being influenced by coworkers at the base. Those who worked at fire-based agencies discuss eating together as part of the culture, and that crews often cooked dinners together.

Participant #7: There's definitely like that peer pressure like hey we're putting in a pizza order, what do you want ... so I feel like I eat out way more [at] work than I ever would at home, we very rarely eat out at home.

3.3. Physical Environment

Factors that influenced the physical environment included geographic location, and the use of ambulance posting. Providers stated that during a shift, their food choice was dependent on availability, which varied based on location and base conditions. Providers working in urban areas had access to more food options, however, they often have a higher call volume, which they mentioned as a barrier to eating due to lack of time, inability to return to the base between calls, and limited options available in the ambulance. Some hospitals have breakrooms with snacks and beverages for providers, but availability is unreliable, and variety is limited. Food availability was particularly problematic for those who worked the night shift, so they often rely on fast food or gas stations.

Participant #8: So your choices get incredibly limited at night there's a there's a nice ... chain here called price chopper market 32 ... where they have a nice food court and you know place where you can get stuff but that closes at 7 pm ... So most of the time it's just a gas station or 711 or some of the fast foods do late night.

Participant #9: And then, if we ran night calls all night, I would just stop you know mcdonald's is like the only thing open for some reason everything else in [location] shuts down early so. That kind of be our go to ... that and gas stations.

Returning to a base between calls was discussed as a facilitator to eating during a shift compared to ambulance posting, which was discussed as a barrier. Having a base increases availability of snacks and ability to cook, store, and reheat food during a shift. However, call volume still precludes cooking during a shift in many cases. The potential to be interrupted by a call was mentioned by providers as a barrier to cooking and purchasing food and led to preference for convenient food options.

Participant #10: But when you're trying to cook something that was our biggest problem at [agency], we would do like spaghetti dinners and stuff, we get everything all cooked and all of a sudden you're getting ready to eat and a call would go out.

> *Participant #11: Well we're lucky, because we can we can go back to the station ... and we have a refrigerator which is awesome, a refrigerator and a microwave, which is another factor to what's so nice there, because if you work in an ambulance you don't have access to a microwave or refrigerator and you know working 12 h days ambulance could get hot too...*

3.4. Organizational Environment

The organizational environment includes factors specific to the EMS system that influence eating patterns such as agency policy and culture. Some policies in place to increase productivity impair ability to eat during a shift. Providers often do not have an official meal break and workload was mentioned as a common barrier to eating.

> *Participant #12: There's no like 30 min lunch break you're just working throughout the entire day you're always doing something; training, doing paperwork, going on calls ... it'd be nice if we were allowed to, but when there's only two people at the station, you and your partner and that's it covering the entire town, you really can't take a break when you want to so you can't have a set time where you're not working and you can dedicate that time to having a nice healthy meal. You just can't do it.*

EMS culture was influenced by the agency organization, management, and coworker support, and discussed by providers as a factor influencing eating patterns. Unsupportive management was discussed as a factor preventing eating during a shift leading to burnout and high rates of employee turnover.

> *Participant #2: yeah and there's a lot of pressure to take open shifts and it's hard to not feel guilty, because you want to help your coworkers right, because if you don't take that open shift that's more work on them*

> *Participant #13: yeah I don't know, and I think they just work, so much so, they don't have time to work out or like care for themselves, like mentally or physically ... There's like no gym there's no like incentive for anybody to work out ...*

> *Participant #14: yeah the stress level can be elevated because of the business ... we got supervisors breathing down our necks sometimes you know, trying to make us clear, so we can just go take another call..*

4. Discussion

EMS providers experience increased risk of chronic disease compared to the general population [33,34]. The purpose of this study was to understand factors related to eating patterns among EMS providers based on their lived experiences by conducting semi-structured interviews with providers throughout the United States. We expanded previous findings by describing each theme in the context of EMS, specifically within the United States. We also developed a conceptual model based on the social ecological model of health to inform future interventions in this population.

The social ecological model of health was developed based on the understanding that health is affected by the interaction between the individual, the community, and the physical, social, and political environment [26,35]. It acknowledges the role of context in the development and treatment of health problems. We adapted the social ecological model to include factors specific to EMS at each of the following levels: physiological, psychosocial, physical environment, and organizational environment. Ideally, interventions in this population should include action at each level to improve eating patterns and overall health, however, operations level changes may be difficult to achieve in this profession.

Physiological factors included fatigue and hunger. Previous research in animals and humans report that food intake increases after sleep loss [36,37]. Fatigue is a common problem noted among EMS providers [1], and previous qualitative work in nurses [38] report fatigue as a factor hindering ability to prepare healthy meals. Fatigue may interfere with cooking, meal planning, and lead to reliance on convenience foods in addition to increasing preference for calorie dense, high carbohydrate foods [37]. In this study, providers reported that hunger level influenced food choice and preference. Sleep loss [39], in addition to short term food deprivation when providers are too busy to eat, may lead to overcompensation of energy intake. Interventions at this level should acknowledge that fatigue may interfere with cooking and meal planning throughout the week, so thoughtful use of nutritionally balanced, easy to prepare meals and snacks should be encouraged. Providers should also receive information regarding the impact of fatigue, what to expect, and how to address it, to give them tools to overcome this unavoidable aspect of the job.

Psychosocial factors include the individual effect and the interaction between psychological and social influence. We identified stress and peer influence as common psychosocial factors. Stress impacts food choice through neurocircuitry and hormonal pathways [40] and has been associated with intake of more pro-inflammatory diets [41]. It is also known that eating is strongly influenced by social context [42]. These factors influence eating patterns and may be an opportunity for intervention by using social interactions to support healthy dietary patterns. Interventions may include group nutrition education classes or training specific to the conditions in EMS. Group nutrition interventions have been successful at improving mental health symptoms, including stress, among participants who consumed a Mediterranean diet high in vegetables, legumes, nuts, and fruit [43]. This type of intervention may be beneficial in EMS providers.

The physical environment was shaped by agency location and ambulance posting. These challenges vary significantly between agencies and may not be modifiable depending on the type of EMS agency and the terms of the contract with the municipality. However, agencies may consider making nutrient dense snacks available at the base or in the ambulance. Future studies should investigate the impact of food deprivation on alertness and productivity, as this could support allocation of funds toward employee nourishment. Work environment directly and indirectly impacts employees' health behaviors [44], and due to the unique, inconsistent physical environment in EMS, further studies should address the impact of environment on eating patterns. Specifically, studies should consider the impact of ambulance street posting on the health and wellbeing of providers.

The organizational environment was shaped by work culture and agency policy. The collective attitudes toward eating and other health behaviors, lack of meal breaks, and intense work and schedule demands influenced eating patterns. Managerial support has been reported to reduce the risk of mental health problems [45], which may improve health behaviors [46,47]. Education at the management level to cultivate a positive work environment may reduce turnover. Further, previous studies in paramedics have found that those who have more control over their schedule are able to rest and recover better from demanding situations [48]. Sleep deprivation and fatigue in EMS leads to increased injury rates, compromised patient care, burnout, and poor health for providers, and increases employee turnover. Schedules designed to allow for adequate recovery between shifts could reduce fatigue, and impact food choice and health outcomes among providers and patients. The approach will differ based on agency type, which should be considered when designing an intervention.

Increased strategies for achieving adequate nutrition would improve employees' health and quality of care as providers report severe hunger levels affecting patient care. Providers struggle with barriers to healthy eating during a shift and targeting these barriers in an intervention may improve adherence to lifestyle modifications. Providers are often in situations where they must rely on convenience foods that are low in nutrients and high in energy, and when paired with high stress and sleep deprivation, this may increase metabolic and cardiovascular disease risk [49–51]. Interventions should address factors at each level to improve employee wellness and retention.

This study had several strengths including the nationally representative sample. This allowed us to examine the experience of EMS providers who respond to calls in various locations including in urban, rural, and backcountry areas. Our participants also worked various schedules ranging from 8–144 h (six 24h shifts in a row), days, nights, and a combination of both. The diversity of our sample, in terms of experience, allowed us to understand what factors were specific to EMS, and those that varied based on location. We were also able to understand the challenges associated with different schedule schemes. However, we were not able to quantify these differences, which is one limitation, and something that should be investigated in future studies with the goal of improving conditions to promote the health status of EMS providers. Another limitation of this study is the lack of ethnic and racial diversity. According to the 2020 National EMS Assessment, providers identifying as Asian, Black, African American, American Indian, and Alaska Native make up 17.7% of the workforce throughout the US [52], and future studies must focus on representation of all racial and ethnic groups. This was a major limitation of this study.

5. Conclusions

The overall rate of turnover in EMS is 10.7% and the median cost of turnover is $86,452.05 for paid agencies [1]. These data are over 10 years old and has likely increased over that time as medical calls have gone up by 32% between 2010 and 2019 (NFPA Fire Experience Survey). The data from the current study, combined with earlier quantitative work, suggest that more work is needed to improve conditions for EMS providers to allow for a sustainable lifestyle and prevention of chronic disease, burnout, and employee turnover. Future studies should build on this work by testing interventions aimed at increasing healthy eating patterns, adjusting shift schedules to improve sleep quality and allow for recovery between shifts, and reconsidering organizational policies. These strategies could improve health and wellbeing among EMS providers and reduce employee turnover costs for agencies and physical health and increase the quality of life for EMS providers.

Supplementary Materials: The following supporting information can be downloaded at: https://www.mdpi.com/article/10.3390/nu14224884/s1, Table S1: Interview guide for semi-structured interviews with 40 EMS providers throughout the United States regarding sleep and eating patterns. The interview questions were determined based on research questions. Probes such as "can you explain what you mean by that" and "can you tell me more about that" were used to gain further insights on topics of discussion.

Author Contributions: T.M., J.L.T., B.M.C. and D.H. designed the research; T.M. conducted all the interviews; T.M., G.G., E.D. and L.H. reviewed the transcripts for accuracy; T.M., G.G., R.B. and L.H. coded the transcripts and contributed to interpretation of the results; T.M. wrote the paper; J.L.T., B.M.C. and D.H. contributed intellectually to the manuscript. All authors have read and agreed to the published version of the manuscript.

Funding: This research did not receive any specific grant from funding agencies in the public, commercial, or not-for-profit sectors.

Institutional Review Board Statement: The study was conducted according to the guidelines of the Declaration of Helsinki, and approved by the Institutional Review Board of The University at Buffalo (STUDY00005153 1/12/2021).

Informed Consent Statement: Informed consent was obtained from all subjects involved in the study.

Data Availability Statement: The transcripts presented in this study are available on request from the corresponding author. The transcripts are not publicly available due to privacy restrictions.

Conflicts of Interest: The authors report no conflict of interest.

References

1. Patterson, P.D.; Weaver, M.D.; Frank, R.C.; Warner, C.W.; Martin-Gill, C.; Guyette, F.X.; Fairbanks, R.J.; Hubble, M.W.; Songer, T.J.; Callaway, C.W.; et al. Association between poor sleep, fatigue, and safety outcomes in emergency medical services providers. *Prehosp. Emerg. Care* **2012**, *16*, 86–97. [CrossRef] [PubMed]
2. Frakes, M.A.; Kelly, J.G. Sleep debt and outside employment patterns in helicopter air medical staff working 24-hour shifts. *Air Med. J.* **2007**, *26*, 45–49. [CrossRef] [PubMed]
3. Anstey, S.; Tweedie, J.; Lord, B. Qualitative study of Queensland paramedics' perceived influences on their food and meal choices during shift work. *Nutr. Diet.* **2016**, *73*, 43–49. [CrossRef]

4. Holmback, U.; Forslund, A.; Forslund, J.; Hambraeus, L.; Lennernas, M.; Lowden, A.; Stridsberg, M.; Akerstedt, T. Metabolic responses to nocturnal eating in men are affected by sources of dietary energy. *J. Nutr.* **2002**, *132*, 1892–1899. [CrossRef] [PubMed]
5. Johnston, J.D. Physiological responses to food intake throughout the day. *Nutr. Res. Rev.* **2014**, *27*, 107–118. [CrossRef]
6. Kohsaka, A.; Laposky, A.D.; Ramsey, K.M.; Estrada, C.; Joshu, C.; Kobayashi, Y.; Turek, F.W.; Bass, J. High-fat diet disrupts behavioral and molecular circadian rhythms in mice. *Cell Metab.* **2007**, *6*, 414–421. [CrossRef]
7. Buxton, O.M.; Cain, S.W.; O'Connor, S.P.; Porter, J.H.; Duffy, J.F.; Wang, W.; Czeisler, C.A.; Shea, S.A. Adverse metabolic consequences in humans of prolonged sleep restriction combined with circadian disruption. *Sci. Transl. Med.* **2012**, *4*, 129ra43. [CrossRef]
8. Al-Hammad, F.A.; Raheel, H.; Al-Baiz, L.E.; Al-Otaibi, A.M. The effect of shift work on psychological stress, sleep pattern and health of nurses working at a tertiary hospital, riyadh. *Middle East J. Nurs.* **2012**, *6*, 14–20.
9. Brum, M.C.B.; Filho, F.F.D.; Schnorr, C.C.; Bottega, G.B.; Rodrigues, T.C. Shift work and its association with metabolic disorders. *Diabetol. Metab. Syndr.* **2015**, *7*, 45. [CrossRef]
10. Canuto, R.; Pattussi, M.P.; Macagnan, J.B.; Henn, R.L.; Olinto, M.T. Metabolic syndrome in fixed-shift workers. *Rev. Saude Publica* **2015**, *49*, 30. [CrossRef]
11. Gale, J.E.; Cox, H.I.; Qian, J.; Block, G.D.; Colwell, C.S.; Matveyenko, A.V. Disruption of circadian rhythms accelerates development of diabetes through pancreatic beta-cell loss and dysfunction. *J. Biol. Rhythm.* **2011**, *26*, 423–433. [CrossRef] [PubMed]
12. Gan, Y.; Yang, C.; Tong, X.; Sun, H.; Cong, Y.; Yin, X.; Li, L.; Cao, S.; Dong, X.; Gong, Y.; et al. Shift work and diabetes mellitus: A meta-analysis of observational studies. *Occup. Environ. Med.* **2015**, *72*, 72–78. [CrossRef] [PubMed]
13. Guo, Y.; Rong, Y.; Huang, X.; Lai, H.; Luo, X.; Zhang, Z.; Liu, Y.; He, M.; Wu, T.; Chen, W. Shift work and the relationship with metabolic syndrome in Chinese aged workers. *PLoS ONE* **2015**, *10*, e0120632. [CrossRef]
14. Lawn, S.; Roberts, L.; Willis, E.; Couzner, L.; Mohammadi, L.; Goble, E. The effects of emergency medical service work on the psychological, physical, and social well-being of ambulance personnel: A systematic review of qualitative research. *BMC Psychiatry* **2020**, *20*, 348. [CrossRef]
15. Sterud, T.; Ekeberg, Ø.; Hem, E. Health status in the ambulance services: A systematic review. *BMC Health Serv. Res.* **2006**, *6*, 82. [CrossRef] [PubMed]
16. Hegg-Deloye, S.; Brassard, P.; Jauvin, N.; Poirier, P.; Tremblay, A.; Corbeil, P. Current state of knowledge of post-traumatic stress, sleeping problems, obesity and cardiovascular disease in paramedics. *Emerg. Med. J.* **2014**, *31*, 242–247. [CrossRef]
17. Bigham, B.L.; Jensen, J.L.; Tavares, W.; Drennan, I.R.; Saleem, H.; Dainty, K.N.; Munro, G. Paramedic self-reported exposure to violence in the emergency medical services (EMS) workplace: A mixed-methods cross-sectional survey. *Prehosp. Emerg. Care* **2014**, *18*, 489–494. [CrossRef]
18. Job Description—New York State Department of Health. Available online: https://www.health.ny.gov/professionals/ems/pdf/srgemt.pdf (accessed on 8 November 2022).
19. Becerra-Tomás, N.; Blanco Mejía, S.; Viguiliouk, E.; Khan, T.; Kendall, C.W.C.; Kahleova, H.; Rahelić, D.; Sievenpiper, J.L.; Salas-Salvadó, J. Mediterranean diet, cardiovascular disease and mortality in diabetes: A systematic review and meta-analysis of prospective cohort studies and randomized clinical trials. *Crit. Rev. Food Sci. Nutr.* **2020**, *60*, 1207–1227. [CrossRef]
20. Souza, R.V.; Sarmento, R.A.; de Almeida, J.C.; Canuto, R. The effect of shift work on eating habits: A systematic review. *Scand. J. Work Environ. Health* **2019**, *45*, 7–21. [CrossRef]
21. Nea, F.M.; Pourshahidi, L.K.; Kearney, J.M.; Livingstone, M.B.E.; Bassul, C.; Corish, C.A. A qualitative exploration of the shift work experience: The perceived effect on eating habits, lifestyle behaviours and psychosocial wellbeing. *J. Public Health* **2018**, *40*, e482–e492. [CrossRef]
22. Nea, F.M.; Kearney, J.; Livingstone, M.B.; Pourshahidi, L.K.; Corish, C.A. Dietary and lifestyle habits and the associated health risks in shift workers. *Nutr. Res. Rev.* **2015**, *28*, 143–166. [CrossRef] [PubMed]
23. Mansouri, T.; Hostler, D.; Temple, J.L.; Clemency, B.M. Eating and Physical Activity Patterns in Day and Night Shift EMS Clinicians. *Prehosp. Emerg. Care* **2021**, *26*, 700–707. [CrossRef] [PubMed]
24. Cone, D. *Emergency Medical Services: Clinical Practice and Systems Oversight*; John Wiley & Sons: Hoboken, NJ, USA, 2021.
25. Patterson, P.D.; Weaver, M.D.; Hostler, D. EMS provider wellness. *Emerg. Med. Serv.* **2015**, 211–216. [CrossRef]
26. Israel, B.A.; Coombe, C.M.; Cheezum, R.R.; Schulz, A.J.; McGranaghan, R.J.; Lichtenstein, R.; Reyes, A.G.; Clement, J.; Burris, A. Community-based participatory research: A capacity-building approach for policy advocacy aimed at eliminating health disparities. *Am. J. Public Health* **2010**, *100*, 2094–2102. [CrossRef] [PubMed]
27. Sallis, J.; Owen, N.; Fisher, E. Ecological Models of Health Behavior. *Health Behav. Health Educ.* **2008**, *5*, 43–64.
28. Wallerstein, N.; Duran, B.; Oetzel, J.G.; Minkler, M. On community-based participatory research. *Community-Based Particip. Res. Health Adv. Soc. Health Equity* **2017**, *3*, 3–16.
29. Harris, P.A.; Taylor, R.; Thielke, R.; Payne, J.; Gonzalez, N.; Conde, J.G. Research electronic data capture (REDCap)—A metadata-driven methodology and workflow process for providing translational research informatics support. *J. Biomed. Inform.* **2009**, *42*, 377–381. [CrossRef]
30. Cane, J.; O'Connor, D.; Michie, S. Validation of the theoretical domains framework for use in behaviour change and implementation research. *Implement. Sci.* **2012**, *7*, 37. [CrossRef]
31. Braun, V.; Clarke, V. Using thematic analysis in psychology. *Qual. Res. Psychol.* **2006**, *3*, 77–101. [CrossRef]

32. Golden, S.D.; Earp, J.A. Social ecological approaches to individuals and their contexts: Twenty years of health education & behavior health promotion interventions. *Health Educ. Behav.* **2012**, *39*, 364–372.
33. Hegg-Deloye, S.; Brassard, P.; Prairie, J.; Larouche, D.; Poirier, P.; Tremblay, A.; Corbeil, P. Prevalence of risk factors for cardiovascular disease in paramedics. *Int. Arch. Occup. Environ. Health* **2015**, *88*, 973–980. [CrossRef] [PubMed]
34. Rębak, D.; Suliga, E.; Grabowska, U.; Głuszek, S. The prevelance of metabolic syndrome on the sample of paramedics. *Int. J. Occup. Med. Environ. Health* **2018**, *31*, 741–751. [CrossRef] [PubMed]
35. Wallerstein, N.; Duran, B. Community-based participatory research contributions to intervention research: The intersection of science and practice to improve health equity. *Am. J. Public Health* **2010**, *100*, S40–S46. [CrossRef] [PubMed]
36. Spiegel, K.; Tasali, E.; Penev, P.; Van Cauter, E. Brief communication: Sleep curtailment in healthy young men is associated with decreased leptin levels, elevated ghrelin levels, and increased hunger and appetite. *Ann. Intern. Med.* **2004**, *141*, 846–850. [CrossRef] [PubMed]
37. Koban, M.; Sita, L.V.; Le, W.W.; Hoffman, G.E. Sleep deprivation of rats: The hyperphagic response is real. *Sleep* **2008**, *31*, 927–933.
38. Phiri, L.P.; Draper, C.E.; Lambert, E.V.; Kolbe-Alexander, T.L. Nurses' lifestyle behaviours, health priorities and barriers to living a healthy lifestyle: A qualitative descriptive study. *BMC Nurs.* **2014**, *13*, 38. [CrossRef]
39. Nedeltcheva, A.V.; Kilkus, J.M.; Imperial, J.; Schoeller, D.A.; Penev, P.D. Insufficient sleep undermines dietary efforts to reduce adiposity. *Ann. Intern. Med.* **2010**, *153*, 435–441. [CrossRef]
40. Yau, Y.H.; Potenza, M.N. Stress and eating behaviors. *Minerva Endocrinol.* **2013**, *38*, 255–267.
41. Attlee, A.; Saravanan, C.; Shivappa, N.; Wirth, M.D.; Aljaberi, M.; Alkaabi, R.; Bataineh, M.F.; Hebert, J.R. Higher Dietary Inflammatory Index Scores Are Associated With Stress and Anxiety in Dormitory-Residing Female University Students in the United Arab Emirates. *Front. Nutr.* **2022**, *9*, 814409. [CrossRef]
42. Higgs, S.; Thomas, J. Social influences on eating. *Curr. Opin. Behav. Sciences.* **2016**, *9*, 1–6. [CrossRef]
43. Patterson, P.D.; Weiss, L.S.; Weaver, M.D.; Salcido, D.D.; Opitz, S.E.; Okerman, T.S.; Smida, T.T.; Martin, S.E.; Guyette, F.X.; Martin-Gill, C.; et al. Napping on the night shift and its impact on blood pressure and heart rate variability among emergency medical services workers: Study protocol for a randomized crossover trial. *Trials* **2021**, *22*, 212. [CrossRef] [PubMed]
44. Kamarulzaman, N.; Saleh, A.A.; Hashim, S.Z.; Hashim, H.; Abdul-Ghani, A.A. An Overview of the Influence of Physical Office Environments Towards Employee. *Procedia Eng.* **2011**, *20*, 262–268. [CrossRef]
45. Donnelly, E.; Siebert, D. Occupational Risk Factors in the Emergency Medical Services. *Prehospital Disaster Med.* **2009**, *24*, 422–429. [CrossRef] [PubMed]
46. Ströhle, A. Physical activity, exercise, depression and anxiety disorders. *J. Neural Transm.* **2009**, *116*, 777–784. [CrossRef]
47. Rosenbaum, S.; Vancampfort, D.; Steel, Z.; Hashim, H.; Abdul-Ghani, A.A. Physical activity in the treatment of Post-traumatic stress disorder: A systematic review and meta-analysis. *Psychiatry Res.* **2015**, *230*, 130–136. [CrossRef]
48. Sofianopoulos, S.; Williams, B.; Archer, F. Paramedics and the effects of shift work on sleep: A literature review. *Emerg. Med. J.* **2012**, *29*, 152–155. [CrossRef]
49. Nedeltcheva, A.V.; Imperial, J.G.; Penev, P.D. Effects of sleep restriction on glucose control and insulin secretion during diet-induced weight loss. *Obesity* **2012**, *20*, 1379–1386. [CrossRef]
50. Pendergast, J.S.; Branecky, K.L.; Yang, W.; Ellacott, K.L.; Niswender, K.D.; Yamazaki, S. High-fat diet acutely affects circadian organisation and eating behavior. *Eur. J. Neurosci.* **2013**, *37*, 1350–1356. [CrossRef]
51. Tsismenakis, A.J.; Christophi, C.A.; Burress, J.W.; Kinney, A.M.; Kim, M.; Kales, S.N. The Obesity Epidemic and Future Emergency Responders. *Obesity* **2009**, *17*, 1648–1650. [CrossRef]
52. Officials NAoSE. National Emergency Medical Services Assessment 2020. Available online: https://www.ems.gov/pdf/2020_National_EMS_Assessment.pdf (accessed on 9 November 2022).

nutrients

MDPI

Article

Socioeconomic Patterns in Budget Share Allocations of Regulated Foods and Beverages in Chile: A Longitudinal Analysis

Guillermo Paraje [1,*], Daniela Montes de Oca [2], Camila Corvalán [2] and Barry Popkin [3]

[1] School of Business, Universidad Adolfo Ibáñez, Avenida Diag Las Torres 2640, Santiago 7941169, Chile
[2] Instituto de Nutrición y Tecnología de los Alimentos (INTA), Universidad de Chile, Santiago 7830490, Chile
[3] Department of Nutrition, University of North Carolina at Chapel Hill, 123 W Franklin St, Suite 210, CB 8120, Chapel Hill, NC 27516, USA
* Correspondence: guillermo.paraje@uai.cl; Tel.: +56-2-2331-1380

Abstract: Chile has enacted stringent legislation regulating food and beverage labeling and advertising. This study assesses the changes in the average relative allocations of food and beverage budgets for regulated versus not regulated products in households of different socioeconomic and demographic backgrounds. A household fixed effect before–after model is estimated and the marginal effects in the changes of levels and trends in budget shares and purchased volumes after the implementation of the regulations are examined. The results highlight how impactful food policies can shift consumption toward healthier products.

Keywords: budget share allocation; food labeling; food regulation; Chile

1. Introduction

In 2016 the Chilean government enacted Law 20,606 to curb high levels of people overweight or with obesity. The regulations in the law include front-of-package octagonal warning labels on manufactured foods and beverages high in added sugars, sodium, saturated fats, and calories if they surpassed predefined cutoffs [1]. These "high-in" cutoffs became increasingly stringent over a 4-year period of enacting the law in 3 phases: phase 1 from 27 June 2016; phase 2 from 27 June 2018; and phase 3 from 27 June 2019. In addition, the law banned sales of products with any front-of-package label in schools and very comprehensively banned marketing these products to children (using cartoons, toys, etc.). These regulations aimed to provide easy-to-understand nutritional information for food and beverage products and protect children under the age of 14 from labeled products' advertising and availability in schools.

A growing body of literature has shown that the population, especially mothers of young children [2,3], received these measures well and that the regulations produced significant decreases in the volume of certain food categories purchased. For instance, the volume of sugar-sweetened beverages (SSBs) purchased decreased by approximately 25% [4]. Unhealthy food purchases declined significantly overall [5], and many food categories, such as breakfast cereals, decreased strongly [6,7]. Product reformulations were also extensive and significant, as the proportion of products with any high-in label decreased from 51% to 44% [8]. These findings are in line with what other countries have experienced. A recent meta-analysis found that food labeling is effective in reducing consumers' intakes of energy, total fat, and other unhealthy options while increasing industry reformulations to decrease sodium and trans fat content [9].

Though these regulations were effective in reducing the intake of regulated ingredients, they did not affect labor market outcomes. Studies have found that after the implementation, neither aggregate employment nor real wages in the affected sectors changed when compared to their evolution in nonaffected sectors [10,11]. Other variables, such as capital expenditures and physical production, in the affected sectors did not significantly change in levels or in trends after the implementation of the law when compared to nonaffected sectors [12].

However, the evidence does not reveal how households changed their budget allocations in monetary terms after the implementation of Law 20606. The law's impact on relative budget allocations between labeled foods and beverages and non-labeled products is unknown. In principle, a decrease in the physical quantities of labeled products purchased, as found elsewhere [5], could have been compensated by an increase in the relative prices of such items, resulting in an increase in those items' household budget shares. In such a case, it could be said that the implementation of Law 20606 had a negative financial impact on households and that the impact could be relatively higher on poorer households. However, preliminary results show that the regulations did not change relative prices of labeled versus unlabeled products for poorer households [13].

If lower socioeconomic households do not change their budget allocations between labeled and unlabeled products, while higher socioeconomic households do, it may imply that the former do not have ready unlabeled alternatives to do so or that they are relatively more expensive. Studying changes in budget allocations may show whether regulations have differential impacts and provide more evidence of regulations' outcome inequalities.

This manuscript assesses the changes in the average relative food and beverage budget allocations for labeled versus non-labeled products in households of different socioeconomic and demographic backgrounds during the first stage of the implementation of Law 20606 between July 2016 and December 2017. In addition, and as a byproduct, it analyzes the changes in the average volume of foods and beverages households of different socioeconomic characteristics purchased.

This study is the first to investigate the relationship between Law 20606 and household budget allocations for foods and beverages. We are not aware of studies of this relationship in other countries. Our working hypotheses are that the enactment of the regulations were associated with a decrease in the volume of labeled products purchased and a decrease in the budget shares allocated to labeled products. We have no evidence of price changes associated with the regulations; consequently, changes in volumes would translate into changes in budget shares. In addition, we expect no significant differences in these changes by socioeconomic status (SES) levels as we find no evidence of SES differences in the availability of healthy products in Chile.

2. Materials and Methods

2.1. Data

We used longitudinal information that Kantar Worldpanel collected on food and beverage purchases at the household level from 1 January 2014 to 31 December 2017. This data set has been used elsewhere to evaluate different aspects of Law 20606 [4,5,8]. Kantar Worldpanel also collected household SES data, including size, ages and genders of members, education level of the head of the household, household assets, and access to services for 2573 households. Kantar Worldpanel presents households in the panel for a median time of 18 months and on average includes 1936 households per month. The sample is representative of urban areas with more than 20,000 habitants, about 74% of the urban population.

Kantar Worldpanel bases household SES on access to a list of goods and services and the education level of the head of the household. The ABC1 group is the highest SES level, representing about 15% of the sample; the DE group is the lowest, representing about 32% of the sample; and the C2C3 group is the middle, representing about 53% of the sample. In addition, Kantar Worldpanel provides a life cycle variable based on the household's demographic structure, categorized as (a) households without children; (b) couples with the youngest child up to 5 years old; (c) couples with the youngest child 6 to 12 years old;

(d) couples with the youngest child 13 to 17 years old; (e) couples with the youngest child 18 to 29 years old; and (f) monoparental households with children.

Kantar Worldpanel interviewers visited households weekly to collect data on food and beverage purchases using a handheld barcode scanner. The data include volume in milliliters (mL) or weight in grams (g), price per unit, brand (with a unique barcode), package size, and date of purchase. Our analysis period registered 92,962 household-month observations and 163 purchased product categories. As described elsewhere [5,14], each product's nutrition facts panel was linked to household purchases using barcode, brand, and product description, and a team of trained nutritionists reviewed each product to determine if it was high in sugars, sodium, or saturated fats or exceeded phase 1's calorie threshold. In this way, every product a household purchased before phase 1 of the implementation of Law 20606, January 2014–June 2016, was categorized as high or not high in regulated ingredients based on the criteria on 27 June 2016, when implementation began.

2.2. Statistical Methods

The outcome variable we considered is the monthly budget share of labeled products. For the analyses we defined several groups of products: (a) unlabeled (no label); (b) labeled (with at least 1 label); (c) high in calories (with at least that label); (d) high in sodium (with at least that label); (e) high in sugars (with at least that label); and (f) high in saturated fats (with at least that label). Groups are not mutually exclusive (apart from unlabeled versus labeled products, which are mutually exclusive) and products are assigned to all the groups that apply to them. For example, a product with 2 labels is assigned to the labeled group and the 2 groups representing its labels.

We defined the budget share of labeled products as the proportion of the average household food and beverage budget allocated to labeled products. That variable is constructed as the ratio between the monthly expenditures on labeled products and the monthly expenditure on the complete food and beverage basket:

$$B_t^H = \frac{\sum_{i=1}^{163} P_{i,t}^H Q_{i,t}^H}{M_t} \tag{1}$$

where B_t^H represents the budget share of labeled products in month t; $P_{i,t}^H$ is the price in month t of the labeled product i (not all of our 163 purchased product categories were labeled products); $Q_{i,t}^H$ is the quantity purchased in month t of the labeled product i; and M_t is the monthly total budget allocated to all foods and beverages consumed at home.

Exploiting the panel data, we estimated a household fixed effect before–after model taking the following form:

$$\begin{aligned} B_{jt} = \alpha + \beta_1 Law_t + \beta_2 T_t + \beta_3 Law_t * T_t + \sum_{i=1}^{2} \gamma_i SES_{ijt} \\ + \sum_{k=1}^{2} \gamma_k SES_{kjt} * Law_t + \\ \sum_{l=1}^{2} \gamma_l SES_{ljt} * T_t + \sum_{m=1}^{2} \gamma_m SES_{mjt} * Law_t * T_t + \sum_{n=1}^{5} \phi_n Cycle_{njt} + \\ \sum_{o=1}^{5} \phi_o Cycle_{ojt} * Law_t + \sum_{p=1}^{5} \phi_p Cycle_{pjt} * T_t + \sum_{q=1}^{5} \phi_q Cycle_{qjt} * Law_t * T_t + \\ \sum_{s=1}^{3} \delta_s HH_{sjt} + \sum_{u=1}^{11} \rho_u D_{ut} + c_j + u_{jt} \end{aligned} \tag{2}$$

where B_{jt} is the budget share of labeled products for household j in month t as defined in (1); Law_t is a dichotomous variable with a value of 1 from July 2016 onward and 0 otherwise; T_t is a monthly trend; SES_{jt} is a set of dichotomous variables recording the SES level of household j at month t (ABC1 is the reference category); $Cycle_{jt}$ is a set of dichotomous variables recording the life cycle variable of household j at month t (household without children is the reference category); HH_{sjt} is a set of household variables that includes the size of the household, the age of the household head, and the proportion of household members overweight or obese; and D_{ut} is a set of dichotomous variables for calendar months. The term c_j is a household fixed effect to control for households' unobserved characteristics.

We estimated a similar model for the purchased monthly total volume of labeled solid foods (g) and beverages (mL). The dependent variable is simply the sum of the volume (g or mL) of labeled products. This breakdown is important as beverage volumes are much greater than those of food and beverage volume shifts can hide food volume changes in the total volume analysis. The results of the models for volume purchases are in the Supplemental Online Material.

We used the "xtreg" command in Stata 17 to estimate models. We used the "margins" command in Stata 17 to estimate marginal effects in the changes of levels after the implementation of Law 20606 and trends after that moment compared to previous existing trends. We estimated such margins for the SES and life cycle variables. To compare marginal effects across SES levels and/or across life cycle categories, we performed standard *t*-tests for equality of marginal effects (*m*) using the delta method [15–17]:

$$Z = \frac{\mathrm{m}_1 - \mathrm{m}_2}{\sqrt{\left(se_{m1}^2 + se_{m2}^2\right)}}$$

3. Results

Table 1 shows the characteristics for the total sample and by SES level. The average household size of the sample was 4.12 members. The ABC1 group, the highest SES level, averaged 3.82 members and the DE group, the lowest SES level, averaged 4.36 members. More than 40% of the households were in Santiago, 11% were in Valparaíso, 12% were in the central south region, 11% were in the Biobío region, 12% were in the south, and 11% were in the north. Households with no children were 21% of the total sample and were more prevalent in the ABC1 group, whereas households with at least one child younger than five were 27% of the sample and were more prevalent in the DE group.

Table 1. Characteristics and distribution of the total sample and by SES level.

		ABC1	C2C3	DE	Average Number of Total Households (Monthly)
Monthly average number of households		292.91	1014.45	626.08	1933.45
		(8.67)	(23.13)	(16.53)	(31.71)
Distribution		0.15	0.53	0.32	
		(0.36)	(0.50)	(0.47)	
Region	North	0.10	0.12	0.11	0.11
		(0.30)	(0.31)	(0.31)	(0.32)
	Central south	0.90	0.88	0.89	0.88
		(0.30)	(0.33)	(0.31)	(0.32)
Female head of household		0.39	0.42	0.46	0.43
		(0.49)	(0.49)	(0.60)	(0.50)
Head of household's age	Mean	58.29	57.38	53.46	56.25
		(14.47)	(15.26)	(15.42)	(15.32)
Household size	Mean	3.85	4.06	4.36	4.13
		(1.47)	(1.67)	(1.72)	(1.68)
Monthly average of households per life cycle					
No children		0.27	0.23	0.15	0.21
		(0.44)	(0.42)	(0.36)	(0.41)
Couple with children < 5 years		0.17	0.25	0.36	0.27
		(0.37)	(0.43)	(0.48)	(0.45)
Couple with children 6–12 years		0.17	0.18	0.16	0.17

Table 1. *Cont.*

	ABC1	C2C3	DE	Average Number of Total Households (Monthly)
	(0.38)	(0.38)	(0.37)	(0.38)
Couple with children 13–17 years	0.13	0.10	0.08	0.09
	(0.34)	(0.29)	(0.26)	(0.29)
Couple with children 18–29 years	0.19	0.13	0.08	0.12
	(0.39)	(0.34)	(0.27)	(0.33)
Monoparental with children	0.08	0.12	0.17	0.13
	(0.27)	(0.32)	(0.38)	(0.34)

Standard deviations in parentheses.

The budget share allocated to foods and beverages was constant across this period in real terms. Figure 1 displays the evolution of the average real budget share allocated to foods and beverages, regulated or not, between January 2014 and December 2017. All prices are converted from current Chilean pesos to Unidades de Fomento (UF), a constant currency unit adjusted daily for inflation used in Chile to update values like wages, mortgages, and loans. July 2016 was the first full month of phase one of the regulations. Our before–after analysis showed no change in either levels or trends for the real expenditures on foods and beverages (not shown but available from the authors). This may indicate that, keeping expenditures constant, any changes are reallocations between labeled and non-labeled products.

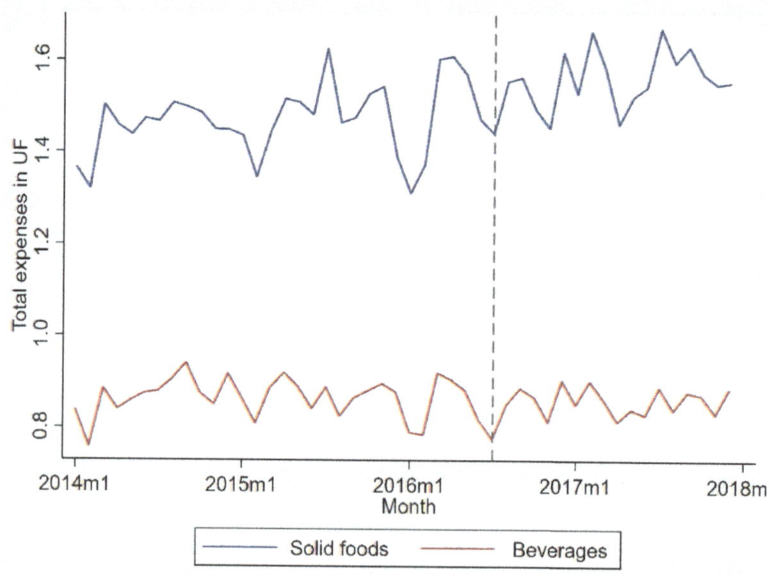

Figure 1. Total real expenditures allocated to foods and beverages.

Table 2 shows the average budget share allocated to labeled products preintervention, January 2014–June 2016, and postintervention, July 2016–December 2017, for the total sample and by SES level. In the preintervention period, more than 57% of an average household's food and beverage budget was allocated to products that would not have had any labeling and it increased to 67% after the intervention, a statistically significant difference. Similarly, the food and beverage budget allocated to any labeled products decreased after the intervention, driven by products with labels for saturated fats, sodium, and sugars. We observed minor increases in products with labels for calories. All SES levels exhibited this pattern though with different intensities.

Table 2. Average monthly budget share allocated to labeled products by period and differences of means, total sample, and by SES level.

	Total Sample					
	No Label	**Any Label**	**Calories**	**Saturated Fats**	**Sodium**	**Sugars**
Preintervention average	0.5740	0.4260	0.1390	0.1330	0.0860	0.2670
	(0.0140)	(0.0140)	(0.1100)	(0.0040)	(0.0040)	(0.0150)
Postintervention average	0.6670	0.3330	0.1430	0.1160	0.0300	0.1900
	(0.0120)	(1220)	(0.0050)	(0.0030)	(0.0020)	(0.0110)
Difference of means	0.0890	−0.0930	0.0040	−0.0170	−0.0550	−0.0770
Standard error	0.0040	0.0040	0.0030	0.0010	0.0010	0.0040
	ABC1 households					
	No Label	Any Label	Calories	Saturated Fats	Sodium	Sugars
Preintervention average	0.5999	0.4001	0.1533	0.1441	0.0782	0.2299
	(0.1333)	(0.1333)	(0.0796)	(0.0804)	(0.0626)	(0.1235)
Postintervention average	0.6998	0.3001	0.1583	0.1249	0.0265	0.1379
	(0.1294)	(0.1294)	(0.0887)	(0.0801)	(0.0372)	(0.0990)
Difference of means	0.0999	−0.0999	0.0050	−0.0192	−0.0518	−0.0921
Standard error	0.0023	0.0023	0.0015	0.0014	0.0010	0.0020
	C2C3 households					
	No Label	Any Label	Calories	Saturated Fats	Sodium	Sugars
Preintervention average	0.5772	0.4228	0.1466	0.1376	0.0821	0.2608
	(0.1442)	(0.1442)	(0.0836)	(0.0813)	(0.0662)	(0.1371)
Postintervention average	0.6736	0.3264	0.1488	0.1177	0.0277	0.1808
	(0.1392)	(0.1392)	(0.0921)	(0.0768)	(0.0393)	(0.1201)
Difference of means	0.0964	−0.0964	0.0022	−0.0199	−0.0544	−0.0800
Standard error	0.0013	0.0013	0.0008	0.0007	0.0005	0.0012
	DE households					
	No Label	Any Label	Calories	Saturated Fats	Sodium	Sugars
Preintervention average	0.5686	0.4314	0.1290	0.1295	0.0905	0.2753
	(0.1597)	(0.1597)	(0.0817)	(0.0822)	(0.0711)	(0.1549)
Postintervention average	0.6553	0.3447	0.1356	0.1161	0.0331	0.2052
	(0.1525)	(0.1525)	(0.0927)	(0.0803)	(0.0415)	(0.1405)
Difference of means	0.0866	−0.0866	0.0065	−0.0134	−0.0574	−0.0701
Standard error	0.0019	0.0019	0.0010	0.0010	0.0007	0.0018

Standard deviations in parentheses.

Table 3 shows the marginal effects for the total sample. Regarding Equation (2), the table shows the derivative of the dependent variable over the variable law. Complete results for Equation (2) are in Supplemental Material Table S1. The change in the level of the budget share allocated to labeled products decreased 9.6 percentage points ($p < 0.01$) right after the intervention (July 2016). The decrease was 1.2 percentage points ($p < 0.01$) for products with at least the label for calories, 3.0 percentage points ($p < 0.01$) for those with at least the label for saturated fats, 5.3 percentage points ($p < 0.01$) for products with at least the label for sodium, and 7.2 percentage points ($p < 0.01$) for products with at least the label for sugars. Results are in Supplemental Material Table S2.

After the implementation of the front-of-package label regulations, the budget share allocation trends changed significantly. Preintervention, the positive trend in spending more on foods and beverages that would have had warning labels was equal to 0.0004 ($p < 0.0100$) per month. Postintervention, the trend became negative, equal to −0.0005 ($p < 0.0100$). Products at least labeled for calories had a preintervention trend of growth in budget share allocations but postintervention experienced a significant decrease. The trend in products at least labeled for sugars was already decreasing preintervention and decreased further postintervention. Results are in Supplemental Material Table S2. Products labeled for saturated fats saw an increase in the positive postintervention trend relative to the preintervention one. Those labeled for sodium showed no change between pre- and postintervention trends.

Table 3. Marginal effect on budget shares and trends before and after the intervention.

	Change in Level Postintervention	Trend		
		Preintervention Trend	Postintervention Trend	Difference between Post- and Preintervention Trends
Any label	−0.0962 *** (0.0026)	0.0004 *** (0.0001)	−0.0005 *** (0.0002)	−0.0009 *** (0.0002)

*** $p < 0.01$. Standard errors in parentheses.

Table 4 displays the marginal effects of changes in levels and trends over SES groups. In all cases, budget shares of labeled products fell with the intervention from 9.2 percentage points for the C2C3 group to 10.1 percentage points for the ABC1 group. However, differences among groups are not statistically significant. Trends in budget share allocations for labeled products did not change with the intervention in the ABC1 group, which remained flat. For the other 2 groups, trends in budget share allocations for labeled products decreased similarly ($p < 0.01$ in both cases) with the intervention.

Table 4. Marginal effects on the budget shares and trends before and after the intervention by SES level.

	Change in Level ABC1	Change in Level C2C3	Change in Level DE
Any label			
	−0.1013 *** (0.0060)	−0.0927 *** (0.0034)	−0.1000 *** (0.0046)
Difference	ABC1 vs. C2C3	C2C3 vs. DE	ABC1 vs. DE
	−0.0086 (0.0067)	0.0072 (0.0056)	−0.0014 (0.0074)
	ABC1	C2C3	DE
Preintervention trend	−0.0001 (0.0002)	0.0002 ** (0.0001)	0.0009 *** (0.0001)
Postintervention trend	−0.0001 (0.0004)	−0.0008 *** (0.0002)	−0.0002 (0.0003)
Difference between post- and preintervention	−0.0001 (0.0004)	−0.0011 *** (0.0002)	−0.0011 *** (0.0003)

** $p < 0.05$, *** $p < 0.01$. Standard errors in parentheses.

Regarding products labeled for specific nutrients, in the ABC1 group the only statistically significant trend change was for saturated fats ($p < 0.05$), which moderately increased after the intervention. Results are in Supplemental Material Table S3. In the C2C3 group, only products labeled for calories showed a significant trend change ($p < 0.01$), which decreased with the intervention. The DE group showed decreases in the trends for calories ($p < 0.10$) and sugars ($p < 0.05$) and an increase in the trend for saturated fats ($p < 0.10$).

Table 5 shows the marginal effects of the implementation of the law over the life cycle variable. Households with at least one child younger than five had the largest decrease in the budget share allocated to labeled products. Right after the intervention, the share fell 11.9 percentage points ($p < 0.01$). Households with children 6–12 years old and 13–17 years old also decreased their budget shares allocated to labeled products by more than 10.0 percentage points. In trend changes, monoparental households with children showed the largest trend reductions in budget shares allocated to labeled products.

Table 5. Marginal effects on budget shares and trends before and after the intervention by life cycle.

	Households without Children	Couple with Children < 5 Years Old	Couple with Children 6–12 Years Old	Couple with Children 13–17 Years Old	Couple with Children 18–29 Years Old	Monoparental with Children
Change in level	−0.0861 ***	−0.1190 ***	−0.1052 ***	−0.1079 ***	−0.0866 ***	−0.0949 ***
	(0.0041)	(0.0181)	(0.0057)	(0.0080)	(0.0053)	(0.0065)
Preintervention trend	0.0004 ***	−0.0001	0.0004 ***	0.0001	0.0002	0.0009 ***
	(0.0001)	(0.0005)	(0.0002)	(0.0002)	(0.0002)	(0.0002)
Postintervention trend	−0.0003	−0.0001	−0.0005	−0.0002	−0.0011 ***	−0.0005
	(0.0003)	(0.0009)	(0.0003)	(0.0004)	(0.0003)	(0.0004)
Difference between pre- and postintervention	−0.0007 **	0.0000	−0.0009 **	−0.0003	−0.0013 ***	−0.0015 ***
	(0.0003)	(0.0010)	(0.0004)	(0.0005)	(0.0004)	(0.0005)

** $p < 0.05$, *** $p < 0.01$. Standard errors are in parentheses.

When we analyzed per label, the largest changes were in high-in sugar products, and the smallest were in high-in calories products. That was true for all SES levels. Results are in Supplemental Material Tables S2 and S3.

Results for volume are in Supplemental Material Tables S4–S10. Labeled products saw significant decreases in volume purchases, while unlabeled products registered the opposite. Monthly purchases of labeled solid foods decreased by 1.5 kg after the intervention, while monthly purchases of labeled beverages decreased by 3.6 L. In addition, after the intervention the trend in monthly purchases of labeled solid foods and beverages decreased significantly ($p < 0.01$). For instance, the preintervention trend in volume purchases of labeled beverages implied a monthly decrease of 50 mL and that trend accelerated to 93 mL with the intervention. Marginal effects of volume purchases also show changes across SES groups, all of which had statistically significant decreases in volume purchases after the implementation of regulations. Statistical comparisons among groups show that decreases in volume purchases were higher for the ABC1 group when compared to the DE group in all cases. Finally, all family types show decreases in volume purchases of labeled products, though the highest drops were in households with children 6–12 and 13–17 years old.

4. Discussion

Using methods different from those of previous studies, we confirmed in this study that the enactment of Law 20606 significantly impacted household purchases of foods and beverages with warning labels [5]. Using a household-fixed effects panel data model to estimate before–after marginal effects of the regulations implemented at the end of June 2016, we found that Chileans immediately decreased both the volume of labeled products purchased and the proportion of households' budgets allocated to them. The reductions were statistically significant and generally a reduction in the trends of monthly purchases followed. We found no statistical differences in the magnitude of the reduction in budget shares allocated to labeled products across SES groups. Budget shares changed in a context of constant real household expenditures, which in practical terms means that households decreased real expenditures on regulated foods and beverages.

Results should be considered in the context of changes in firms' marketing strategies and product reformulations [3,8]. In response to the regulations, firms may have reduced and changed marketing campaigns, reformulated products to avoid the regulations, or changed prices of both regulated and nonregulated products. For instance, in the case of marketing, evidence shows that after the regulations, children's exposure to high-in food media advertisements decreased by 44% for preschoolers and 58% for adolescents with significant decreases in child-directed appeals, such as cartoons [18]. TV ads for high-in products decreased significantly. Before the regulations, 42% of food advertisements on TV were for high-in products compared with 15% after the regulations [19]. The prevalence of child-directed appeals on packages of certain products, such as breakfast cereals, decreased significantly after the implementation of the law [20].

Additionally, the product reformulations that were extensive at least during phase one of the law's implementation [8] could have impacted costs and prices, though a recent study conducted with the same database we used found that prices of reformulated products did not change vis-à-vis non reformulated products [13]. Constant relative prices between regulated and nonregulated foods and beverages suggest that decreases in the volumes purchased account for almost all of the regulations' effects on household budget shares.

Though decreases in purchased volumes were significant, they do not seem to be enough to reverse the high levels of people overweight and obesity in Chile, which is currently 75% of the population [21]. Law 20606 achieved many of its goals, including educating the population about regulated ingredients, prompting reformulation of products, and restricting child-oriented marketing, among others. However, further decreasing consumption of products high in regulated ingredients may require measures that affect relative prices, such as taxes. Currently, SSBs are the only food or beverage taxed and have a relatively low excise taxes that have minor effects on consumers' purchases [22].

A frequent concern about imposing taxes on food and beverage products is the negative financial impact (i.e., regressivity) that increased prices may have on lower income households [23]. A counterargument is that overweight/obesity is more prevalent among lower SES households and reduced consumption of unhealthy products would lower present and future expenditures on health care. Chile has a clear negative gradient between years of education and overweight/obesity [21]. Studies on the distributive effects of SSB taxation have found that taxes are progressive, as lower income households' positive effect of lower health care expenditures outweigh any financial burden due to higher taxes [24–26].

Our results show no large SES differences in how households reacted to food regulations. A recent umbrella review found, apart from taxation that reduces SES inequalities, no compelling evidence of food regulation effects on inequalities [27]. Our results show that in terms of budget shares and volumes, the policies adopted in Chile had a uniform socioeconomic effect despite arguments that less-educated individuals and families would not change their habits in response to regulations.

Although we found no changes in budget allocation patterns based on SES after the intervention, this does not mean that other kinds of regulations, such as taxes on unhealthy foods and beverages, will not impact those patterns. Future research should investigate how these policies could affect household choices.

This analysis has some limitations. First, Law 20606 is a package of regulations, including labeling and advertising bans, and the individual effects of each regulation on households' expenditures cannot be separated. Second, the basket in the Kantar Worldpanel database corresponds to one-third of the total food and beverage basket, mostly from supermarket purchases, that the Institute of National Statistics considers because the Kantar Worldpanel data set does not include information on purchases of bulk products, such as fruits, vegetables, meats, and breads. We have no evidence that the regulations changed the proportions of foods and beverages bought from supermarkets, smaller stores, or other sources. As such, one can assume that the regulations did not alter the patterns of purchases and that the changes reported here effectively reflect changes at the population level. Third, there has been a significant time gap with the situation described here and the current situation. In that period, there was not only COVID but also a political shock due to social unrest in Chile (from October 2019 to the appearance of COVID in March 2020). We are not claiming that changes in budget allocation produced by the initial implementation of the Law remained until today. We acknowledge that that is unlikely and that many other factors may have affected such allocation. However, such factors (COVID, social unrest, etc.) are not related to the implementation of the Law (exogenous factors) and, as such, should not be considered in an enquire about the effects of the Law.

5. Conclusions

The enactment of Law 20606 has been called "the world's most ambitious attempt to remake a country's food culture" [28,29]. It decreased volume purchases of products with warning labels and incentivized product reformulations while having no discernible effects on aggregate levels of employment or real wages. This article shows that the enactment of the law was associated with changes in households' budget allocations as they reduced the shares spent on labeled products. The reduction was similar across households' SES levels and demographic compositions.

Supplementary Materials: The following supporting information can be downloaded at: https://www.mdpi.com/article/10.3390/nu15030679/s1, Table S1: Complete results for the estimation of Equation (2) for budget share; Table S2: Marginal effect on the budget shares and trend before and after the intervention by type of labels; Table S3: Marginal effect on the budget shares and trend before and after the intervention by type of labels and SES level; Table S4: Average monthly volume purchased of high in- products by period and by SES level; Table S5: Marginal effect of the intervention on the volume purchased of labelled products and trends before and after the intervention; Table S6: Marginal effect of the intervention on the volume purchased and trend before and after the intervention by label and by SES level; Table S7: Marginal effect of the intervention on the volume purchased and trend before and after the intervention by "life cycle"; Table S8: Marginal effect of the intervention on the monthly volume purchased in labelled products and trends before and after the intervention by type of label; Table S9: Marginal effect of the intervention on the volume purchased and trend before and after the intervention by type of label and by SES level; Table S10: Marginal effect of the intervention on the volume purchased and trend before and after the intervention by label and by life cycle.

Author Contributions: Conceptualization, G.P. and B.P.; Methodology, G.P. and D.M.d.O.; Validation, G.P., D.M.d.O. and C.C.; Formal Analysis, G.P. and D.M.d.O.; Data Curation, D.M.d.O.; Writing—Original Draft Preparation, G.P. and D.M.d.O.; Writing—Review and Editing, G.P., B.P., C.C. and D.M.d.O.; Visualization, G.P. and D.M.d.O.; Supervision, G.P., C.C. and B.P.; Funding Acquisition, B.P. All authors have read and agreed to the published version of the manuscript.

Funding: This research was funded by Bloomberg Philanthropies, grant number 46129, and the National Institutes of Health, grant to Carolina Population Center P2C HD0509.

Institutional Review Board Statement: Not applicable.

Informed Consent Statement: Not applicable.

Data Availability Statement: The data used in the study are licensed and not publicly available.

Conflicts of Interest: The authors declare no conflict of interest.

References

1. Gobierno de Chile. *Ley 20606: Sobre Composición Nutricional de los Alimentos y su Publicidad*; Gobierno de Chile: Santiago, Chile, 2016.
2. Subsecretaría de Salud Pública. *Informe de Evaluación de la Implementación de la Ley Sobre Composición Nutricional de los Alimentos y su Publicidad*; Ministerio de Salud: Santiago, Chile, 2017.
3. Correa, T.; Fierro, C.; Reyes, M.; Carpentier, F.R.D.; Taillie, L.S.; Corvalan, C. Responses to the Chilean law of food labeling and advertising: Exploring knowledge, perceptions and behaviors of mothers of young children. *Int. J. Behav. Nutr. Phys. Act.* **2019**, *16*, 21. [CrossRef] [PubMed]
4. Taillie, L.S.; Reyes, M.; Colchero, M.A.; Popkin, B.; Corvalán, C. An evaluation of Chile's Law of Food Labeling and Advertising on sugar-sweetened beverage purchases from 2015 to 2017: A before-and-after study. *PLoS Med.* **2020**, *17*, e1003015. [CrossRef] [PubMed]
5. Taillie, L.S.; Bercholz, M.; Popkin, B.; Reyes, M.; Colchero, M.A.; Corvalán, C. Changes in food purchases after the Chilean policies on food labelling, marketing, and sales in schools: A before and after study. *Lancet Planet. Health* **2021**, *5*, e526–e533. [CrossRef] [PubMed]
6. Araya, S.; Elberg, A.; Noton, C.; Schwartz, D. Identifying Food Labeling Effects on Consumer Behavior. *Mark. Sci.* **2022**, *41*, 982–1003. [CrossRef]
7. Vatter, B.; Barahona, N.; Ortero, C.; Ortero, S.; Kim, J. Equilibrium Effects of Food Labeling Policies. In Proceedings of the 10th Annual Conference of the American Society of Health Economists, Online, 21–23 June 2021.

8. Reyes, M.; Smith Taillie, L.; Popkin, B.; Kanter, R.; Vandevijvere, S.; Corvalán, C. Changes in the amount of nutrient of packaged foods and beverages after the initial implementation of the Chilean Law of Food Labelling and Advertising: A nonexperimental prospective study. *PLoS Med.* **2020**, *17*, e1003220. [CrossRef] [PubMed]
9. Shangguan, S.; Afshin, A.; Shulkin, M.; Ma, W.; Marsden, D.; Smith, J.; Saheb-Kashaf, M.; Shi, P.; Micha, R.; Imamura, F.; et al. A Meta-Analysis of Food Labeling Effects on Consumer Diet Behaviors and Industry Practices. *Am. J. Prev. Med.* **2019**, *56*, 300–314. [CrossRef] [PubMed]
10. Paraje, G.; Colchero, A.; Wlasiuk, J.M.; Sota, A.M.; Popkin, B.M. The effects of the Chilean food policy package on aggregate employment and real wages. *Food Policy* **2021**, *100*, 102016. [CrossRef]
11. Paraje, G.; Montes de Oca, D.; Wlasiuk, J.M.; Canales, M.; Popkin, B.M. Front-of-Pack Labeling in Chile: Effects on Employment, Real Wages, and Firms' Profits after Three Years of Its Implementation. *Nutrients* **2022**, *14*, 295. [CrossRef] [PubMed]
12. Corvalán, C.; Correa, T.; Reyes, M.; Paraje, G. *Impacto de la ley Chilena de Etiquetado en el Sector Productivo Alimentario*; Food and Agricultural Organization: Rome, Italy; Instituto de Nutrición y Tecnología Alimentaria, Universidad de Chile: Santiago, Chile, 2021.
13. Paraje, G.; Montes de Oca, D.; Corvalán, C.; Popkin, B. Evolution of food and beverage prices after the front-of-package labeling regulations in Chile. 2022; *manuscript*.
14. Kanter, R.; Reyes, M.; Corvalán, C. Photographic Methods for Measuring Packaged Food and Beverage Products in Supermarkets. *Curr. Dev. Nutr.* **2017**, *1*, e001016. [CrossRef] [PubMed]
15. Van Ours, J.C.; Williams, J. Cannabis prices and dynamics of cannabis use. *J. Health Econ.* **2007**, *26*, 578–596. [CrossRef] [PubMed]
16. Paternoster, R.; Brame, R.; Mazerolle, P.; Piquero, A. Using the correct statistical test for the equality of regression coefficients. *Criminology* **1998**, *36*, 859–866. [CrossRef]
17. Clogg, C.C.; Petkova, E.; Haritou, A. Statistical Methods for Comparing Regression Coefficients Between Models. *Am. J. Sociol.* **1995**, *100*, 1261–1293. [CrossRef]
18. Carpentier, F.R.D.; Correa, T.; Reyes, M.; Taillie, L.S. Evaluating the impact of Chile's marketing regulation of unhealthy foods and beverages: Pre-school and adolescent children's changes in exposure to food advertising on television. *Public Health Nutr.* **2019**, *23*, 747–755. [CrossRef] [PubMed]
19. Correa, T.; Reyes, M.; Taillie, L.S.; Corvalán, C.; Dillman Carpentier, F.R. Food Advertising on Television Before and After a National Unhealthy Food Marketing Regulation in Chile, 2016–2017. *Am. J. Public Health* **2020**, *110*, 1054–1059. [CrossRef] [PubMed]
20. Stoltze, F.M.; Barker, J.O.; Kanter, R.; Corvalán, C.; Reyes, M.; Taillie, L.S.; Carpentier, F.R.D. Prevalence of child-directed and general audience marketing strategies on the front of beverage packaging: The case of Chile. *Public Health Nutr.* **2017**, *21*, 454–464. [CrossRef] [PubMed]
21. Ministerio de Salud de Chile. *Encuesta Nacional de Salud 2016–2017. Primeros Resultados*; Ministerio de Salud de Chile: Santiago, Chile, 2017.
22. Caro, J.C.; Corvalán, C.; Reyes, M.; Silva, A.; Popkin, B.; Taillie, L.S. Chile's 2014 sugar-sweetened beverage tax and changes in prices and purchases of sugar-sweetened beverages: An observational study in an urban environment. *PLoS Med.* **2018**, *15*, e1002597. [CrossRef] [PubMed]
23. Hattersley, L.; Thiebaud, A.; Silver, L.; Mandeville, K. *Countering Common Argumentw against Taxes on Sugary Drinks*; Health, Nutrition and Population Global Practice Knowledge Brief; World Bank: Washington, DC, USA, 2020.
24. Fuchs, A.; Fernanda, M.; Icaza, G. *The Welfare and Distributional Effects of Taxing SSB to Reduce the Risks of Obesity in Ukraine*; Unpublished Report; World Bank: Washington, DC, USA, 2021.
25. Fuchs, A.; Mandeville, K.; Alonso-Soria, A. *Health and Distributional Effects Taxing Sugar-Sweetened Beverages: The Case of Kazakhstan*; Poverty and Equity Notes 24; World Bank: Washington, DC, USA, 2020.
26. Thow, A.M.; Downs, S.M.; Mayes, C.; Trevena, H.; Waqanivalu, T.; Cawley, J. Fiscal Policy to Improve Diets and Prevent Noncommunicable Diseases: From Recommendations to Action. *Bull. World Health Organ.* **2018**, *96*, 201–210. [CrossRef] [PubMed]
27. Løvhaug, A.L.; Granheim, S.I.; Djojosoeparto, S.K.; Harrington, J.M.; Kamphuis, C.B.M.; Poelman, M.P.; Roos, G.; Sawyer, A.; Stronks, K.; Torheim, L.E.; et al. The potential of food environment policies to reduce socioeconomic inequalities in diets and to improve healthy diets among lower socioeconomic groups: An umbrella review. *BMC Public Health* **2022**, *22*, 433. [CrossRef] [PubMed]
28. Shekar, M.; Popkin, B. *Obesity: Health and Economic Consequences of an Impending Global Challenge*; World Bank: Washington, DC, USA, 2020.
29. Jacobs, A. In Sweeping War on Obesity, Chile Slays Tony the Tiger. *New York Times*, 7 February 2018. Available online: https://www.nytimes.com/2018/02/07/health/obesity-chile-sugar-regulations.html (accessed on 18 December 2022).

MDPI AG
Grosspeteranlage 5
4052 Basel
Switzerland
Tel.: +41 61 683 77 34

Nutrients Editorial Office
E-mail: nutrients@mdpi.com
www.mdpi.com/journal/nutrients

www.ingramcontent.com/pod-product-compliance
Lightning Source LLC
Chambersburg PA
CBHW061613210926
51850CB00009B/2312
* 9 7 8 3 7 2 5 8 5 8 8 9 7 *